S0-BXE-239

Forensic Neuropathology

FORENSIC NEUROPATHOLOGY

Lesions of the Brain and Spinal Cord
of Medicolegal Importance

CYRIL B. COURVILLE, M. D.
Consultant in Neuropathology
Office of Medical Examiner, Los Angeles County
Director of Cajal Laboratory of Neuropathology
Los Angeles County Hospital
Professor of Neurology
School of Medicine, Loma Linda University
Los Angeles, California

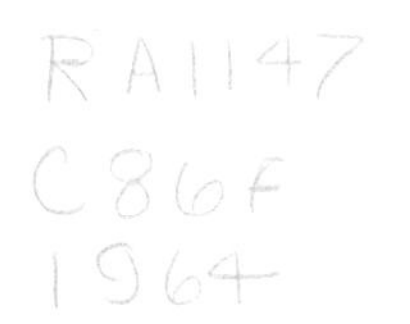

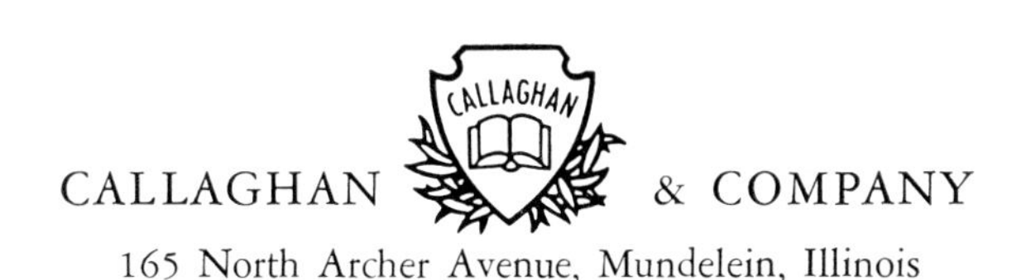

CALLAGHAN & COMPANY
165 North Archer Avenue, Mundelein, Illinois

LIBRARY OF CONGRESS CATALOG CARD NUMBER 64–17546

Dedicated to the Memory of

DR. A. F. WAGNER

Who Introduced the Author to the

Problems of Forensic

Neuropathology

Preface

Soon after beginning his service on the staff as Resident in Neurology and Neurosurgery at the Los Angeles County Hospital, the present writer was faced with the importance of Forensic Pathology. He had been given the additional responsibility of a small laboratory of Neuropathology in order to evaluate the nature of brain lesions from tissues secured at biopsy as well as autopsy. Because of Dr. Carl W. Rand's current interest in brain injury, it was necessary to keep in more or less constant contact with the Coroner's Office in order to secure material for these studies. In spite of the heavy work load carried by Dr. A. F. Wagner, then the County Coroner, this kindly soul was never too busy to arrange autopsies at a time when the busy young resident could get downtown to see the nature and extent of brain damage in fatal cases. Since these early investigations were concerned with acute trauma, we were anxious to compare histological changes with the clinical manifestations in patients cared for in the wards of the hospital. It was on occasion of these visits that many gems of information regarding such injuries were collected, information which furnished a solid basis of knowledge for what proved to be a long continued education in this field. As with Dr. Wagner, so it was with his associates and successors. Not once has the writer experienced anything but constant courtesy and willing answers to his queries from those who have carried the responsibility for performing autopsies of forensic importance in this community. No doubt this factor has contributed greatly to his present interest in this branch of Neuropathology.

But the factors which have led to the writing of this brief study on Forensic Neuropathology are of an entirely different origin. Because of the writer's interest in craniocerebral injury, as well as in certain other details of medicolegal concern (i. e., asphyxia), he has been obliged to testify in many courts of law throughout this area and beyond. He has been grieved, if not stirred to wrath by the gross ignorance of some purported pathologists who failed to recognize a traumatic lesion of the brain when they saw one. Moreover they also seemed indifferent to the fact that this ignorance was the basic reason for putting innocent people "behind the bars" for as serious a sentence as murder. This information was particularly disconcerting when the alleged pathologist was apparently working in collusion with a politically ambitious official who was willing to gain power through injustice. After a series of such experiences the writer was impelled to spell out some of the rudiments of the pathology of craniocerebral trauma to be published in sources available to any pathologist. Hence the invitation to record these observations before medical neurologists (in Tice's Practice of Medicine), and before pathologists concerned with forensic science (Gradwohl's "Legal Medicine") has been welcomed. The latest opportunity has come through Dr. Samuel A. Levinson, capable editor of the Journal of Forensic Sciences, who has permitted the publication of a series of articles on the several phases of "Forensic Neuropathology." The interest in this series of articles not only in this country but abroad, has led to the publication of these essays in the form of this small monograph. The united efforts of Dr. Samuel Levinson of the Journal and of Mr. Rae Smith of Callaghan & Company have made possible its production.

One is obliged to give credit to many local pathologists, too many to list by name for his continuing education, as well as his associates in the Neuropathology Laboratory. Much credit is also due to our tissue technicians (particularly Miss Alice Scott) and hospital photographers (especially Mr. Lloyd Matslovsky) who have made so many elegant illustrations. But it is especially fitting to remember the successive laboratory secretaries who have literally typed "reams of records" on these cases. Mrs. Doreen Iwata has been responsible for acting as the chief liaison officer between the Coroner's-Medical Examiner's Office and our Laboratory. Mrs. Lois Dodds and Mrs. Janice Zamudio have had the responsibilities for preparation of the original manuscripts and seeing the completed book through its final stages.

It is to be hoped that this book will prove to be a ready source of information to many pathologists, especially in the smaller communities where relatively infrequent contacts are made with the problems of Forensic Pathology. It is also the deep-seated desire of the writer that his efforts in this direction will keep innocent men from wasting their lives in "durance vile" because some of his fellows sworn to uphold the law are either ignorant or dishonest.

Cyril B. Courville, M.D.

Foreword

For centuries, and in most countries, the work of a Coroner has been recognized to be of great public importance. This was clearly pointed out in an ancient Chinese book entitled Hsi-yüan-lü, literally translated as the "Record of the Washing Away of Wrongs" or more freely interpreted as a "Book of Instructions for Coroners." This book was first published early in the XIII century (1241–1253 A.D.) during the reign of Emperor Shun Yu. As a basis for the responsibilities of those who were commissioned to examine bodies found under suspicious circumstances, this book noted that "There is nothing more important than human life; there is no punishment [for a murderer] greater than death." For both reasons, the greatest care was demanded in the examination of the body of a victim so that no detail that might shed light on the nature of the fatal wound be overlooked. It also indicated that vital wounds were often found about the head (in 12 out of 22 possible locations). A form was also provided for the exact localization of such an injury. A fracture of the skull with escaping brain tissue was always regarded as a mortal wound, usually resulting in death within three days. Even the confession of a crime was to be checked by an examination of the wound, for the one was to be established by the other. Since in this volume so much emphasis was placed on wounds of the head, the ancient Chinese adage would suggest the great importance of Forensic Neuropathology:

> A difference of a hair will be
> the difference of a thousand *li*.*

Since a *li* is the Chinese measure of a third of a mile, the importance of understanding the true nature of even minor lesions of the brain is clearly implied.

---

* See Herbert A. Giles, Proc. Roy. Soc. Med. Section of the History of Medicine Vol. 17:59–107 (Feb. 20) 1924.

Table of Contents

Chapter I. Introduction—Technical Matters*

Introduction

It is now generally recognized that the various lesions of the central nervous system tend to present a characteristic pattern, both grossly and microscopically, which is typical of this system. Of necessity, therefore, there has arisen a special group of pathologists who have limited their attention and interest to lesions of the brain and spinal cord. However, the general pathologist engaged in the performance of medicolegal autopsies is not infrequently called upon, not only to describe gross lesions of the nervous system, but also to interpret the mechanism of their production and their possible clinical effect in terms of morbidity and mortality. The relation of such lesions as a cause of mortal clinical states calls for a nicety of judgment which is often vital to legal opinion.

It has been the writer's unhappy experience to learn that all too often a misinterpretation or erroneous evaluation of a cerebral lesion has led to a gross miscarriage of justice. This has been particularly true in criminal cases, to the end that a number of innocent individuals have been given prison sentences, up to life imprisonment, charged with manslaughter or even murder, because the nature or degree of a cerebral lesion alleged to be feloniously afflicted was misinterpreted. This has been due to the insufficient knowledge of the medical

---

* It is advisable for any pathologist who is called upon to do medicolegal autopsies, to have available at least a small textbook of Neuropathology so that a description of lesions of the central nervous system which are of spontaneous origin can be studied for comparison. A small volume by the present author entitled *Essentials of Neuropathology* is a suitable companion volume for this purpose. It is published by the San Lucas Press, 316 North Bailey Street, Los Angeles 33, California. It can be ordered through your regular bookseller or directly from the San Lucas Press.

examiner regarding the fundamentals of neuropathology, or what is even worse, to his *refusal to recognize his error in the face of incontrovertible evidence to the contrary!* Such experiences give one cause to wonder what has happened to the medical ethics of such physicians when the Hippocratic oath is so abused as to assault the basic rights of mankind.

Such happenings have stirred the present writer to outline a series of studies of some of these fundamentals as they apply to medicolegal affairs for publication in the Journal of Forensic Sciences. It is hoped that by this means those who have not had the opportunity of special training in neuropathology will have access to necessary information in evaluating serious lesions of the nervous system. It is hoped that this effort will eliminate some of the injustice due to lack of knowledge on the part of general pathologists in the smaller communities who serve as part-time medical examiners.

It is proposed to outline briefly in this first study proper methods of examination (both grossly and microscopically) of the brain and spinal cord. If these suggestions are followed, not only will an adequate preliminary study of the specimen be possible, but also from an adequate dossier of the record and preserved tissues a complete review of the essential problem can subsequently be made by any trained neuropathologist who may be called upon to review it.

In future studies attention will be given to a number of important neuropathological problems of importance to the medical examiner.

Handling the Intact Brain

In the majority of instances, the brain can best be studied *after* the body has been embalmed.[1] The specimen should be

[1] Exceptions do occur. If the individual has succumbed because of a suppurative disease of the central nervous system (subdural abcess, meningitis, brain abcess, etc.) and a *culture* is desired, the specimen must be removed before embalming. When an *aneurysm* of the large arteries at the base of the brain is suspected to be the cause of a severe basal subarachnoid hemorrhage (clinically represented by signs of meningeal irritation and a nontraumatic, diffusely bloody cerebrospinal fluid), a nonembalmed brain permits easy evacuation of the blood in the basilar cisterns and a better opportunity to separate the lobes and convolutions so as to quickly trace out the vessels forming the circle of Willis.

removed after an interval of two or more hours after embalming to allow for adequate fixation *in situ*. This will give the observer an opportunity to see it in its proper anatomical shape and relationship. The brain should then be carefully removed from the cranial cavity, avoiding damage to its lateral aspects by saw cuts through the calvarium. Care should also be made to section the optic nerves close to the optic foramen, to cut the tentorium close to the petrous ridge and to sever the medulla well down within the foramen magnum.

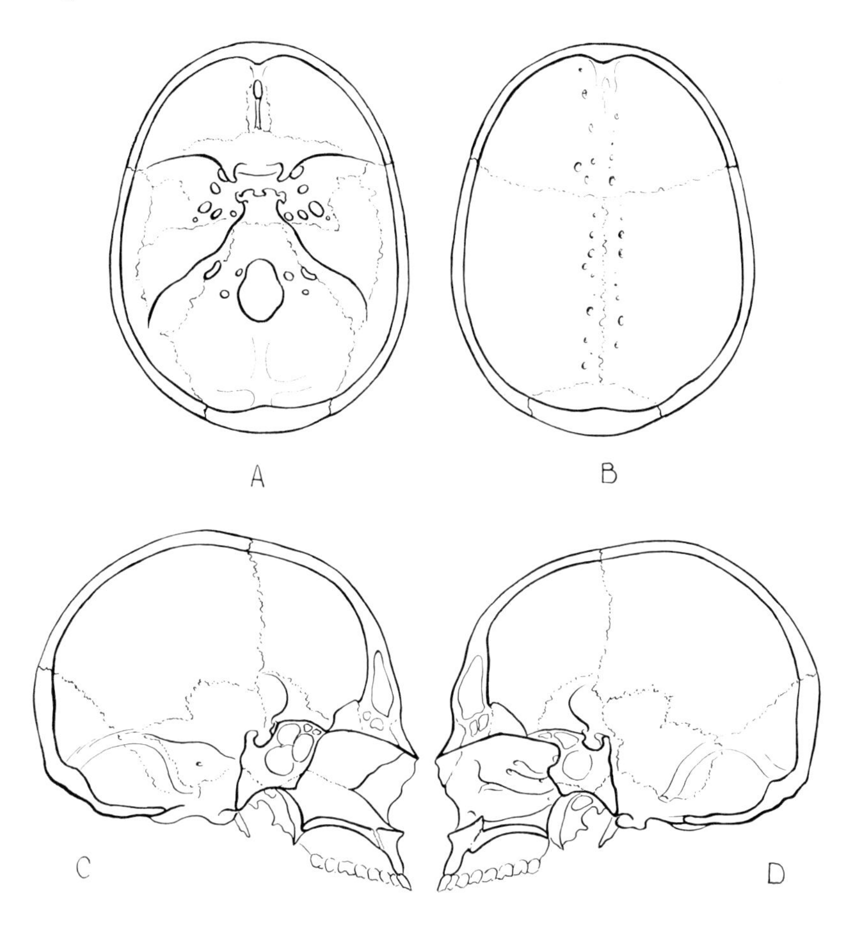

Fig. 1—Diagrams of interior of skull to record nature and course of fracture lines.

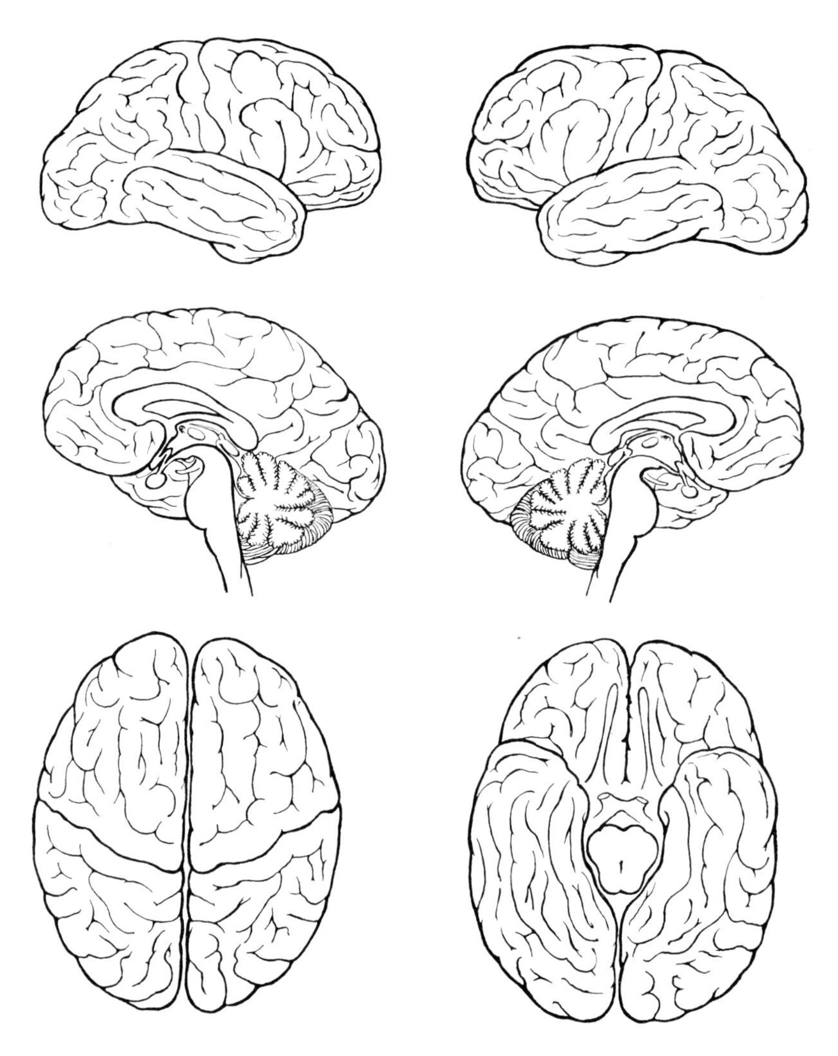

Fig. 2—Diagrams of exterior of brain to record lesions occupying or reaching the cerebral or cerebellar cortex.

After the brain has been removed, the dura mater should be inspected for external or subdural hemorrhage, lacerations, punctures or surgical wounds, thrombosis of the venous sinuses, etc. This membrane should then be torn loose from the cranial base, a detail easily accomplished by a firm grip with a rough towel on this membrane. The vault and base of the skull should then be carefully inspected (in traumatic cases) for fracture lines. If present, the location, nature and extent of such fractures should be indicated on an appropriate outline of the interior of the skull (Fig. 1).

The intact brain should then be immersed in a sufficiently large vessel containing 10 per cent formalin for further fixation and examination when time permits.[2]

If possible, any significant external lesions of the brain should be photographed as a matter of record for such a picture is worth many words of cold description. If this is not possible, the location and extent of these lesions can at least be indicated on an appropriate outline of the exterior of the brain and this be made a part of the permanent record (Fig. 2).

Sectioning the Brain

The gross specimen should be cut in a systematic fashion so that any internal lesions disclosed can be accurately localized by appropriate description, photograph, or at least by recording its shape, size and location on a series of printed outlines to correspond with important internal structures of the brain (Fig. 3). In this way the association of the lesion or lesions with clinical symptoms can be readily accomplished. This will be of importance to attending physicians who may be called upon to testify in the case.

The best method to achieve this objective is one in which parallel sections through the cerebral hemisphere are made after the brain stem and cerebellum have been removed by a cut through the cerebral peduncles. These sections should be made with a large flat-bladed knife held at right angles to the base of the brain (see inset in lower right hand corner of Fig. 3). Such sections should be made through (1) the base of the frontal lobe one inch in front of the tips of temporal

[2] Such as the Tupperware jumbo cannister (No. 8) with cover and cariolier (No. 9).

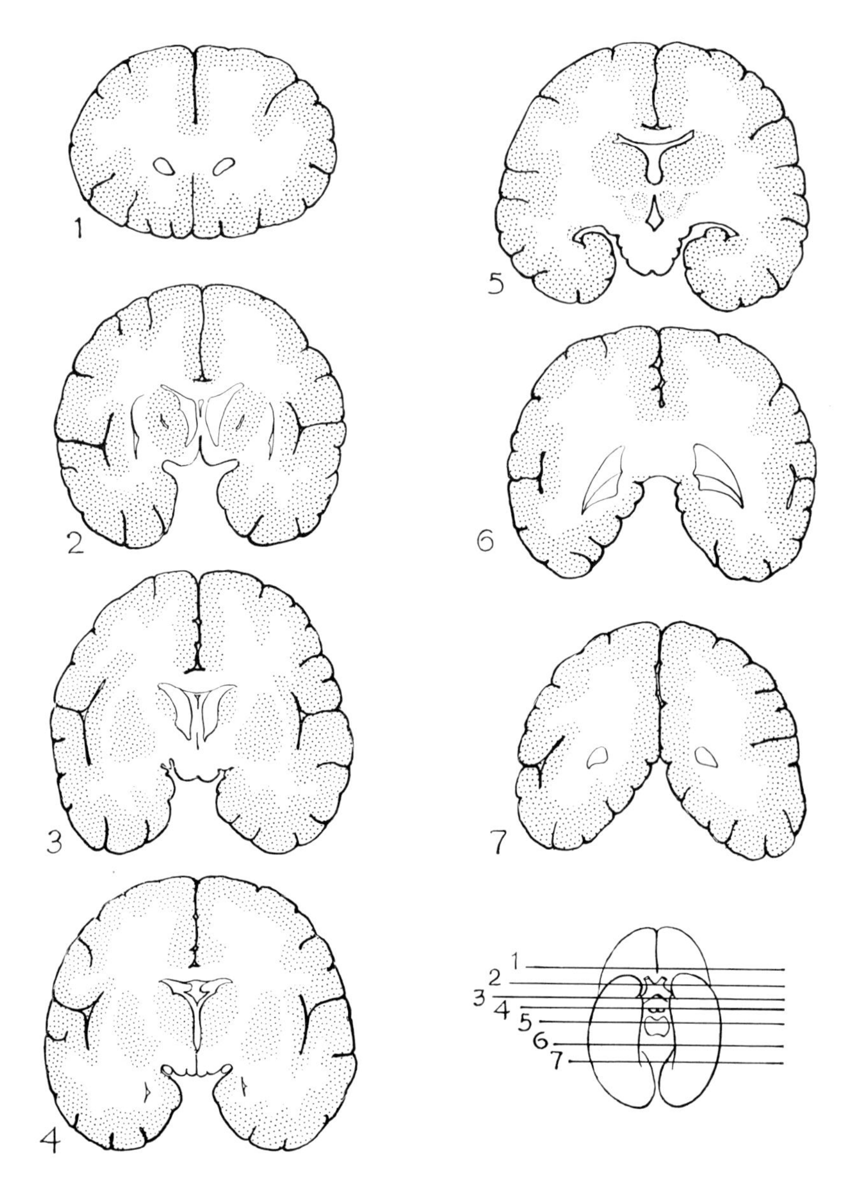

Fig. 3—Cross sections of the brain at specific levels to show important internal structures. See inset for levels of the individual sections.

lobe, (2) the optic chiasm, (3) the infundibulum, (4) the mammillary bodies, (5) the cerebral peduncles, (6) the splenium of corpus callosum and (7) the temporo-parietal region. These cross sections (shown in Fig. 3) are "standard" in the sense that the location of the important internal structures of the cerebral hemispheres are clearly indicated. The outlines of lesions found, as well as associated swellings and deformations can be drawn either in red on the outline printed in black, or in black on an outline printed in some lighter color.[3, 4]

This extra effort at indicating the precise size, extent and location of the lesion takes very little time and creates a record of permanent value.

Application of Plan to Hypothetical Case

A practical application of these methods in describing and graphically reporting may be shown in a purely hypothetical case, the essential features of which are indicated as follows.

A Caucasion male of middle age was found by patrol officers early one morning lying on the sidewalk in a stuporous state. Because the odor of alcohol on his breath suggested drunkenness, the man was placed in the back of the patrol car and taken to regional emergency hospital for examination. From there he was taken to the city hospital, because of multiple focal contusions about his body and head and a laceration of the scalp in the right parieto-occipital region. In the hospital, the patient was found to have a dilated left pupil and an increase in the deep reflexes on the right side which led to the diagnosis of a left subdural hemorrhage. A left temporal burr hole by members of the neurosurgical staff disclosed a recent widespread subdural hemorrhage associated with underlying contusions of the temporal cortex and marked edema

---

[3] The outlines shown in this article may be reproduced by anyone wishing to make use of them without obtaining permission from the author.

[4] Extent of lesions can be indicated by use of vertical or horizontal lines or by crosshatching; use of colored pencils also has advantage by indicating type of lesion by specific color (*red* for contusions or hemorrhage; *orange* for old contusions; *yellow* for infectious lesions; *blue* for tumors). These two systems can be integrated with still further advantage (red for hemorrhage, but lines and crosshatching for bleeding in the various locations, such as solid for intracerebral, crosshatching for subarachnoid and lines for subdural, etc.).

of this lobe. The patient failed to regain consciousness, went downhill and died 36 hours later.

Autopsy by a deputy medical examiner disclosed, in addition to the sutured laceration in the right parieto-occipital region and the underlying operative cranial defect, an effusion of blood in the regional scalp. On opening the skull, a fracture line extending downward and forward into the posterior fossa associated with a small amount of extradural blood was also discovered. There was also a layer of subdural blood clot 2 cms. thick over the entire left cerebral hemisphere, extending onto the under surface of the left frontal lobe. When this clot was washed away, the dorsolateral cortex of the frontal lobe was found to be somewhat atrophic. Contusions of the cortex of the under surface of the left frontal lobe and the tip of the left temporal lobe were also discovered. The left frontal and temporal lobes were edematous resulting in flattening of the regional convolutions. Blood in the subarachnoid space had extended into the meninges in the region of the contusions. On sectioning the brain in a coronal fashion, the contusions were found to be limited to the cortex. A blood clot the size of a walnut was also found in the centrum of the left frontal lobe. The left lateral ventricle was reduced in size due to edema of this hemisphere and the entire ventricular pattern as seen on cross section was dislocated toward the right side.

Aside from the fracture of the right radius, an enlargement of the liver, and pulmonary congestion, the autopsy revealed nothing unusual. The essential cranial and intracranial findings are recorded on the accompanying montage (Fig. 4).

According to the police report, the victim and a male companion had been drinking in a neighborhood bar the evening before the victim had been found on the sidewalk. The barkeeper had also reported that the two had been quarreling before they left his premises. According to the companion, the victim had tripped over an uneven place in the sidewalk and had fallen and struck the back of his head on the concrete. Because he was unable to explain why he left the victim lying on the sidewalk, he was booked as a homicide suspect being accused of striking the deceased on the head with a club.

With this information available it was possible to make the following evaluation of the case: The injury to the brain was most likely the result of a fall, since linear fractures of the skull in the occipital bone and extending into the base are more likely to be due to falls than to any other mechanism. This is in keeping with the cortical contusions and intracerebral hemorrhage on the left side of the brain (*contrecoup* mechanism with lesions on the opposite side of the brain to

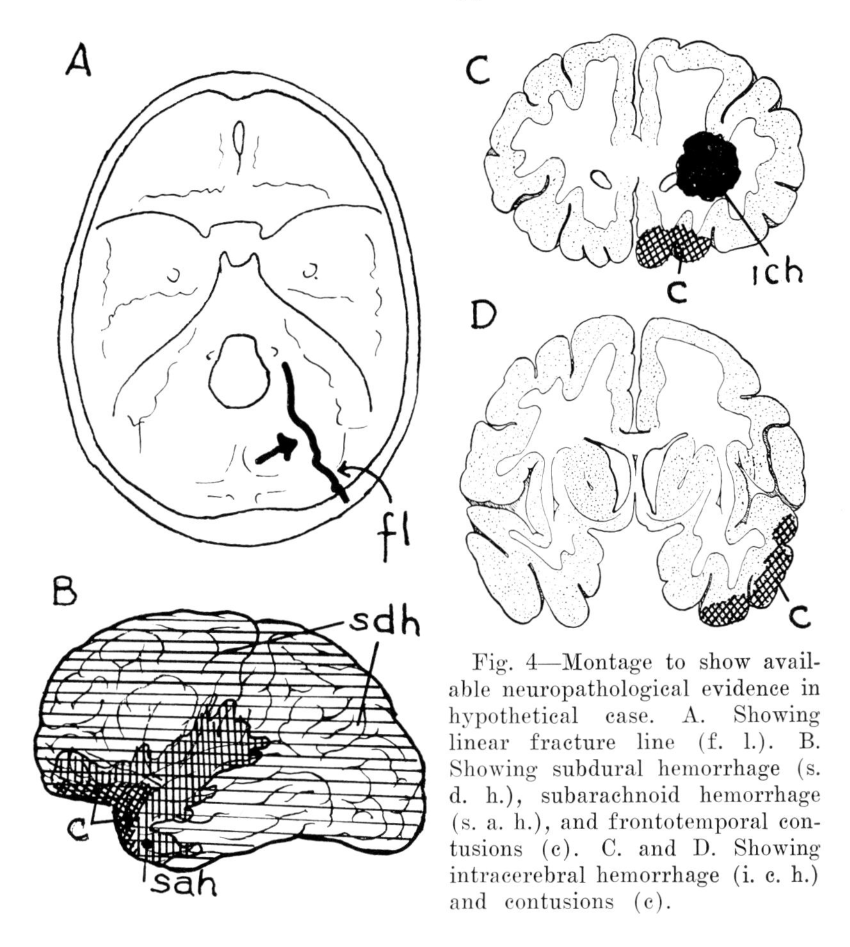

Fig. 4—Montage to show available neuropathological evidence in hypothetical case. A. Showing linear fracture line (f. l.). B. Showing subdural hemorrhage (s. d. h.), subarachnoid hemorrhage (s. a. h.), and frontotemporal contusions (c). C. and D. Showing intracerebral hemorrhage (i. c. h.) and contusions (c).

the point of impact of the skull, the injury being sustained with the head in motion).[5] Both of these points speak against an injury of the brain resulting from a blow to the quiescent

[5] The mechanisms of this and other types of craniocerebral injury will be discussed in Chapter III.

head with a club. The excessive bleeding in the meninges and brain suggest that the victim was under the influence of alcohol at the time of his injury (blood alcohol proved to be 0.18 at the time of autopsy). Atrophy of the dorsolateral frontal cortex (as well as enlargement of the liver) in a man of 37 also suggests that the victim was a chronic alcoholic (verified from data subsequently received). On the basis of this analysis, the victim's companion was released from custody.

Selection of Blocks for Microscopic Study

No other detail of a routine examination of the brain is usually so poorly done in so many pathology laboratories as is that of a microscopic study of brain tissues. The sections are usually too small, are taken hit-or-miss through any area under suspicion and at such an angle as to make localization impossible. Such sections are often almost entirely useless. This is particularly true if the sections are also imperfectly cut from a poorly embedded paraffin block of tissue and inadequately stained (too often overstained with eosin or understained with hematoxylin). This is the chief cause of inconclusive examinations of the nervous tissues.

How Many Blocks and from What Areas? In the case of gross lesions found on sectioning the brain, the problem of selection of blocks is relatively simple. In case of tumors, blocks taken from a well-defined border of the growth will usually give a correct impression of its average architecture and cytology. In cortical contusions, a sizeable block, made to fit the full width of the glass slide, and including at least one edge of the contusion and adjacent cortex, is necessary. The same may be said for vascular lesions of the cortex, taking in this case as large a block as possible from the margin of the lesion, to show the possible causative vascular changes. In case of hemorrhages into the brain, blocks should be taken from the *medial* or *ganglionic* side of the lesion to determine the presence of possible degenerative (arteriosclerotic) or inflammatory (syphilitic) changes in the vessels. In case of such hemorrhages, their margins should also be carefully searched for small anomalous vessels which are so easily overlooked grossly. Blocks should be taken, if necessary, from several locations.

It is in specimens without evident gross lesions that the greatest problems arise with respect to the proper selection of blocks. Rules for every case cannot be laid down, but cortical-subcortical blocks from the midfrontal area in cases of clinical evidence of mental deterioration (especially when frontal cortical atrophy is grossly present); from the contralateral motor cortex or any evident lesions of the motor pathway when paralysis has occurred during life; from the relevant motor cortex (face, arm, leg) and uncus or hippocampus in cases of epilepsy without gross lesion; from the cortex about calcarine cortex as well as from the optic chiasm and tract in cases of visual failure; from the cerebellar cortex and centrum (including the dentate nucleus) and medulla (inferior olivary nucleus), as well as block from spinal cord in cases with acute antemortem ataxia; from the thalamus, midbrain, pons, medulla and upper spinal cord in sudden death in a febrile state (to look for signs of poliomyelitis or encephalitis).

In any case in which no specific localization in the brain is indicated by the clinical record, multiple blocks may need to be taken. To avoid using multiple containers, the *shape* and *size* of the blocks can be made to determine the exact location from which they are taken. Square blocks, cortical or subcortical, suggest the frontal lobe (with *deep* rectangular block instead to indicate the motor strip), a *flat* rectangular block indicates one from the parietal lobe, a triangular block the occipital lobe (usually with a width of the visual cortex about the calcarine fissure), while an elongated block from the hippocampus, a triangular block from the lenticular nucleus or cerebellar cortex, or a deep vertical block from the thalamus and subthalamus which can be readily located and distinguished from others of the same shape by their characteristic architectural markings.

If blocks need be taken from identical areas of both sides of the brain, the larger block is always taken from the left side (which is usually the major hemisphere). If more than one block is taken from a single lobe, one or more small notches are cut in the base of the section, appropriate notations being made in the written report to indicate the exact area selected (Fig. 5). All of these blocks, therefore, can be

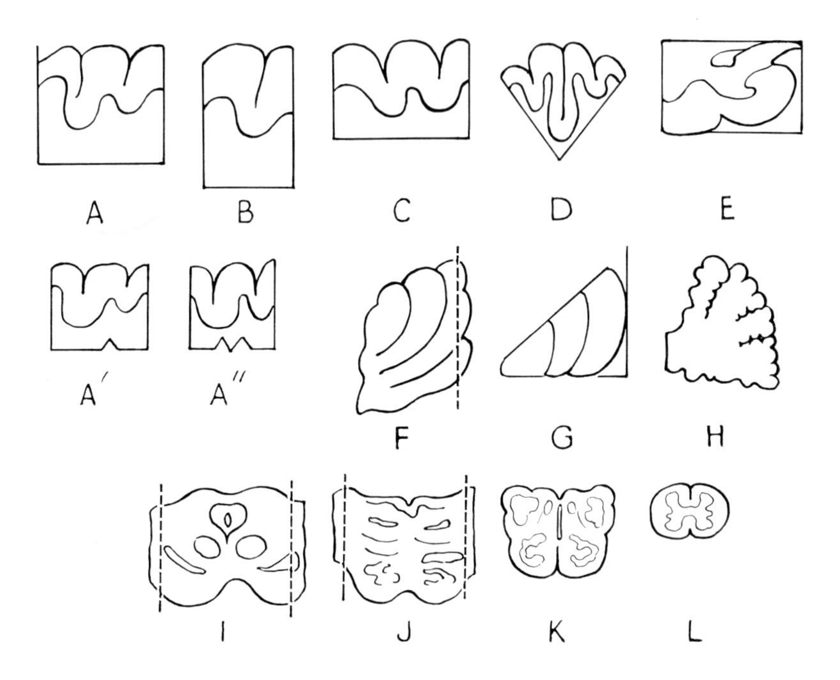

Fig. 5—Drawing showing shape and relative size of sections from various parts of the brain. A. Frontal lobe. B. Motor cortex. C. Parietal lobes. D. Occipital (visual) cortex. E. Hippocampus (or other parts of temporal lobe). A′, A″. Two blocks taken from the right frontal lobe (as compared to the larger block A from the left frontal lobe (major hemisphere). F. Block from thalamus. G. Block from lenticular nucleus. H. Block from cerebellar cortex. I, J, K, L. Blocks from brain stem and spinal cord. Dotted lines indicate how larger blocks can be trimmed to fit ordinary 1″ x 3″ glass slide.

stored in a single bottle pending their sectioning. If frozen, as well as paraffin sections may be subsequently needed for special stains or metallic methods, thick blocks should be taken and then split for this purpose. These blocks take up very little room for storage and can be properly disposed of after the reasonable length of time.[6]

The location of sections from the brain stem when taken at right angles through the long axis of this structure can always be readily identified by their characteristic internal architecture.

It must be recognized that in many instances, neither gross examination nor adequate histological studies can give a satisfactory answer as to the cause of death, even though general autopsy fails to do so. In some instances death from an acute cause suggestive of brain involvement may be on a *chemical* or *physiological* basis, from causes which are not reflected in any significant gross or microscopic alteration. In such instances, a critical review of the clinical findings of attending physician or of the terminal event or circumstances of the individual's demise as described in the hospital record may be necessary to settle this point.

Summary

Lack of fundamental knowledge as to nature and sequence of pathological processes taking place in the central nervous system not infrequently leads the medical examiner to reach erroneous conclusions, especially when he attempts to establish an actual cause of death. When such findings are misinterpreted in civil medicolegal cases injustice is often done; in criminal cases, an even greater tragedy occurs when innocent individuals are often punished more or less severely for alleged felonies.

In the writer's experience such miscarriage of justice not infrequently occurs in the smaller urban centers. It is the purpose of this and subsequent studies to review the basic

---

[6] Not infrequently the entire brain is temporarily preserved in our laboratory until a satisfactory conclusion has been reached. This is especially advisable when a study of additional sections is likely to be necessary and *always* when the case is in litigation. Under such circumstances disposal of the specimen by the medical examiner should be reason for the suspicion that important evidence has thus been destroyed.

aspects of Forensic Neuropathology in an effort to avoid such tragedies. This introductory study is concerned with some simple technical methods which make possible accurate, adequate and appropriate conclusions in medicolegal autopsies.

Chapter II. Significance of Traumatic Extracranial and Cranial Lesions*

The title of this study suggests that while cranial and extracranial lesions of traumatic character may have little to do with the cause of death in an individual with severe craniocerebral injuries, such lesions may be of vital importance in the interpretation of these intracranial lesions and therefore should not be overlooked. It might also be said that a lesion of the scalp indicates what the nature of the traumatic intracranial lesion will be. Moreover, the nature of the cranial lesions are likely not only to indicate the mechanism of the intracranial lesions but also to separate those produced with criminal intent from those which are of purely accidental origin. In any case, the total and most accurate analysis of the chronology and mechanism of the traumatic process must include all three, the extracranial, the cranial, and the intracranial components of the pathological picture.

Extracranial Components

The accompanying lesions of the scalp are usually vitally related to the injury which proves to be fatal as far as the brain is concerned. At times, however, they are purely incidental and may even be misleading, such as in the case of a patient who falls in the course of an apoplectic stroke. The

---

* It is perhaps needless to emphasize the necessity of considering the external evidences of injury (scratches, "brushburns," punctures, cuts, indriven dirt and foreign bodies), but such lesions give the examiner an insight into the nature of the impact of the head and to some extent also the nature of the surface upon which the head was impinged. It also suggests the manner of the impact, whether at right angles or as a glancing blow. The direction in which the head was traveling (in blunt injuries) by the direction of the scratch marks. Hence the exact location and the pattern of these external marks should be indicated.

contusion about the scalp or face may in such circumstances be entirely misleading. On the other hand, a relatively minor and often overlooked lesion of the scalp, as from a penetrating or perforating object, may be of vital importance in evaluation of the total injury. It is therefore important for the medical examiner to be certain that such lesions are not overlooked by being hidden in the hairy portion of the scalp.

As in other parts of the body, external injuries in the scalp are to be grouped as (1) abrasions, (2) contusions, (3) lacerations, (4) incised wounds or cuts, (5) puncture or stab wounds, and (6) pattern wounds. Defense wounds which are the result of the patient trying to fend off an assailant or prevent himself further injury by falls, and so forth, while significant with respect to the extremities, have no important part to play as far as scalp wounds are concerned.

Abrasions may be defined as superficial injuries produced by a traumatizing object moving roughly parallel to the surface of the skin, or by an individual whose head is moving parallel to such a surface. This type of injury causes removal of the superficial layer of the skin. Such abrasive lesions may include scratches, grazes, brush burns, impact abrasions, and pressure, or punctate abrasions. The significant feature of an abrasion is that it implies a direction of movement of the traumatizing object or the head at the time the injury was sustained. This in itself gives a clue to the mechanism of the injury.

Contusions or bruises constitute local injury due to abrupt force applied more or less at right angles to the injured surface. They cannot be differentiated, of course, from the impact of a moving head against an exposed prominence. The nature of a contusion with its characteristic coloration is due to the escape of blood into the loose tissue of the scalp or face. Such a traumatic wound may be simulated or aggravated by certain hemorrhagic processes. In the case of the skull they are usually superficial, since the thickness of the scalp is of minor degree. However, in certain portions of the scalp, particularly in the temporal regions where not only the scalp, but the temporal muscle is of greater thickness, a deep contusion may occur without being noticed. An antemortem contusion should be distinguished from a postmortem one by the presence of actual tissue responses, such as exudation of fluid and infiltration of blood into loose tissues, as well as by the superficial damage to the skin. If possible, it is also helpful to know the age of such lesions, particularly whether or not there has been any change in the hemoglobin of the blood which is extravasated into the surrounding tissues.

Lacerations, which are splits or tears in the surface, are of special significance in scalp wounds. They are often irregular and are produced by moving objects with an edge or a blunt implement. They may be due in reverse, of course, to the impact of the moving head against such an object. Where a laceration occurs at the top of the head it suggests at once its production by a moving object, or a blow by an appropriate implement. Under such circumstances, it is often associated with an underlying depressed fracture. When lacerations occur from falls, they are particularly apt to be found on the posterior part of the head, and here, too, they may be associated with fractures of linear type. The shape and character of the laceration often suggests the nature of the traumatizing implement. Lacerations have been classified (Camps, 1954) (1) as (1) stellate, produced by a blunt, round-headed implement, with the underlying fracture characterized by radiating fissures; (2) crescentic shaped, produced by a blunt object with a similar margin, the underlying injury to bone assuming an identical shape; (3) Y-shaped, produced by a Y-shaped linear round object with the underlying fissure or groove in the brain corresponding to it; (4) cut-out linear, with Y-shaped ends, produced by a linear object with an edge; and finally (5) small penetrating, which may be produced by a sharp-pointed object.

Incised wounds are made by cutting implements or objects and are apt to be applied with criminal intent except when produced by flying glass. In the latter case, one may find multiple short incised wounds in the frontal location of the scalp or about the face. On the other hand, a single incised wound may be produced by a single piece of glass, such as a fragment of windshield, which may even be driven into the skull.

Stab or puncture wounds are usually obvious from their more or less characteristic appearance. A stab wound may be produced by a single or double-edged weapon (knife). A puncture wound is more often due to a rounded or pointed object rather than one with a sharp blade. Although infrequent, stab wounds of the scalp and skull do occur, and if the blade of the knife is broken off, may go entirely unnoticed until the scalp is reflected (Courville, 1955) (2).

Pattern wounds, which may be found anywhere about the body, including the scalp, are suggested by the repeated occurrence of characteristic patterns which in themselves suggest the nature of the implement used. Occasionally the occurrence of multiple wounds of a given type about the head may be used to predicate the nature of the traumatizing implement. The pattern may also be reproduced in the cranial vault, at least in its external table. Particular significance should therefore be attributed to such pattern wounds.

As stated in the original report on technique, the precise location, arrangement, and size of any superficial wound of the scalp should be reported on appropriate diagrams, or, whenever possible, photographed to be made a part of the record. This is doubly true whenever foul play is suspected.

Location of Wounds and Injuries About the Head

The combination of scalp wounds and underlying fractures also has meaning, particularly in view of the location and nature of the scalp wound, which is to be associated with the underlying fracture. For example, an anterior group of contusions of the scalp with an underlying linear fracture suggests a fall forward and downward. Less likely, it may result from the impact of a blunt implement in an assault. Bilateral temporal contusions of the scalp associated with a crushing type of fracture may mean the squeezing of the head between approximating objects. A unilateral contusion suggests a fall on the lateral aspect of the head, particularly when associated with a deep contusion of the temporal muscles and an underlying linear fracture. A posteriorly placed contusion of the scalp, often not seen until the scalp is reflected in the course of the autopsy, when associated with a linear fracture running downward into the posterior fossa, usually indicates a fall on the back of the head. An indented or depressed area may indicate either a true depressed fracture of the central depression or a hematoma of the scalp sometimes seen in children. The so-called "ping-pong" type of fracture in the newborn is also characterized by a local rounded depression. A depressed fracture, of course, always suggests either the impact of a small object traveling with some force, or impact of the moving head against an irregular projection. Comminuted and compound fractures may be produced in many ways and in themselves can only imply a local type of injury as just described. Local bruises with linear fractures or fracture by diastasis can also occur with blunt injuries, especially from blows by objects of considerable size. The separation of sutures is frequently an extension of a linear fracture.

Fracture of the orbital plates may not be associated with any external contusion other than a small opening in the upper eyelid, when it signifies an object penetrating the intracranial cavity in this direction. Such fractures, either unilateral or bilateral, may also follow a fall on the back of the head, thus having contrecoup significance. It may also follow a gunshot wound of the head in which the muzzle of the weapon is placed tightly against the skull so that the force of the explosion is expended within the skull. Falls on the lateral aspect of the head may be associated with linear fractures running into the middle fossa of the skull, especially when the impact of the head is in the temporal region. Fractures resulting from falls on the back of the head are not only linear but are usually found to pass either anteriorly in the direction of the foramen magnum or more laterally to cross the petrosal ridge. "Ring fractures" of the occipital bone may also occur without any external wound, representing the forcible impact of the forehead against a stationary object while the head is in motion. Such fractures are most often seen as a result of football injuries.

Significance of Fractures of the Skull

Fractures of the skull, hitherto mentioned only in connection with superficial wounds, are significant in several aspects. In previous times it was the fracture itself that counted most, and no diagnosis was considered complete until the demonstration of a fracture, or lack of a fracture, in an individual suspected of having a craniocerebral injury was accomplished. In ancient times, the demonstration of a fracture was so important that efforts were made to outline it by rubbing a dark colored dye on the exposed outer surface of the bone to demonstrate its presence. This was done because one of the important objects of therapy was to remove the line of fracture itself as well as any resultant fragments.

This philosophy has continued into the third decade of this century. The victims of even severe craniocerebral injuries were hustled onto the x-ray table at any cost, while anxious relatives awaited with bated breath the outcome of the roentgenologic examination. They were immediately relieved if no fracture was found, for even the medical attendants were often unaware that fatal injuries could occur without such a fracture. At the present time, however, it is recognized that a cranial fracture, or absence of one, may have little to do with the outcome of a given case. Severe fractures are not imcompatible with life, although fatal injuries may occur without them.

On the other hand, the genuine significance of fractures should not be overlooked. In the first place, the presence of a fracture indicates something of the severity of the original injury, because a force sufficient to fracture the skull must of necessity be greater than one which has failed to do so. In the second place, the type, location, and direction of a fracture contribute much to an understanding of the mechanism of injury. Thirdly, the presence of a fracture may forewarn of complicating intracranial hemorrhage, particularly when found in certain locations. Finally, the presence of a fracture in certain locations may indicate the danger of infectious complications within the cranial vault. Such complications may not be immediate, but may occur even in the remote future, particularly when fractures involve the nasal sinuses or auditory apparatus. Certain fractures, notably seriously depressed ones, constitute an immediate indication for emergent surgery. Each of these situations will be considered in detail in subsequent sections.

Classification of Fractures of the Skull

Medical observers throughout history have had a peculiar fascination for fractures of the skull, and from ancient times have applied a variety of terms to the numerous types. As long ago as 2500 B. C., according to the Edwin Smith Surgical Papyrus (Elsberg, 1931) (3), the ancient Egyptian writer described them as either "splits" (linear fractures) or "smashes" (compound comminuted fractures). Hippocrates also classified fractures of the skull, but in a more detailed manner. He identified fissures (linear fractures), contusions of bone, depressed fractures, indentations (*hedra*) with or without fractures, and finally, contrecoup fractures. One would conclude that the fractures which Hippocrates saw were more likely those of civilian, rather than of military life, although some have considered otherwise. As reflected in modern terminology, fractures vary considerably, some being less important than others. In accordance with our present postulates, these fractures should be considered as (1) depressed fractures, (2) linear fractures, and (3) fractures of a specific type. It should be recognized that it is not always possible to correlate the specific types of fracture with the types of cerebral injury (this will be discussed in detail later). For example, depressed fractures are usually an isolated type, while special fractures may be associated with incised wounds, stab wounds, puncture wounds, and missile wounds. Moreover, fractures may be compound, a complication involving almost any type. For instance, linear fractures may occur around the missile exits in gunshot wounds or radiating from the margins of depressed fractures.

Depressed Fractures.—A depressed fracture usually results from the local impact of a moving object on the cranial vault. It is characterized by a circumferential break in the bone, with depression of the enclosed fragment into the intracranial space. The enclosed fragment of bone is often broken (comminuted). Such fractures are often compounded by laceration of the overlying scalp incident to the impact of the traumatizing object. This superficial lesion is often associated, in severe cases, with laceration of the dura mater, contusion or laceration of the subjacent brain tissue, and often with hemorrhages incident to laceration of the regional blood vessels.

Mechanism of Depressed Skull Fracture.—The changes in the bone resulting from a depressed skull fracture depend upon the size and shape of the traumatizing object, the force with which it is applied to the skull, and the thickness of the bony vault (infant vs. adult skull). The least important of these fractures (first degree) is an indentation of the outer table of the skull into the less dense diploe. This indentation of the skull is what Hippocrates would call *hedra*. The second degree of depressed fracture is a simple depression of both the inner and outer table into the intracranial space. Radiating away from the circumferential break may be short lines of fracture caused by the original modification of the surrounding area of bone. Teevan (1865) (4) described the mechanism of this type of wound and divided it into several stages (Fig. 6, A). The first stage consists of a depression of the outer table of the skull against the inner table. With the continuation of the traumatizing force, the inner table is fractured, resulting in a greater degree of shelving of this inner table. The outer table, continuing along its line of force, drives the inner table through the dura and into the underlying brain. In other words, the fragments of bone from the outer table also act as a traumatizing agent as far as the inner table is concerned, thus resulting in further fragmentation of this table. The second degree does not go so far as to lacerate the dura, but simply results in a mild degree of depression. The third degree of depressed fracture, however, does result in laceration of the dura and damage to the underlying brain in the form of contusion or laceration. This third degree, of course, may vary considerably in degree, from a simple superficial contusion, even one of microscopic character, to one in which the underlying brain may be severely torn.

Of greater importance are the larger depressed fractures usually produced by the forceful impact of some flying object on the cranial vault. The size and shape of the depressed fragment often suggests the nature of the object (i. e., the head of a hammer produces a characteristic lesion of the bone as well as of the scalp), while the degree of depression is at least a rough indication of the force applied. Such fractures are usually found at the crown of the head, while similar fractures resulting from injuries to the moving head are often found about the parietes—frontal, temporal or occipital.

Depressed fractures may be *simple* or *complex.* Simple fractures are shallow depressions (*ca* the thickness of the cranial vault) without laceration of the underlying dura. Complex fractures, on the other hand, are often compound, and the depressed bone is broken into several fragments. Such fragments with sharp points and edges often lacerate the dura mater and underlying brain, at times complicating the original lesions with an immediate hemorrhage or delayed infection from indriven infectious material. Immediate complications have already been considered; delayed complications will be dealt with in the next study.

These several features of depressed fractures are indicated in the accompanying drawing (Fig. 6).

Linear Fractures.—By far the greatest number of cranial fractures are linear in character. They may be due to the impact of the moving head, either in a fall to the ground or projection against some solid object. Linear fractures may be classified as *primary,* being the direct effect of such an impact, or *secondary,* being associated with other and more complicated types of traumatic lesions (i. e., radiating fissures about depressed fractures or about the wounds of exit in missile wounds). Linear fractures may also be classified on the basis of their position as *vertical fractures* and *transverse fractures,* running either horizontally or anteroposteriorly in the lateral aspects of the skull. Therefore, "basal" fractures may also be horizontal, when the side of the head is impacted against the edge of a beam or box. Under these circumstances, the fracture may be described as "circumferential", partially enveloping the top of the cranium.[1] Fractures of this location and type may cause an extensive horizontal laceration of the cerebral convolutions, because of dislocation of the top of the cranium against the brain.

Patterns of Linear Fractures.—Most fractures resulting from blunt injuries (Group C), particularly in falls, may be divided into two groups, as shown by Rand and Nielsen (1925) (5). The first group of these fractures is a *lateral* one, in which fractures result from a lateral impact of the

[1] Smaller circumferential fractures of different connotation may also occur about the wounds of exit in through-and-through missile wounds.

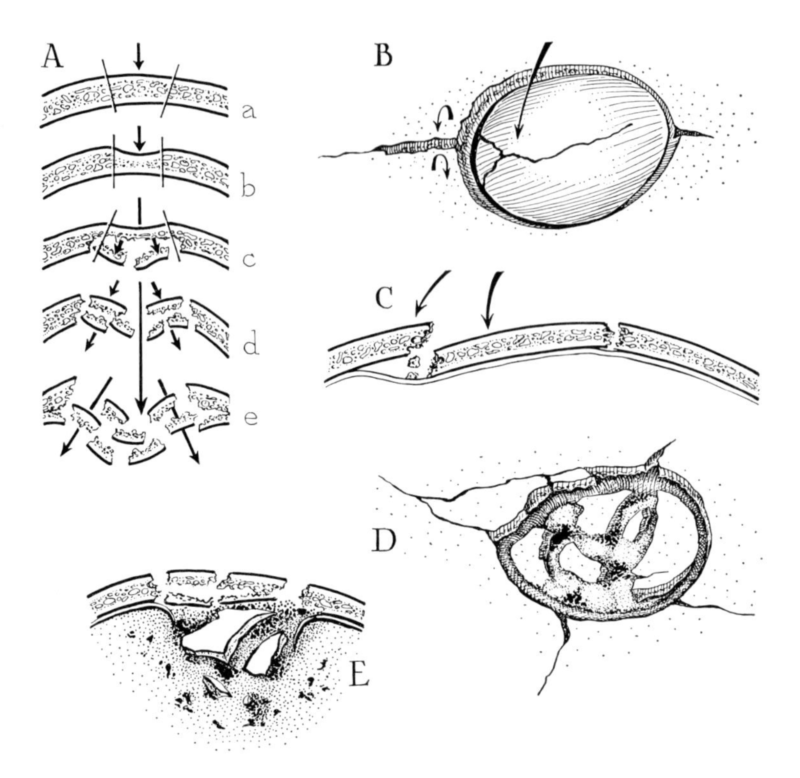

Fig. 6—Depressed fractures of the skull. A. Teevan's theory of stages of development of focal depressed fracture showing how primary depression of outer table tends to cause "shelving" and shattering of inner table. B. and C. Mechanism of simple depression without indriven fragments. D. and E. Complex depressed fracture with laceration of the dura, indriven fragments, and laceration of the brain.

head. As observed on a lateral roentgenographic view, the fracture lines usually begin in the parietal region, run downward and forward, tending to be parallel to the frontal buttress of the skull. Such fractures may cause extradural hemorrhage by laceration of the middle meningeal artery, or may lacerate the cortex of the lower portion of the temporal lobe.

Fractures in the *posterior* group usually result from a fall on the posterior or posterolateral aspect of the head. They usually begin in the posterior parietal or occipital regions, and tend to course downward and either medially (toward the foramen magnum) or laterally (toward the petrous bone). The basilar surface of the cerebellum may be lacerated by such fractures. (Such fractures may also lacerate the lower temporo-occipital cortex. Laceration of the lateral sinus may occur, especially in infants or children, although this is rare.) The more laterally placed fractures may extend across the posterior fossae of the skull, often entering the petrous bone, damaging the delicate auditory or labyrinthine structures in this region.

The locations of these two groups of linear fractures, as well as other scattered fractures, are indicated in the accompanying illustration (Fig. 7) redrawn from a figure in the contribution of Rand and Nielsen (1925) (5).

This pattern of linear fractures, as suggested by their tendency to localize in certain areas, is probably accounted for by the anatomical structure of the skull (reinforcing buttresses). Therefore, one cannot draw too concise conclusions from these "pattern fractures," other than an estimate of the area of impact of the causative blow. On the other hand, a horizontal fracture line involving the crown of the cranium indicates not only the location of the impact but also suggests that the head struck some horizontally placed object with a relatively sharp edge. Such fractures are significant because they may result in an extensive laceration of the upper cerebral cortex.

Evaluation of Forces in Production of Linear Fractures.—By using an ingenious technique, Gurdjian and Lissner (1947) (6) made an analytical study of forces resulting in cranial fractures. By coating skulls recently recovered from the autopsy room (still "green" from their organic content) with a special type of varnish (Stresscoat), these investigators determined the location and direction of stresses resulting from the impact of these skulls when in motion. The covering material will crack along lines of stress, thereby suggesting the mechanism of injuries causing fractures. A summary of their findings is given in the accompanying drawing (Fig. 8). A comparison of the data disclosed in their study shows a remarkable correlation to the location and course of fractures as discovered by Rand and Nielsen (1925). These articles should be studied further by anyone especially interested in this subject.

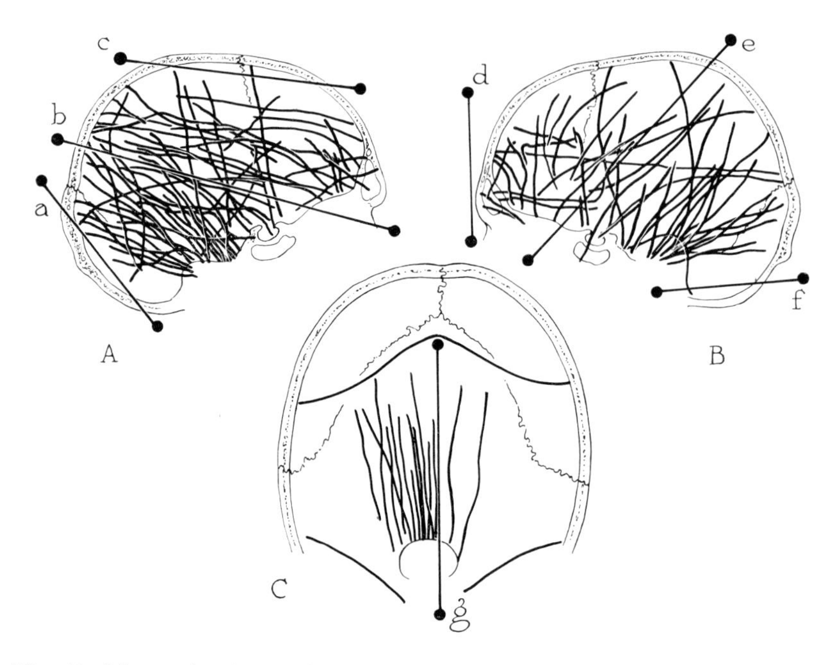

Fig. 7—Linear fractures of the skull. A, B, and C. Location of linear fractures in a series of 171 cases (145 cases with examples of linear fractures) of cranial injury studied by Rand and Nielsen (1925). Adjacent heavy broken lines indicate direction of fracture lines (figure was redrawn from their study).

The extension of fractures of the vault into the base of the skull, a factor of double importance, will be discussed at greater length elsewhere. Their course points out the direction of force which caused the cranial injury. These fractures thereby help in evaluation of the nature of any resultant lesions of the brain. This is especially true in coup-contrecoup cases.

Other Types of Fractures.—In addition to the more common types of fractures already enumerated, other less common traumatic lesions of bone should be mentioned. Perhaps the most common of these is known as *fracture by diastasis*. This is a linear fracture which extends into a suture line, occurring most often in an infant or child, but which is also found

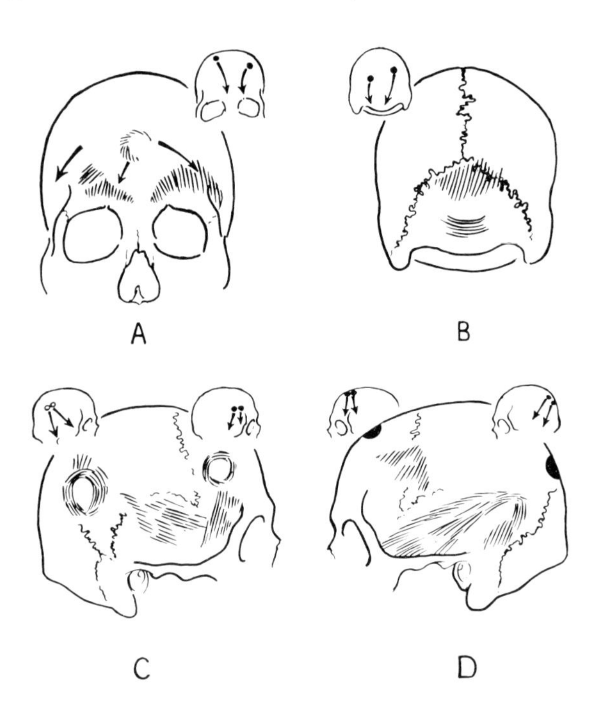

Fig. 8—Mechanical factors responsible for linear fractures. Black dot indicates point of impact; arrow shows direction of force and shaded areas show effect of stress on cranial vault. Comparison of these figures with those of Rand and Nielsen are very informative. Figures redrawn from Gurdjian and Lissner (1947).

occasionally in adults. Such a fracture is of no special significance, other than the obvious increased force required to break into and open the involved suture.

Another type of fracture is that known as *meridional fracture,* which occurs at a distance from the point of impact and which is consequent to a crushing type of cranial injury (as a fall from a height). The sudden flattening of the head as a whole tends to cause a fracture of the cranial bones at the meridian of the head. *Bursting fractures* are also the result of extensive crushing injuries, either from compression of the head or its impact in a fall from a height.

True *contrecoup fractures* are rather rare. In the writer's opinion they are more or less limited to fractures of the very thin bones of the orbital roof from a sudden increase in intracranial pressure such as result from falls on the back of the head. They may also result from the explosive effect of gunshot wounds when the weapon is held against the head when fired. In most cases apparent contrecoup fractures are simply the extension of a fracture line from the opposite side of the head, through the cranial basis, to appear finally on the opposite lateral wall.

Specific Types of Cranial Wounds

Not all traumatic lesions of the skull can be correctly or specifically designated as *fractures*. Some lesions, particularly those associated with either blunt or closed injuries cannot be so described. This applies to mild *indentations* of the cranial bones (which the Greeks called *hedra*) and to *abrasions* of the outer table of the skull. An abrasion results from an auto accident in which an injured individual is thrown out of his car, the scalp and outer table of the cranial vault being abraded by scraping along the pavement. Such injuries do not ordinarily produce *intracranial* damage, but street dirt indriven into the opened diploe may lead to the development of an osteomyelitis, with potential secondary intracranial complications.

Bony Lesions in Missile (Gunshot) Wounds of the Skull.—A characteristic gunshot wound of the head results in a round defect in the skull at the point of entrance of the missile. The mechanism of this type of bony lesion is somewhat similar to that of the ordinary depressed fracture (Fig. 9), but the defect is much more limited in size and presents a greater degree of fragmentation of both outer and inner tables of bone. In gunshot wounds of a century ago (such as seen in the American Civil War), the lead missiles of slow velocity were often imbedded in the bones of the skull at the end

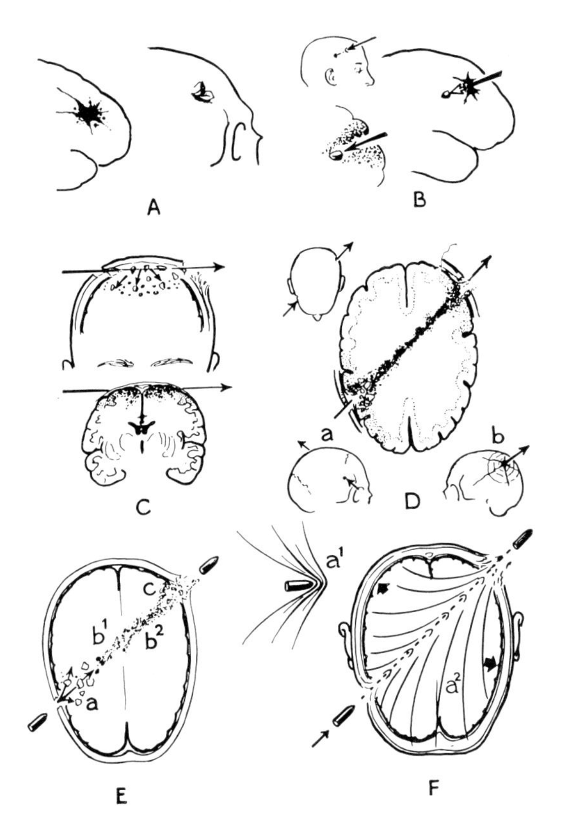

Fig. 9—Effects of missiles on skull. Series of simple drawings showing **cranial defects produced by bullets.** A. Simple wound by missile which remains lodged in skull. B. Penetrating wound of cranial vault with superficial damage to brain tissue. C. Gutter or superficial through-and-through wound with indriven fragments. D. Deep through-and-through wounds with simple perforation of calvarium at wound of entrance (a) and larger complex wound of exit (b) with radiating and circumferential fractures about focal wound made by the missile. Presence of indriven fragments and effects of waves of force on the brain set up by flight of missile are also shown in E and F.

of their trajectory, sometimes actually split against the margin of the defect. On the other hand, in cases of missiles of greater velocity fired with smokeless powder, this seldom occurs, even in the case of lead revolver bullets.

The characteristic missile injury, as will be explained in a subsequent chapter, involves first a cone-shaped laceration of tissue behind the wound of entrance. The fragments of bone which provoke this localized laceration are composed to a greater degree of those from the splintered inner table of the skull, which is characteristically more profoundly shattered than is the outer table.

If the missile traverses the intracranial cavity and emerges from the opposite wall, a second bony defect is produced (perforating wound). The dimensions of this wound are larger, the outer table in this case being more widely damaged than the inner, the mechanism of destruction therefore being reversed according to the rule of Teevan. In severe wounds, this wound of exit is surrounded by one or more circular or circumferential fractures, as well as a number of radiating fractures. The wound in the overlying scalp is larger and more often ragged in appearance.

The pattern of missile wounds as observed in war has been described by Cushing (1918) (7) and more recently by Abbott (1961) (8). Fungus cerebri as a complication of missile wounds of the brain has been discussed by Courville et al. (1956) (9). These lesions will be described in the subsequent chapter.

Incised Wounds.—This type of wound is not ordinarily seen in medicolegal autopsies. They are usually produced by an assault with a tomahawk (in Colonial days), hatchet, ax, or cleaver (in more recent times). In the past, however, such wounds produced by slashes with a sabre were not uncommon in cavalry combat. If the head is struck a glancing blow, not uncommon with sabres in hand-to-hand combat, a portion of the skull may be cut away. This may be completely detached or may continue to hang to the scalp by a bridge of tissue. If the blood supply to the detached bone via the scalp is sufficient, repair of the defect will occur after simple replacement of the bone and its fixation by sutures in the scalp.

The wound in the skull differs somewhat in degree, depending whether or not it has resulted from a glancing blow. If the weapon is sharp, a vertical wound results in a typical incision corresponding to the edge of the weapon used. When the blade of the injuring weapon is wedge-shaped, the skull is split open, resulting in a sharply bordered wound which corresponds in length to the actual contact with the blade, with a terminal split at either end of the incision (Fig. 10).

However, if the cutting edge is blunt, such as is often the case with a hatchet or ax, there results an elongated, irregular, depressed fracture, much as would occur from an elongated implement of any sort. The margins are grossly irregular and the fragments are indriven, resulting in an irregular laceration of the underlying brain. This type of lesion results in considerable hemorrhage. In other words, it is not always possible to identify the cranial wound as an incised wound per se under these circumstances.

If the wound is due to a sharp-edged weapon, an elongated, sharply defined defect in the skull is produced. Healing results in a more or less complete filling in by bridging of newly formed bone from margins of the defect.

Stab Wounds.—Such wounds are now quite rare. In this country, they are usually produced by pocketknives, and in other countries by daggers. They are usually a result of criminal assault. Most such wounds encountered in the Los Angeles County Hospital have been in Negroes, and usually have been inflicted in the course of a drunken assault. Because of the purposeful action of an assailant, the blade is usually driven in at right angles to the surface of the skull. Nevertheless, the blade is often broken off, either in attempt to remove the blade from the skull or by the violent movements of the individual thus assaulted. It is possible, under such circumstances (especially if the injured individual is under the influence of alcohol), for the blade to be broken off, remaining *in situ.* The resultant small flesh wound is sometimes overlooked, so that only sometime later, when convulsions may ensue and roentgenograms of the skull are taken, is the true nature of the wound discovered. The blade ordinarily causes a smooth-edged defect in both bone and brain, oftentimes without any evidence of hemorrhage. When hemorrhage does occur, there forms beneath the superficial wound a cyst-like defect in the brain (Fig. 11, A).

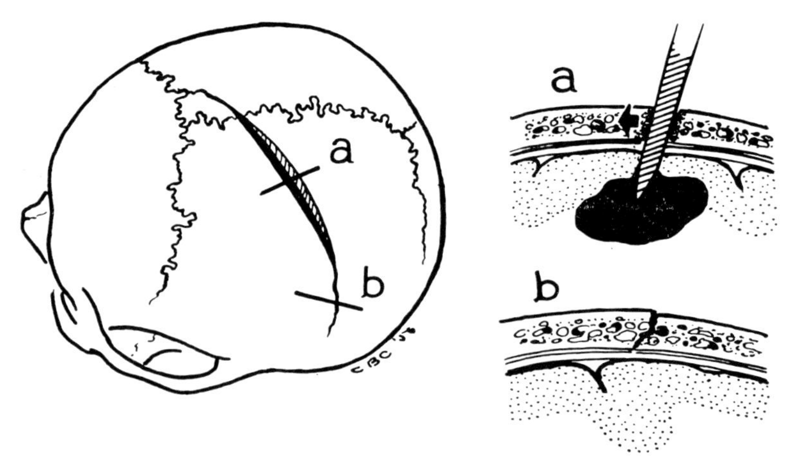

Fig. 10—Incised cranial wounds. Wound made by a *sharply edged* weapon presents a slightly widened defect corresponding to the thickness of the blade (a) and terminal "splits" on either end of the incision (b) due to the wedging effect of the blade.

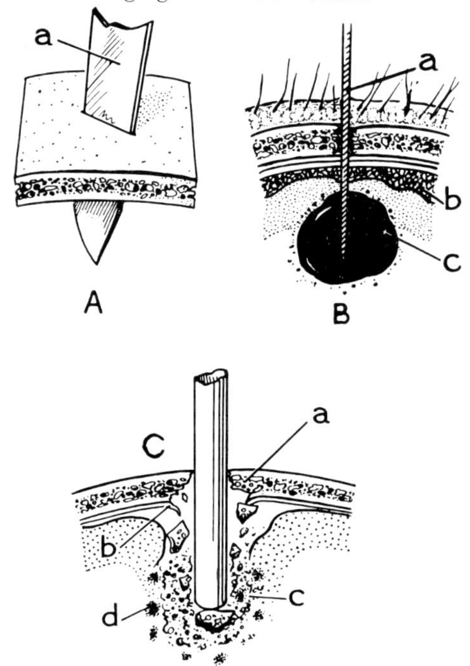

Fig. 11—Puncture wounds (stab and blunt types). A. and B. Stab wounds made by a knife (a) or dagger. Wound of scalp, skull, and brain usually corresponds closely to size of weapon and may actually be overlooked clinically if the weapon has been withdrawn. Hemorrhage (c) may occur if the blade interrupts a vessel of any size. C. Blunt puncture wounds made by rods, etc., produce a rounded defect but with a large wound in the inner table (a) and are more likely to lacerate the dura (b), drive in small fragments of bone (c) and macerate the brain with hemorrhage (d).

With a larger weapon, such as a butcher knife, a small fragment of bone is not infrequently indriven before the point of the weapon. This fragment in itself acts as a lacerating object, and local hemorrhage of more severe degree usually results. In such cases, the bony defect is larger and often more irregular in contour than is the smooth-edged opening produced by an ordinary pocketknife.

Blunt Puncture Wounds.—Such wounds are small, round, or oval, sharply outlined defects, resulting from an indriven sharp stick, rod, or other implement. This type of wound is more often found in children who are injured by falling on the point of the wounding implement. The shape of the defect in the skull corresponds to the end of the injuring weapon (Fig. 11, B). Such wounds resemble the openings made by cone-shaped arrowheads, as seen in ancient Peruvian skulls (Abbott and Courville, 1942) (10), or the stones of a medieval crossbow. A roentgenogram of the skull may show a small bony mass not too deeply indriven into the regional brain.

In addition to the more formal type of cranial fracture and traumatic bony lesions discussed in this connection, almost every neurosurgeon or military surgeon with any great amount of experience with traumatic lesions can add to the great variety of oddities, with which the pertinent literature is replete. This is probably also true of the experienced medical examiner.

Summary

Injuries to the exterior of the head in the forms of abrasions, contusions, and lacerations are not important in themselves as far as mortality is concerned. However, the type, location, and extension of fractures of the skull in such injuries may be helpful in evaluating the nature of the mechanism which produced the more important damage to the brain. It is therefore important for the forensic pathologist to pay critical attention to these accessory injuries, noting carefully their location and type and recording them faithfully as a part of the medical record. It is a source of great satisfaction when a careful evaluation of all of these lesions often proves to be of great help in reaching a correct conclusion as to the mechanism of the total injury.

Perhaps of greater importance is the relation of the different types of fracture of the skull and the occurrence of a variety of intracranial lesions resulting from injury. An evaluation of this group of lesions, complications resulting from fracture, will be considered in another study.

REFERENCES

1. Camps, F. E.: Wounds of the Head and Body and Their Interpretation, in Gradwohl's Legal Medicine, St. Louis, C. V. Mosby Co., 1954, pp 220–259.
2. Courville, Cyril B.: Contribution of the Pathology of Stab Wounds of the Brain. Report of Three Cases Verified at Autopsy. Bull. Los Angeles Neurol. Soc. 20:162–176 (Dec) 1955.
3. Elsberg, C. A.: The Edwin Smith Surgical Papyrus and the Diagnosis and Treatment of Injuries to the Skull and Spine 5,000 Years Ago. Ann. Med. Hist. 3:271, 1931.
4. Teevan, W. F.: An Inquiry into the Causation, Diagnosis and Treatment of Fracture of the Internal Table of the Skull. Brit. & For. M.-Chir. Rev. 36:189–199, 1865.
5. Rand, C. W., and Nielsen, J. M.: Fracture of the Skull; Analysis of 171 Proved Cases; Diagnosis and Treatment of Associated Brain Injury. Arch. Surg. 11:434–458 (Sept) 1925.
6. Gurdjian, E. S., and Lissner, H. R.: Deformation of Skull in Head Injury as Studied by "Stresscoat" Technic. Am. J. Surg. 73:269–281 (Feb) 1947.
7. Cushing, H.: A Study of a Series of Wounds Involving the Brain and Its Enveloping Structures. Brit. J. Surg. 5:558–684, 1918.
8. Abbott, K. H.: Acute Missile Wounds of the Brain. An Atlas of Surgical Pathology. Bull. Los Angeles Neurol. Soc. 26:103–131 (Sept) 1961.
9. Courville, Cyril B., Moyar, J. B., Eberlin, E. W., and Haymaker, W.: Fungus Cerebri as a Complication of Missile Wounds of the Brain. Military Med. 118:437–487 (May) 1956.
10. ———, and Abbott, K. H.: Cranial Injuries of the Precolombian Incas; with Comment on Their Mechanism, Effects and Lethality. Bull. Los Angeles Neurol. Soc. 7:107–130 (Sept) 1942.

Chapter III. Mechanisms of Craniocerebral Injury and Their Medicolegal Significance*

Traumatic lesions of the skull and brain are found so frequently in medicolegal autopsies that it is vitally important for the medical examiner to understand how structural alterations are produced by injuries as well as to know how to record such lesions properly. Only by their proper evaluation can the medical examiner distinguish, for example, between the result of an accident on one hand and a felonious assault on the other. When objective signs of trauma are understood it is surprising how much light can be shed on the medicolegal problems presented thereby.

In the first place, each type of injury results to a considerable degree in its own series of characteristic lesions and sometimes their complications as well. The mechanism of some types of lesions is relatively simple to understand. This is particularly true of those in Group A in which a direct blow to the head by a traumatizing implement or weapon presents no major problem in evaluation. This is also true of the lesions in Group B although differently produced by compression of the head. On the other hand, injuries resulting from traffic accidents or falls (Group C) may be very complex and difficult to interpret. This is certainly true unless one has a clear concept of the mechanism by which such lesions are produced. In Groups A and B, a moving object strikes a quiescent head while in Group C the injury is sus-

---

* It has already been pointed out that traumatic lesions of the scalp and skull also give clues as to the mechanism of a given craniocerebral injury. However, this chapter is concerned with damage to the brain proper which is the serious if not the lethal element to be concerned. In these mechanisms which have to do with penetrating injuries, the penetrating object also plays an important part in the nature and extent of the brain wound.

tained when the head in motion is suddenly halted by an immobile or relatively immobile object. Herein lies the essential difference in their mechanism of production.

Before these three mechanisms are investigated, however, some features in the applied anatomy and physiology of the head and brain as they apply to traumatic lesions should be evaluated.

Applied Anatomy of Cranial Trauma

The skull which envelopes the brain is essentially a globoid bony shell. The upper part of this shell, commonly designated as the *calvarium,* varies somewhat in thickness. The lower part of the skull or the *cranial basis* is irregularly thickened due to the separation of its outer and inner tables by the nasal air sinuses, an increase in width of the diploic spaces, or the structures or spaces constituting the audito-vestibular apparatus. In its fresh state the skull is somewhat elastic, not only because of its shape, but also because of the organic content of the bones which compose it. The domed contour of the calvarium also serves as a protection against the effects of trauma, especially blows which strike the head at an angle. Such blows tend to glance off and the delicate brain structure is protected from injury. The head itself being attached to the torso by means of a flexible neck is therefore quite mobile. Thus the first effect of a blow or impact is considerably modified by this mobility which prevents the force of the injury to be wholly expended on the brain. The hair and soft tissues of the scalp further serve to cushion even direct blows. Therefore, not only the structure of the skull itself, but also its accessory investments as well as its mobility constitute the first line of defense against traumatizing forces.

The otherwise relatively thin cranial vault is moreover reinforced by a series of bony buttresses—two midline thickenings anteriorly and posteriorly and two lateral wedges which separate the frontal from the temporal lobes anteriorly and the basal temporal brain from the cerebellum posteriorly. These buttresses also tend to direct any fracture lines downward into the base where they are dissipated by the complex bony structure in that region (Fig. 12). The diploe, the accessory nasal sinuses and the spaces within the petrous bone containing the audito-vestibular structures further serve to cushion the brain against injury.

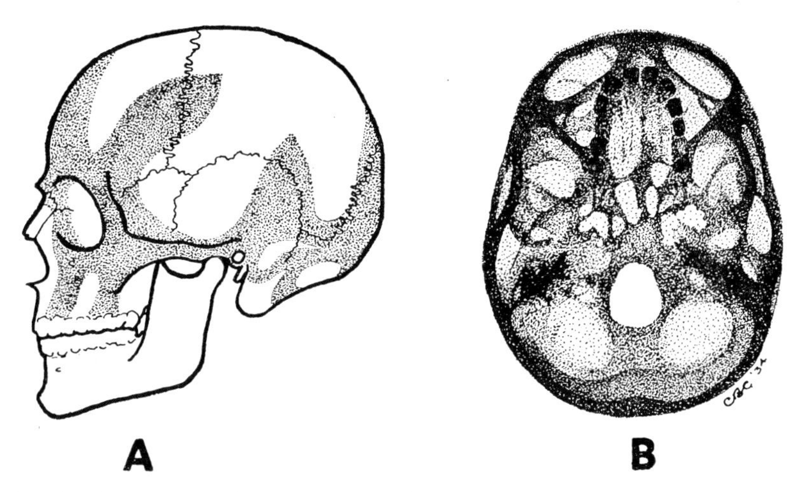

Fig. 12—Buttresses of the skull serving as reinforcements of bony wall. A. Lateral aspect of skull showing thickenings of lateral wall. B. Reinforcements in base of skull shown by transillumination (after Knoblauch).

Additional protection for the delicate nervous tissues is provided by the dura mater, which rounds off the smaller elevations and depressions of the anteroposterior reduplication (the falx cerebri) and a posterior horizontal reduplication (the tentorium cerebelli), both of which tend to subdivide the intracranial space and reduce excessive movements of the brain produced by any unusual degree of jarring. Such movements of the brain are further reduced by an attachment of the cerebral vertex to the dura along the saggital midline by means of the superior cerebral veins and the pacchionian granulations. At the base of the skull the brain is anchored by means of the cranial nerves and the carotid arteries. These points and lines of fixation are of importance in preventing laceration of the entrance and exits of the blood vessels. A final cushioning effect of the cerebrospinal fluid, greatest in degree at the cranial basis (basilar cisterns), between the two cerebral hemispheres (superior longitudinal fissure), and about the sylvian ridges (sylvian cisterns) should also be mentioned.

Thus the various structural aspects of the cranial vault and its external and internal investments form the first line of defense against injury. It is obvious, of course, that serious injuries can and often do produce severe lesions of the cranial vault and base, the dura mater, the leptomeninges, the brain and its blood vessels.

Applied Physiology of Craniocerebral Injury

The application of force to the rounded surface of the calvarium tends to be dissipated by its globoid contour. The effects of this force depends upon the *size* of the traumatizing object, the *speed* with which it is applied to the head and the *angle* of its trajectory. It is therefore obvious that whenever an object strikes the head at right angles, the effect on the brain will be more severe, while the force of glancing blows tends to be dissipated.

The effect of any material impact on the brain varies considerably. With reference to the severity of the blow, it is possible for the function of the brain to be temporarily depressed or even obliterated (cerebral concussion) without producing either a fracture of the skull or a grossly visible lesion of the brain. On the other hand, the brain may be structurally altered at the point of impact by lacerating effect of a linear fracture or by indriven bony fragments consequent to a depressed fracture. The amount of functional depression resulting from cerebral concussion, or the extent of structural damage produced either by the fracture itself or indriven bony fragments depends upon the degree of force which has been applied. The local impact sets up waves of vibration which pass over and through the brain. The immediate effects of cerebral concussion are due to the effects of these vibrations on the cerebral cortex which becomes progressively involved by the wave of excitation and/or depression spreading over the brain. Since the cranial vault is often the first to receive the impact, the motor centers, particularly the leg areas, are first to receive this shock. Hence, the first symptom, even in minor degrees of concussion, is weakness of the legs which may be sufficient to precipitate the victim to the ground. As the wave of excitation passes over the brain it simultaneously tends to upset the function of the delicate labyrinth resulting in a degree of vertigo with loss of balance and production of ataxia. If the degree of force is still more severe, the wave of force will affect the upper brain stem and result in loss of consciousness. This symptom in particular has long been considered as the characteristic sign of cerebral concussion although this is not always the case. All of these symptoms may occur without any consequent structural changes in the brain. However, in the more severe degrees of concussion, particularly those which do not produce immediate death from the effects of shock on the vital (cardiovascular and respiratory) centers, vasomotor effects may influence the intracranial circulation. If this effect is widespread, petechiae may be found throughout the white matter of the cerebral hemisphere in fatal cases. If, on the other hand, the effect of traumatic shock is expended through the cerebrospinal fluid system, extending from the lateral and third into the fourth ventricle, focal subependymal hemorrhages may be found in the floor of the fourth ventricle (Duret's hemorrhages). One or both of these lesions are to be expected in most fatal cases of cerebral concussion (Courville, 1935; 1953) (1).

Residual effects of concussion may also be manifested in the form of disturbances in the cerebrospinal fluid circulation. This effect may also be reflected in the cerebral nerve cells. These nerve cell changes are probably incident to functional disturbances in the cerebral circulation. They occur as a loss of tigroid material from the cell cytoplasm and/or minute alterations in their nuclei (Courville, 1953) (1).

These introductory remarks should make it apparent that changes in cerebral function, not explained by any gross or microscopic alterations in cerebral structure, may occur. Such changes may even result in a fatality (severe cerebral concussion), but more often continue on as a group of symptoms known collectively as the post-concussion syndrome. These symptoms include various "nervous" manifestations (forgetfulness, increased irritability, restlessness, insomnia, etc.), "dizziness," and headaches which constitute the classical post-concussion triad. It is now generally believed that these symptoms are not due to any structural changes in the nervous tissues, but are due rather to an impaired vasomotor control, a residual of the general effects of the impact on the brain. While these manifestations do not often enter into consideration of the forensic pathologist, they must be evaluated along with other post-traumatic clinical manifestations in evaluating the total picture of craniocerebral injury as described in the clinical history of the case.

Evaluation of Necropsy Findings in a Case of Craniocerebral Injuries

The first study of this series dealt with the matter of making complete and accurate records of the various central nervous system lesions found in a medicolegal autopsy. The importance of developing such a dossier cannot be overemphasized if the medical examiner is to serve the public efficiently. Since correct conclusions are at best often difficult to draw, the problem should not be complicated by defective records or by incorrect interpretations of complete ones.

When a history of an injury to the head is elicited in the case of an individual who has died under questionable circumstances, all possible physical evidence of such injury should be noted, including not only that of the head, but also of the entire body. The *size, location* and *nature* of contusions, lacerations, cuts or abrasions and their approximate age should be noted. In case of injuries to the head, it is also important to locate extravasations of blood in the tissue of the scalp and temporal muscles, which information often aids in determining the mechanism of the causative trauma.

The location and amount of extradural hemorrhage (usually associated with a fracture) as well as subdural hemorrhage or hematoma should be recorded. An impression of the age of the effusion (especially of subdural hematomas obtained by microscopic section of its capsules) is quite often helpful in evaluating the total picture.

It is also most important to make a careful search for fracture lines presenting themselves on the interior surface of the cranial vault after the dura has been removed. Such fracture lines often give valuable clues as to the point of impact and the direction of the traumatizing force producing contusions or lacerations of the brain. For example, the direction of a fracture line coursing across the base of the skull *usually follows the direction of the line of force applied to the head* (Fig. 13).

Traumatic lesions of the leptomeninges and brain should also be indicated on appropriate diagrams (see previous study), giving their approximate location and size so as to be available for reference. When this is correctly done, a more or less complete reconstruction of the traumatic episode can be made.

General Manifestations of Craniocerebral Injury

In addition to the purely functional disturbances produced by craniocerebral injury, more severe degrees of force produce certain other general effects altering the structure of the brain. These alterations are often overlooked unless they are specifically searched for. Nevertheless, they form an integral part of the total picture of craniocerebral damage. These alterations include *congestion* and *edema.*

Congestion. In individuals who die within a short time after their injury, the brain is found to be generally congested. The degree of congestion depends largely upon the degree of the traumatizing force as well as other attendant circumstances (particularly acute alcoholism). In this state, which implies a paralysis of the vasomotor centers, the capillary pattern of the brain becomes conspicuous by the presence of increased amounts of blood in these channels. Congestion is at first commensurate with the degree of concussion. However, it may extend into the subacute or chronic stage. It does not ordinarily leave any permanent residuals insofar as any structural change is concerned. After severe degrees of concussion, however, the associated vasomotor instability may be responsible for the microscopic areas of pallor which are observed in the cortex days or weeks following a severe craniocerebral injury (Rand and Courville, 1936) (2).

Cerebral Edema. Post-traumatic cerebral edema has been a matter of considerable controversy throughout the years. It has often been observed in decompressive operations as a

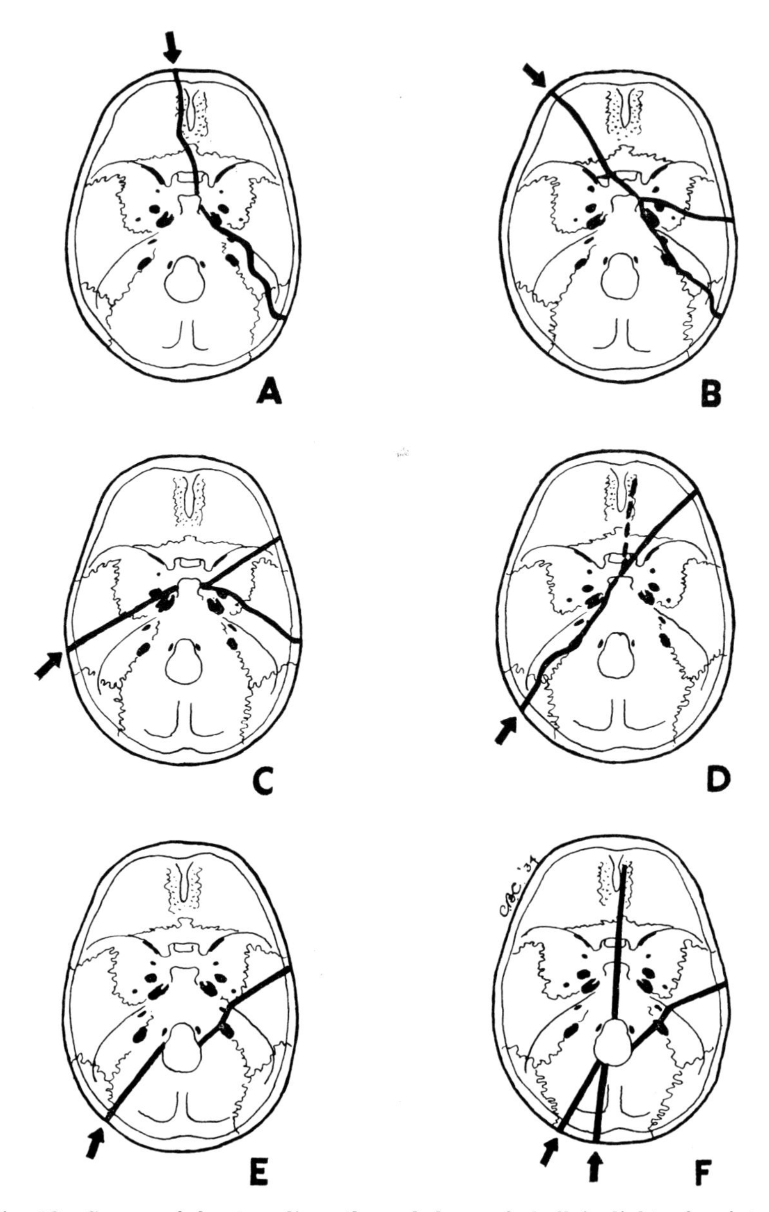

Fig. 13—Course of fracture lines through base of skull in light of point of application and direction of force causing craniocerebral injury (after Rawling).

"wet brain" or as accumulations of subarachnoid or subdural fluid. This excess of free fluid is found in individuals who have sustained a fairly severe degree of craniocerebral injury from automobile accidents or falls (Group C). The findings indicate an outpouring of fluid both into the ventricles (from choroid plexus) and cerebral tissues (into perivascular spaces) from whence it extends ultimately into the subarachnoid or subdural spaces. It evidently represents an increased transudation of fluid through the walls of the veins rather than the arteries. At least there is an associated passive engorgement of the veins rather than an active congestion of the arteries (Courville, 1942) (3).

This generalized edema is manifested grossly by a swelling of the nervous tissues and is characterized by the flattening of the dorsolateral convolutions of the cerebral hemispheres and associated with a corresponding narrowing of the ventricular cavities. Its exact significance, however, is not so well demonstrated in fatal cases in the brain of embalmed bodies.

Local edema resulting from contusions, lacerations or hemorrhages has an entirely different significance. As is true of traumatic lesions of any part or organ, a swelling of the regional nervous tissues is associated with a structural lesion. This is perhaps best exemplified in a swelling of the temporal lobe in the presence of a severe cortical-subcortical contusion. This localized edema is therefore commensurate with the degree of damage to brain tissue and results in swelling of one or more lobes or, in severe cases, of an entire cerebral hemisphere. Note should be made of the degree of this local swelling so that it is recognized as a part of the total picture of cerebral damage in any given case.[1]

[1] The phenomena of cerebral congestion, as well as cerebral edema, appears to be much more marked as a general result of trauma in patients who have sustained injuries of the Group C type. This would therefore imply that injuries sustained when the head in motion strikes an immobile or relatively immobile object is much more potent as a mechanism in producing such changes. These changes are very limited in direct injuries to the head. The element of movement, therefore, seems to be especially significant. This principle of movement of the brain which has been recognized for two centuries or more before the highly significant and praise-

Brain Movement in Craniocerebral Injury

As long ago as 1749 Le Dran (4) and others observed that patients who sustained injuries to the head incident to falls suffered from greater degrees of concussion than did those who were struck on the stationary head. These early observers concluded correctly that movement of the head had something to do with the severity of concussion, a factor which has been recently demonstrated objectively by the physiological studies of Denny-Brown and Russell (1941) (5). The various theories which have been postulated to account for the so-called coup-contrecoup injuries of the brain included some degree of movement of the brain to account for the contusions resulting therefrom, a lesion which is characteristic of these injuries.

Thus it will be seen that there are two factors responsible for injury of the brain itself. The first we have just mentioned, namely *movement of the brain* within the cranial vault found typically in Group C injuries in which the head in motion strikes an immobile or relatively immobile object. It is also recognized that in any head injury of material degree there is probably some movement of the brain. In most cases, however, such movement per se is not capable of producing gross damage to the brain. A second factor which comes into play is the *direct effect of force* applied to the skull. This may result in a simple linear fracture of the vault which assumes a horizontal course or which extends vertically towards the base. These vertical fractures tend to produce damage in the subfrontal region or the lower temporal or occipital cortex, but are particularly apt to lacerate the basilar surface of the cerebellum. In most instances, however, any serious injury to the brain resulting from fracture itself occurs as a consequence of a comminuted depressed bony lesion in which indriven fragments of bone lacerate the dura mater and the superficial portion of the brain itself. This matter will be discussed more in detail in a subsequent section.

---

worthy work of Denny-Brown and his associates has been pointed out as explaining the occurrence of two possible mechanisms in cerebral concussion as well as the influence of acceleration and deceleration.

Essential Mechanisms of Cerebral Injury

Thus far in this discussion it has been anticipated that cranial injury tends to fall into three well defined types, based upon the mechanism by which the injury has occurred (Fig. 14). In the first group (Group A) injury to the skull and brain results from the impact of a moving object on the head. This group can be subdivided into four subgroups. Subgroup 1 results from the impact of a relatively large object traveling at slow velocity. When such an object strikes the skull with sufficient force, a local depressed fracture will result. The nervous tissues may be damaged secondarily through the intervention of fragments driven into the cranial cavity with resulting compression, contusion or actual laceration of the underlying brain. In Subgroup 2, the cranial injury results from the entrance at a relatively slow velocity of a pointed implement. The area of impact on the skull is usually limited to a small point or narrow slit (stab wound). In Subgroup 3, the traumatizing object or weapon has a sharp edge which produces an incised cranial wound, often with a "splitting fracture" at either end of the incision. Subgroup 4 is characterized by the penetration of the cranial vault by small objects, usually of metallic character traveling at high velocity. These missiles result in a penetrating or perforating type of injury.

In the second group of wounds (Group B) there is compression of the skull between two relatively broad surfaces tending to approximate one another. This group is also divided into two subgroups. In Subgroup 1 the movement of the two approximating bodies is usually slow but progressive, as occurs in compression of the fetal head between the blades of an obstetrical forcep. Under this circumstance, injury of the brain is usually limited to pressure by consequent subdural hemorrhage, although a depressed fracture with laceration of the cortex may rarely occur. Subgroup 2 occurs in adult life, the head being compressed either between two large approximating surfaces or by one surface compressing the head against a second unyielding surface. Such mechanisms tend to produce severe crushing injuries of the skull with gross damage to the brain.

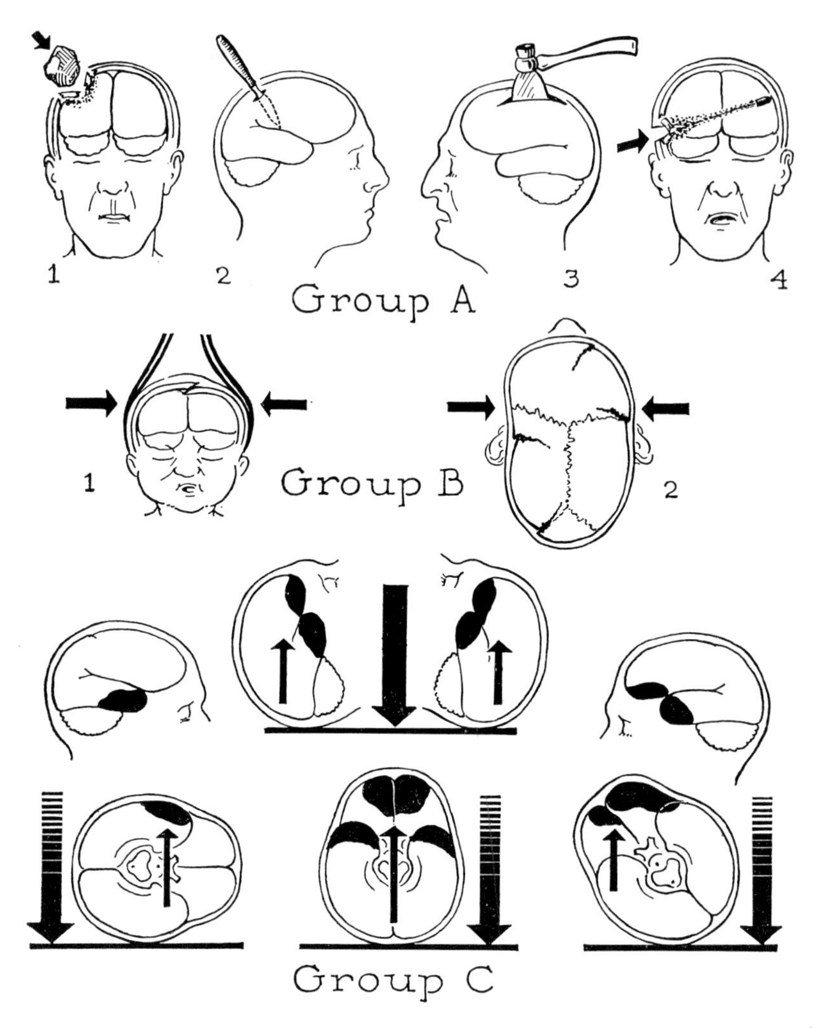

Fig. 14—Diagrammatic representation of types of craniocerebral injury. Group A. Injuries sustained when various types of objects fall on quiescent head. 1. Focal injury with comminuted depressed fracture from falling object. 2. Stab wound. 3. Incised wound. 4. Missile wound. Group B. Compression injuries. 1. Compression of infant's head by obstetrical forceps. 2. Compression of adult head. Group C. Coup-contrecoup injuries sustained when head in motion strikes a quiescent object (traffic accidents and falls).

The third group of injuries (Group C) are those sustained when the head in motion strikes an immobile or relatively immobile object. These injuries, which are the most common ones experienced in civilian life (Courville, 1937) (6), typically result as a consequence of traffic accidents or falls. The great importance of this group lies in their frequency. They also produce a classical series of intracranial lesions such as subdural hemorrhage (or hematoma), subarachnoid hemorrhage, cortical or cortical-subcortical contusions, and intracerebral hemorrhages. These lesions are the result of what is commonly known as a coup-contrecoup mechanism.

Each of these three groups of injuries will be considered separately, attention being paid to the type of lesions which are characteristically produced thereby. In each group the nature of the traumatizing objects, their effect on the scalp and skull, as well as the type of damage produced on the intracranial structures will be considered.

Lesions of Group A (from Impact of Moving Bodies)

As noted in the above classification, injuries in Group A (in which a moving object strikes the quiescent head) may be of three types. Injury to the brain tissues per se results when the traumatizing object produces a local depressed fracture of the skull, or when the lesion is modified by entrance of the traumatizing object into the cranial cavity.

Injuries of Subtype 1 are commonly sustained in industrial accidents or in felonious assaults on the victim's head. The nature and degree of injury depends entirely upon several factors involved. In mild injuries the scalp alone may be traumatized in the form of a bruise, abrasion or laceration. If the injury is more severe, the object tends to cause (a) local contusion of bone with depression of the external table into the diploe, or (b) a local depressed fracture which may comminute the bone either of the inner table alone or of both tables. Indriven bony fragments may result in laceration of the dura with compression or laceration of underlying brain. The characteristic intracranial lesions are (1) hemorrhage resulting from laceration of regional vessels and (2) compression, contusion or laceration of the underlying brain. The degree of brain damage is proportional to the extent of the depression and the degree of laceration of the brain by the indriven fragments or entrance of the traumatizing object.

It is important to recognize in this group of cases that *unless the skull is fractured and unless the depression is sufficient to indicate contact with the brain no material degree of gross brain damage will result.* It is sometimes true that a fracture (described as "greenstick") occurs in which a temporary depression of the inner table is followed by restoration of the original contour when the depressed fragments spring back into place. In such cases transitory cerebral symptoms are followed by recovery usually within a few days following the injury.

In a group of cases in Subtype 2, the injury is the same as in Subtype 1 except that the impact diameter of the traumatizing object is relatively small. A puncture-type of wound will then result. This depends upon the force with which the object is projected against the head. In Subtype 3, an edged weapon or sharp bladed implement will produce an incised wound of the skull often with a "split" fracture at either end.[2]

The basic principle of brain damage is the same as in Subtype 1, namely that the brain will not be injured unless the cranial vault has been penetrated. Moreover, the injury sustained must of necessity lie immediately beneath the point (or line) of injury. The amount of brain damage is again dependent upon the size, shape and extent of penetration of the injuring object.

Stab Wounds of the Brain. Puncture wounds of the brain from pointed implements or weapons are not uncommon. They may occur as a result either of an accident (a fall on sharp pointed tool or an implement such as an ice pick) or from a felonious assault (stab wound from a dagger or knife). If exposed at autopsy in their recent phase, a sharply outlined defect is found corresponding to the length and width of the blade. In recent cases, there is usually an associated hemorrhage from severance of meningeal or cerebral vessels; later meningitis may develop from indriven contaminated material. In late cases, the blade of the knife may still be found *in situ* with a variable degree of thin-bordered glial

[2] If the cutting edge of an implement such as an axe or hatchet is too blunt, an elongated depressed fracture will result rather than a true incised wound.

scar about it. Small focal cystic spaces within a dense scar may follow hemorrhages from vessels originally severed by the blade. Convulsive seizures are perhaps the most common complication of individuals who survive such a wound for any great length of time (Courville, 1955) (7).

In wounds of Subtype 4 are those produced by flying missiles usually propelled by gun powder. Formerly designated as gunshot wounds, they have more recently been described as "missile" wounds to include the wounds of war in which fragments of shells, grenades, or bombs, as well as bullets are concerned. Conforming to the pattern, however, the amount of brain damage is dependent upon the depression or fragmentation of the inner table of the skull and indriven bits of foreign material such as bone or by penetration of the missile itself. Such wounds of the skull and brain have been variously classified but the ones involving the brain may be described as (1) *tangential wounds*—in which the scalp and skull may be traumatized together with damages to the underlying brain. (2) A *penetrating wound* is one in which fragments of bone are driven into the cranial cavity by a missile striking more or less at right angles to the surface of the skull, the missile itself as well as these indriven fragments being retained within the skull. Such a wound is characterized by (a) a cone of destruction which consists of a focus of lacerated brain tissue immediately beneath the point of impact, and (b) a second portion of the wound or "track" produced by the missile and by attendant foreign material and blood clot, a linear defect corresponding to the course of the missile. The missile itself is to be found at the end of the track. (3) A *through-and-through wound* is one in which there is a wound of exit as well as a wound of entrance, the missile having extended its trajectory through the opposite side of the skull. There may be a slightly expanded terminal defect in the brain at this point but the other portions of the wound correspond to the penetrating wound. The cranial wound of exit is larger than the one of entrance, and the outer table of the skull rather than the inner one being more extensively fragmented. Other types of wounds depending upon their location and the parts involved have also been described, such as orbito-nasal and auriculo-temporal wounds in which a missile has produced a complex lesion involving a considerable portion of the skull and brain. The surgical pathology of these types of wounds was originally described by Cushing (1918) (8) and more recently by Abbott (1961) (9) and need not be described in detail further.

It should be said, however, that the degree of lethality of such wounds is dependent not only upon the severity of damage to the brain either by the missile or by indriven fragments of bone, but also by the possibility of laceration of blood vessels, the proximity of the path of the missile to the ganglionic areas of the cerebral hemispheres or the vital centers in the brain stem. The possibility of secondary or "late" inflammatory complication incident to indriven foreign material must also be considered.

Group B Wounds—Compression Fractures and Crushing Brain Wounds

The Group B types of craniocerebral injury are not ordinarily of concern in forensic neuropathology. As previously stated two types are possible: (1) the slowly developing compressions in infants due to excessive force in the use of the obstetrical forceps and (2) those of adult life. The second type is so often fatal as to be only of medicolegal concern. The mechanism is usually obvious. The fractures resulting from these compressions tend to occur at right angles to the site of compression (meridional fractures). If this mechanism is carried out to its fullest extent total destruction of the skull and brain results.

Type C Injuries—The Common Civilian Lesions

Injuries of Group C type, namely those resulting when the head in motion strikes an immobile or relatively immobile object results in a characteristic cluster of lesions. This mechanism has long been described as the coup-contrecoup type of injury, a term introduced by early French observers. The characteristic resulting intracranial lesions are subdural hemorrhage (or hematoma), subarachnoid hemorrhage, contusions of the subfrontal region and anterolateral aspect of the temporal lobes, and intracerebral hemorrhages within the frontal, temporal or temporo-occipital centrum. This train of lesions are not found as the result of any other mechanism; therefore their significance should not be mistaken. *Since this group of lesions is found almost exclusively as the result of traffic accidents or falls, there is little excuse for confusing this group of lesions for those produced by direct criminal assault.*

Injuries Sustained with the Head in Motion—The Coup-Contrecoup Mechanism

Since Renaissance times surgeons dealing with cranial injuries, particularly those resulting from falls (since vehicular traffic in that era was usually slow and accidents infrequent), there came to be recognized bruises or contusions of the brain at points diametrically opposite to the point of impact. Description of such injuries was first made by the French surgeons of the eighteenth century. In the latter half of this century in particular, many contributions appeared dealing with the mechanism of contrecoup injuries, although not all the factors involved were then fully appreciated. In fact, it was not until the significant study of Apfelbach (1922) (10) based on a large series of craniocerebral injuries consequent to automobile accidents that a true concept of the mechanism was fully appreciated. This observer made it clear that such injuries occurred when the head was in motion at the time of impact. This asserted mechanism was early put to the test by the present writer in a large series of cases and found to be remarkably consistent in its application. This interpretation of coup-contrecoup injuries proved to be so reliable that it was with assurance that one can readily distinguish injuries sustained in traffic accidents from those produced by blows to the head. A correct evaluation of the results of these mechanisms in a given case, therefore, becomes most important in suspected cases of criminal assault. While a number of theories have been proposed to account for this peculiar manifestation, the lesions are probably dependent upon a number of factors working in combination. A brief survey of the essential factors regarding this group of injuries has been previously outlined (Courville, 1950) (11) and may be referred to if further study on this point is desired.

Because the most common and most characteristic lesion of the coup-contrecoup mechanism is a contusion, it is advisable to consider carefully the mechanism of its production (Courville, 1942, 1950) (12). It is necessary here to mention briefly one theoretical aspect of the problem, since no actual experimental demonstration of the mechanism has been forthcoming. It has been postulated that when the head is in motion (as in the course of a fall) the soft and pliable brain lags behind the movement of the enveloping skull. When the dependent part of the falling head is suddenly stopped by contact with an unyielding object (the ground) the lagging brain is dashed against the hard and irregular internal surface of the opposite wall of the skull. In a strict sense, it is the "pole" of the brain which lies diametrically opposite to the point of impact that is injured in this manner. The brain in the immediate environment of this pole tends to glide away, thereby coming in contact with any bony prominences in this vicinity. The greater the speed of this gliding movement, the larger will be the resulting contusion.

After this "splash" of the brain against the opposite wall, a secondary ebbing wave follows, one which flows back in the opposite direction toward the point of original impact. The brain is now thrust against the inner surface of the skull and glides along its dural lining. If the bony surface is smooth (as in case of the occipital pole) no contusion will result; if the wall happens to show some irregularity, (as in the case of the temporal region) a second but smaller contusion will result. This lesion, occurring at the site of the original impact, is therefore designated as a *coup* lesion although it very likely represents the effect of a resurgence of the first wave of force which traveled through the brain in line with the movement of the head.

In addition to the original mass movement of the brain which has produced the *contrecoup* (and occasionally a *coup*) contusion, a factor of *shearing stress* sometimes plays a role in the production of secondary brain damage (Holbourn, 1943) (13). This effect is observed at the rostrum of the corpus callosum where the midportion of the brain is thrust through the opening beneath the falx cerebri, the adjacent medial surface of the hemisphere being held against this unyielding structure. This factor also accounts for small contusions on the lateral aspect of the gyri in cases of subfrontal injuries on lateral movements of the head.

With this somewhat oversimplified concept in mind, a review of the effects of impacts on various parts of the moving head may now be considered. These areas of impact are shown diagrammatically in the accompanying drawing (Fig. 15). In it are indicated the effect of an impact in the frontal

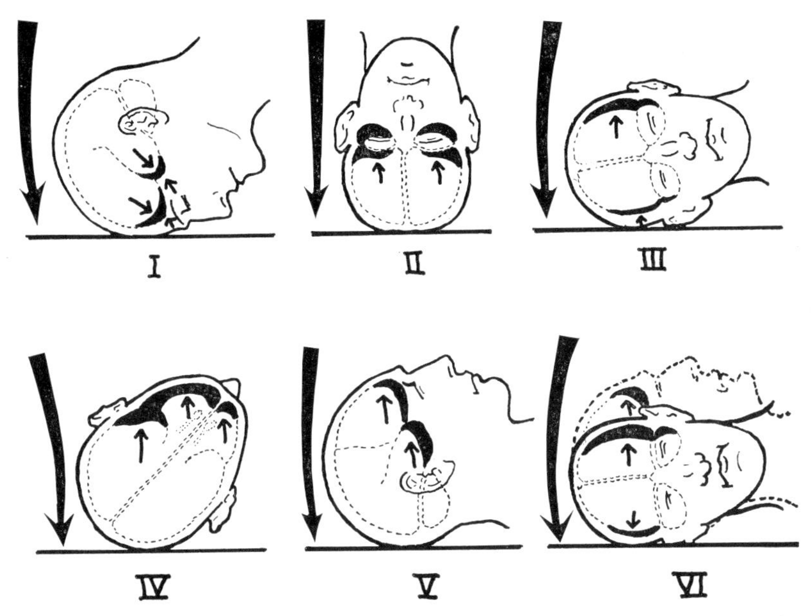

Fig. 15—Location of cerebral contusions based on site of impact of moving head. I. Impact in frontal region (rare *coup* contusions). II. Impact on vertex. III. Impact on lateral aspect of head. IV. Posterolateral impact. V. Impact in midline occipital region. VI. Multiple impacts. Contusions are represented by solid black areas.

region (Group I), falls on the vertex of the head (Group II), falls on the lateral aspect of the head (Group III), falls on the posterolateral aspect of the head (Group IV), falls directly on the back of the head (Group V), and as a final group, the possible effects on the brain of individuals who have multiple impacts of the head (Group VI) in the course of their trajectory. Unfortunately, this last situation is not uncommon and constitutes the most difficult element in the evaluation of lesions resulting from coup-contrecoup mechanism.[3]

One sometimes finds on the medial aspect or one of the other temporo-occipital regions areas of red softening limited largely to the cortex (Courville) (15). This type of lesion can follow an injury sustained with the head in motion (lateral impacts) but are more typically found in patients in whom a subdural hematoma has developed. Progressively and intermittently increasing pressure of the underlying cerebral hemisphere forces the ipsilateral posterior cerebral artery against the edge of the tentorium. In this sense we are dealing not with a true contusion but with red softening due to

---

[3] The occurrence of more than one point of impact of the moving head, as might well take place when an individual is first injured inside a moving vehicle in the course of a collision should be anticipated. The moving head might first be thrown forward and into contact with the windshield or dashboard. This might result in a fracture of the frontal bone (with laceration by this fracture of the anterior and especially the corresponding subfrontal region). A second impact with the door adjacent to the individual could occur secondarily if the vehicle turned on its side (which would result in a gross contrecoup lesion of the opercular region of the brain on the side opposite the impact and possibly a lesser coup contusion on the opposite side). A final impact on the vertex of the head might then occur when the head struck the pavement (with basal contusions of the frontal and temporal lobes). Each of these impacts should be indicated by some bruises of the skin and scalp, as well as hemorrhages into its loose tissues. The more severe impacts could also be marked by regional fractures of the skull. With reasonable attention to the several lesions in such instances, the mechanism of trauma should not readily be mistaken for one of an entirely different type.

In a recent study by Lindenberg and Freytag (1960) (14), a somewhat different approach to the problem of coup-contrecoup injuries is made. In the first place, these investigators consider all lesions occurring at the point of impact, regardless of the mechanism of injury. Such a grouping includes the effects of local skull fracture, either linear or depressed. Even the effects of the "bending" effects of such an injury are included. Moreover, the possibility of multiple mechanisms are not always clear, making analysis of the individual cases somewhat difficult. An appeal to hypothetical factors consequent to the effects of mechanical force furthermore complicate the pictures. However, two aspects of the problem do coincide with the views set forth in this article, (1) the contrecoup effects of falls on the back of the head, and (2) the complex lesions which may occur in case of multiple mechanisms. Any student of the problem of mechanisms of craniocerebral trauma should study this paper carefully.

an intermittent ischemia of this artery. When due to the immediate effects of the force of the injury itself, it may be designated as a true diffuse contusion, but when pressure by edema or hemorrhage causes it, it should be referred to as secondary red softening.

In order to obtain a clear picture of the effects of cerebral contusion by this group of mechanisms, a series of 274 cases of acute brain damage in traffic accidents and falls were reviewed (Courville, 1958) (16). In these cases, 135 examples of contusion were found. The outline of the contused area was then drawn upon a series of separate diagrams of the brain, in each verified case the point of contact of the head with the unyielding object was clearly defined by objective evidence. This composite of a number of unequivocal cases makes it obvious that the location and outline of the resulting contusions have followed a consistent pattern and clearly supports the theory of the coup-contrecoup mechanism herein described. The individual patterns resulting from impacts in the several groups of cases are indicated in the accompanying figure which is clearly labeled (Fig. 16).

In order to demonstrate how well this principle works out on actual autopsy specimen, a series of photographs of the base of the brain with actual contusions are here depicted. The point of impact of the head is shown in each case as well as the direction of the lines of force producing the contusion (Fig. 17). In diagrams used to indicate the location of contusions included in each record, it would be well to indicate the point of impact as well as the location and direction of any basal fracture, so that this mechanism can be clearly and readily made out.

A few points still need to be emphasized. Occasionally (in only two cases of this series) a severe impact in the frontal region has resulted in a *coup* contusion in the subfrontal and anterior temporal cortex. Such lesions must therefore be quite rare; indeed the situation may actually be modified by the presence of fracture of the frontal bone in this region. A second interesting fact which is a corollary to this first one is that while *contrecoup* contusions of the subfrontal and anterior temporal regions are the rule in impact of the moving head in the parieto-occipital regions, *contrecoup contu-*

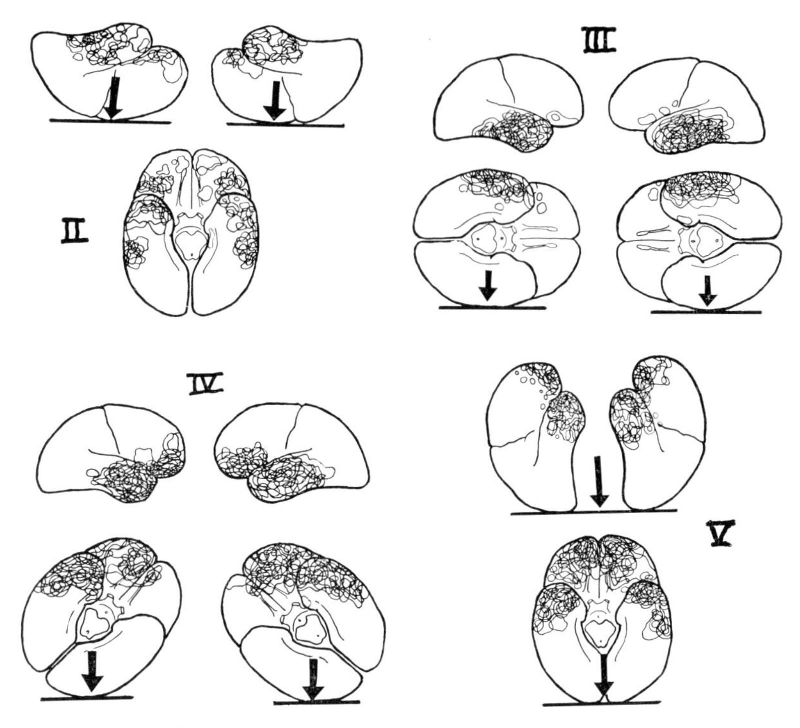

Fig. 16—Composite drawing showing location of contusions of large number of cases with impacts on different parts of head, (II) on vertex of head, (III) on lateral aspect, (IV) on posterolateral aspect, (V) on midline of occipital region.

sions of the occipital lobe from impacts of the frontal region are never known to occur! In impacts on the lateral aspect of the head where the interior of the skull is symmetrical on the two sides, both *coup* and *contrecoup* contusions may occur, but the contrecoup contusion is always the more severe. This last group of lesions emphasize the real importance of the *contrecoup* factor in the production of contusions.

Characteristics of Cerebral Cortical Contusions. Incredible as it may seem, some pathologists serving as medical examiners seem unable to differentiate either old or recent contusions of the cerebral cortex from other lesions typical of vascular etiology, i. e., focal infarctions. This should easily be done if it is but remembered that true traumatic lesions are usually found limited to the subfrontal or anterior tempo-

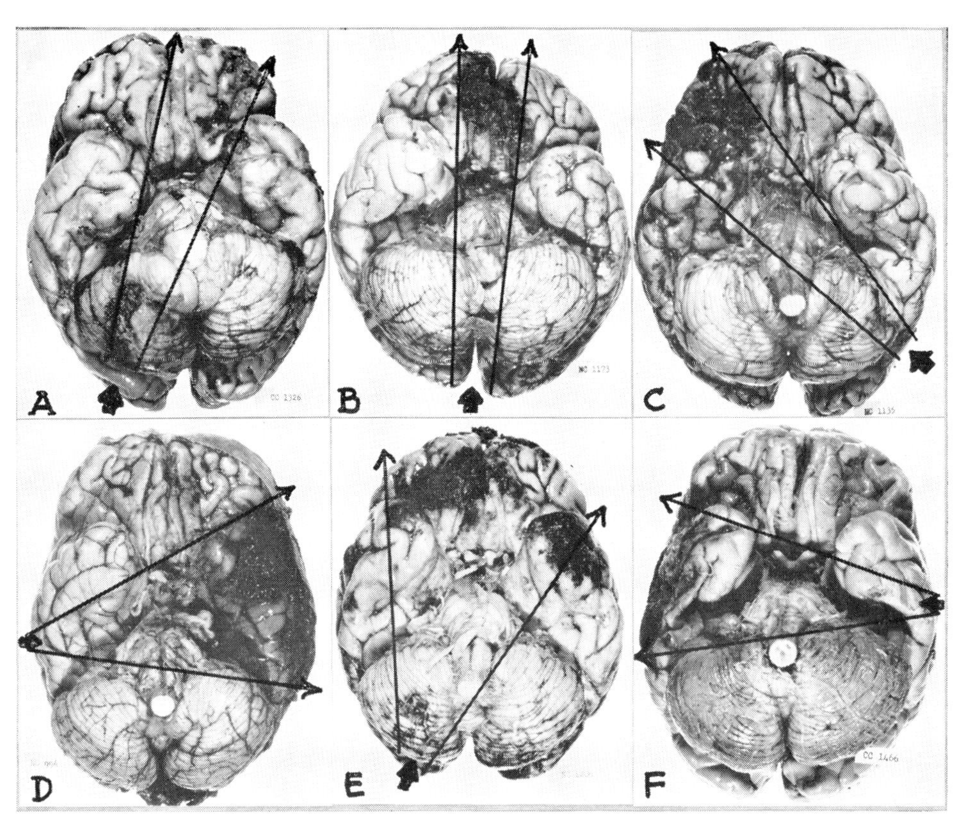

Fig. 17—Mechanism of cerebral contusions as observed in actual cases. A. Impact just to right of posterior midline. B. Posterior midline impact in a fall. C. Left posterolateral aspect. D. Right lateral impact just behind middle of head. E. To right of midline. F. Direct left lateral impact. Contused lacerations of inferior surface of cerebellum mark line of fracture of cranial basis.

ral regions, that the focal hemorrhagic center of the contusion (or old defect) almost invariably involves the apex or ridge of the involved convolution (or convolutions), that on cross section the lesion is wedge-shaped with the tip of the wedge tending to point into the underlying white matter, and that this lesion is sharply circumscribed, not ordinarily being associated with regional zones of ischemia (focal softening marked by endothelial proliferation of regional capillaries). In minimal lesions, there is also noted a narrow zone of unaltered cortex lying just beneath the pia mater. In the fresh state the lesion itself consists of a number of focal circumscribed hemorrhages with destruction of the cortical tissue by lacerating effects of these effusions. The larger central hemorrhagic focus is surrounded by a number of satellite foci, but the zone formed by these hemorrhages is definitely limited. The nerve cells and fibers are well preserved remarkably close to the margin of the wedge-shaped defect.

Cross sections of old lesions are also characterized by a wedge-shaped defect of varying size, involving a single gyrus or multiple adjacent gyri. The margin of the superficial portion of the defect usually has a wisp of arachnoid pointing into it, while the borders are composed of a thin, glial scar made up of fibrous neurological cells enmeshed in fine neuroglial network. In this scar, compound granular corpuscles may be found even after many months. Along the border of the preserved cortex, isolated or clusters of decadent nerve cells encrusted with iron are often present.

In the accompanying figure, the contour of a series of variously-sized recent contusions are shown in cross section (Fig. 18).

As a point of special interest showing the importance of the *contrecoup* as opposed to the *coup* mechanism, the group of cases in which the victim falls striking flatly on one side of the head, the *most severe lesions are invariably contrecoup.* These more widespread frontotemporal contusions are quite superficial in character due to the fact that the bony grooves in which the gyri rest are likewise rather shallow.

It is important to distinguish between lacerations resulting from fracture lines crossing the cranial fossae from true contusions, particularly if the lesion occurs on the basilar surfaces of the frontal and temporal lobes. The explanation of the presence of lacerations in these locations is that these surfaces of the brain are held in close apposition to the cranial basis by the cranial nerves and blood vessels so that the fracture line cuts into the adjacent soft brain, even though the covering dura remains intact. Such lacerations may extend above the inferolateral margin of the cerebral hemispheres if the fracture line also extend onto the sides of the cranial vault. The lacerations so produced may be distin-

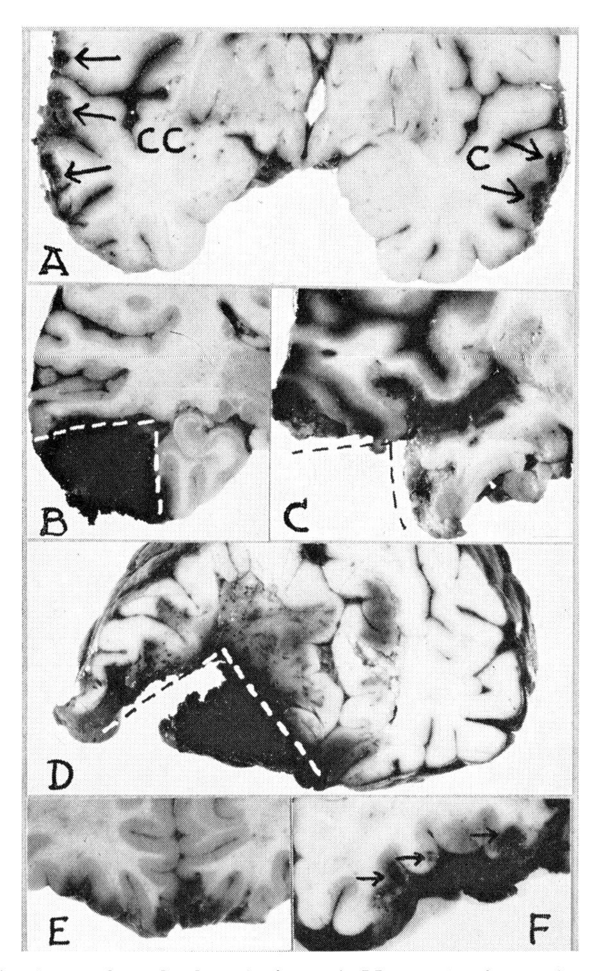

Fig. 18—Anatomy of cerebral contusions. A. More extensive contrecoup superficial contusion on left; focal coup contusions on right. B and C. Wedge-shaped hemorrhage and defect in severe temporal lobe contusions. D. Hemorrhage and wedge-shaped defect in subfrontal contusion. E. Minor subfrontal cortical contusions. F. Contusions of lateral aspect of frontal gyri resulting from shearing stress.

guished by the fact that it lies in line with the fracture, it produces a narrow, more or less continuous line of destruction of tissue, crossing the convolutional ridges and sulci without definite interruption, and may be found where contusions do not usually occur. The true *contusion*, on the other hand, is a more oval lesion which tends to involve the ridges of the convolutions, leaving the margins of the sulci undamaged (unless the lesion is large when the entire central portion of the contusion is disorganized). The presence or absence of a linear fracture line, is of course an important criterion.

The matter of traumatic cerebral hemorrhage is an important one but will be considered more in detail in the next study because the hemorrhagic effusions following trauma must often be distinguished from those of spontaneous origin.

Summary

In order to bring the several aspects of the mechanisms of craniocerebral injury within a limited discussion it may be said that each particular type of injury produces its own train of lesions which are more or less characteristic of that mechanism. A critical study of the craniocerebral lesion complex found at autopsy, therefore makes it possible in most cases to reconstruct the mechanism of the injury. This is true even of the more complicated lesions produced by traffic accidents and falls (coup-contrecoup lesions). Since these accidental injuries must be distinguished from those due to felonious assault, a clear understanding of the causative coup-contrecoup mechanism is of vital importance. Because the lesions resulting from this latter condition are still so typical that there is no excuse for a medicolegal pathologist to confuse them with traumatic lesions of other mechanisms. It should be remembered that a direct blow to the quiescent head will not produce actual brain damage unless the skull itself has been fractured, usually with depression and comminution of bone. The problem of accompanying traumatic intracranial hemorrhage must await further discussion.

A study now in progress is concerned with the effect of the contrecoup mechanism in infants and young children. Some have denied the occurrence of contrecoup lesions in infancy and early childhood, and have used this assumption to deny the whole philosophy. In our current study, however, it has been shown that contrecoup cortical contusions as well as intracerebral hemorrhages do occur but are much more rare before the age of three years. A typical cortical contusion was found in a fatal case of craniocerebral injury at the age of six weeks. The typical adult pattern of contusions (location and relative incidence), does not occur until some time after the age of five years, exact time not having been determined for want of sufficient cases.

REFERENCES

1. Courville, Cyril B.: The Pathologic Aspects of Cerebral Concussion. Arch. Neurol. & Psychiat. 34:1351 (Dec.) 1935. Ibid: The Functional and Structural Basis of Psychic Phenomena Consequent to Cerebral Concussion. J. Nerv. & Ment. Dis. 118:447–454 (Nov.) 1953. Ibid: Commotio Cerebri. Cerebral Concussion and the Post-Concussion Syndrome in Their Medical and Legal Aspects. Los Angeles. San Lucas Press. 1953, pp. 62–80.
2. Rand, C. W., and Courville, Cyril B.: Histologic Studies of the Brain in Cases of Fatal Injury to the Head. VI. Cyto-Architectonic Alterations. Arch. Neurol. & Psychiat. 36:1277–1293 (Dec.) 1936.
3. Courville, Cyril B.: Structural Changes in the Brain Consequent to Traumatic Disturbances of Intracranial Fluid Balance. Bull. Los Angeles Neurol. Soc. 7:55–76 (June) 1942.
4. Le Dran, H. F.: The Operations in Surgery. Tr. by T. Gataker, London, C. Hitch, 1749.
5. Denny-Brown, D. E. and Russell, W. R.: Experimental Cerebral Concussion. Brain 64:93–164 (Sept.) 1941.
6. Courville, Cyril B.: Fatal Craniocerebral Injuries. A Statistical Study. Bull. Los Angeles Neurol. Soc. 2:59–65 (June) 1937.
7. Courville, Cyril B.: Contribution to Stab Wounds of the Brain. Report of Three Cases Verified at Autopsy. Bull. Los Angeles Neurol. Soc. 20:189–192 (Dec.) 1955.
8. Cushing, H.: A Study of a Series of Wounds Involving the Brain and its Enveloping Structures. Brit. J. Surg. 5:558–684, 1918.
9. Abbott, Kenneth H.: Acute Missile Wounds of the Brain. An Atlas of Surgical Pathology. Bull. Los Angeles Neurol. Soc. 26:103 (Sept.) 1961.
10. Apfelbach, C. W.: Studies in Traumatic Fractures of the Cranial Bones. I. Edema of the Brain. II. Bruises of the Brain. Arch. Surg. 4:434 (Mar.) 1922.
11. Courville, Cyril B.: Pathology of the Central Nervous System. A Study Based Upon a Survey of Lesions Found in a Series of Forty Thousand Autopsies. Mountain View, California. Pacific Press Publish. Assn., 3rd ed. pp. 297–298, 1950.
12. Courville, Cyril B.: Coup-Contrecoup Mechanism of Craniocerebral Injuries. Arch. Surg. 45:19–43 (July) 1942. Ibid: The Mechanisms of Coup-Contrecoup Injuries of the Brain. A Critical Review of Recent Experimental Studies in the Light of Clinical Observations. Bull. Los Angeles Neurol. Soc. 15:72–86 (June) 1950.

13. Holbourn, A. H. S.: Mechanism of Brain Injury. Lancet 245:438 (Oct. 9) 1943.
14. Lindenberg, R., and Freytag, E.: The Mechanisms of Cerebral Contusions. Arch. Path. 69:440–469 (Apr.) 1960.
15. Courville, Cyril B.: Diffuse Cortical Contusion of the Occipital Lobe. Arch. Path. 20:523–534 (Oct.) 1935.
16. Courville, Cyril B.: Traumatic Lesions of the Temporal Lobe as the Essential Cause of Psychomotor Epilepsy, in Temporal Lobe Epilepsy, ed. by M. Baldwin and P. Bailey, Springfield, Illinois, Charles C Thomas, 1958, pp. 220–239.

Chapter IV. Intracranial Hemorrhage—Spontaneous versus Traumatic*

In autopsies on medicolegal cases, hemorrhage into the cranial space is one of the most common lesions to be found. The essential problem under such circumstances is to determine whether the hemorrhagic effusion is spontaneous or traumatic. In the great majority of cases, the solution of this problem is not difficult if due attention is given to certain basic postulates. The answer lies in a complete evaluation of the hemorrhage itself as well as the associated lesions. The purpose of this contribution is to point out the essential features in the differential diagnosis between spontaneous and traumatic intracranial effusions. It will first be necessary to present a review of intracranial hemorrhage in general.

Predisposing Factors in Intracranial Hemorrhage.—The factors which determine the cause of hemorrhage include (1) the location of the blood vessels, (2) the size of the blood vessel, (3) the thickness of the vessel wall, (4) the presence of abnormalities in the number and structure of the vessels (vascular anomalies and malformations) or of localized defects in the vessel wall (congenital or saccular aneurysms), (5) diseases of the vessel wall (syphilis, arteriosclerosis), (6) associated diseases or toxic states of the blood, or (7) an excessive degree of intra-arterial pressure. Not all of these factors have any bearing in traumatic hemorrhages, but do play an important role in spontaneous ones.

---

* Gross intracerebral hemorrhage is one of the most common of all brain lesions. Not infrequently the victim of such an insult has his "stroke" under circumstances which suggest a craniocerebral injury as its possible cause. A careful evaluation of the actual etiology of the hemorrhage in the intracranial space will then become an important decision for the pathologist to make.

The Location of Blood Vessels.—Not all vessels are equally susceptible to the effects of trauma, depending upon their exposure to injury. This variation also holds true of spontaneous hemorrhage, as will subsequently be shown. The *size of the vessels* is also one of the important factors. The largest intracranial vessels are not usually affected by trauma, unless torn by involvement in a fracture line or are the seat of serious arterial disease. For example, the carotid arteries are not ordinarily lacerated unless they are torn by a fracture line through the sella turcica. The same factor, however, does not play a part except in case of a penetrating wound, when any size vessel may be severed.

Inherent Thickness of the Arteries.—Very thin vessels (which may be in fact hypoplastic) are naturally more easily ruptured than are arteries of normal thickness. For instance, the writer has seen a fatal extradural hemorrhage with death in a period of three hours, in a little girl who sustained only minor injury to the head from a fall to the sidewalk. The middle meningeal arteries were so hypoplastic as to be scarcely visible in the dura when examined at autopsy.

Congenital Defects.—Such defects are much less predisposed to traumatic bleeding than would be anticipated. Under such circumstances spontaneous rupture is more likely.

Changes in Quality of the Blood.—Blood dyscrasias or other toxic changes in the quality of the blood not infrequently result in spontaneous bleeding. Only rarely, however, does this predispose to hemorrhage incident to trauma. Certain toxic states, especially alcoholism, are much more likely to result in prolonged bleeding, once precipitated by trauma, than to produce it in the first place.

Diseases of Blood Vessel Walls.—The same situation occurs in case of disease of the walls of the blood vessels. For example, it is rare to have a traumatic intracerebral hemorrhage in an old person with arteriosclerosis. This lesion is actually much more common in young adults.

Intra-arterial Tension.—Arterial hypertension likewise does little to favor traumatic hemorrhage although it is the most common cause of spontaneous hemorrhage.

The negative or positive influence of these several factors of intracranial hemorrhage is often misinterpreted in evaluating *hemorrhages* in individuals who have been subject to cranial injury. These factors therefore deserve critical attention whenever there is disclosed a questionable lesion.

Classifications of Cerebral Hemorrhage

The most practical way to classify hemorrhage in the intracranial space is on the basis of its anatomic relationships. The location of such a hemorrhage is an easy matter to decide at autopsy. Moreover, the location itself gives one an early clue as to its cause. These effusions may be classified as (1) extradural hemorrhage or "hematoma" occurring between the dura mater and bone, (2) subdural hemorrhage or hematoma, (3) subarachnoid hemorrhage, either vertical or basilar, (4) intracerebral hemorrhage, and (5) intraventricular hemorrhage. Each type of hemorrhage will now be evaluated on the basis of its location and with respect to its possible etiology.

Extradural Hemorrhage

Extradural hemorrhages other than those of traumatic etiology are extremely rare. The only noteworthy exceptions are the small effusions usually occurring in early infancy and incident to blood dyscrasias. The differential diagnosis in this group of cases is therefore a simple matter. The traumatic hemorrhages are almost invariably associated with a fracture line, which likewise assists in diagnosis. They are due to laceration of one of the larger meningeal arteries, anterior, middle or posterior, less commonly to tears of the dural venous sinuses or to laceration by fracture of the diploic or emissary veins.

There are three common locations where laceration of the meningeal arteries and their accompanying veins may take place. The *frontal meningeal artery* grooves the interior surface of the frontal bone, and a hemorrhage resulting from a regional fracture occurs in this region not far removed from the corresponding frontal pole. The most common temporal group of traumatic extradural hemorrhages is found along the course of the middle meningeal artery, and is the result of a fracture in the middle fossa, or where this vessel crosses the tip of the sphenoidal ridge or along the arterial groove of the artery, on the inner surface of the squamous portion of the temporal bone (Fig. 19). The posterior meningeal artery is found on one side of the posterior fossa and hemorrhages result from linear fractures crossing its groove.

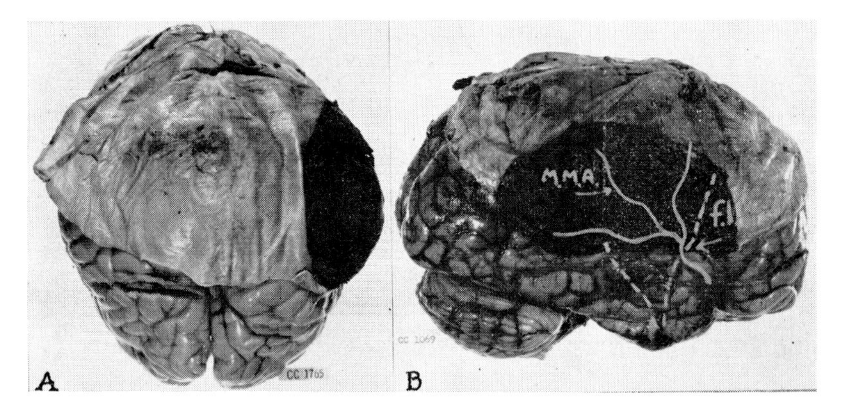

Fig. 19—Traumatic extradural hemorrhage. Marked circumscribed accumulation of blood on the under surface of the right temporal bone. A. Lateral view showing extent of blood clot and B. relation of linear fractures (f. l.) (broken lines) to branches of right middle meningeal artery (m. m. a.).

One of the characteristics of these extradural hemorrhages is that they are fairly well circumscribed. Such hemorrhages are usually fairly rapid in their evolution, often accumulating within 24 hours, with rapidly increasing signs of intracranial pressure, such as headaches, progressive lethargy, and paralysis or convulsions (in the central group). These hemorrhages tend to accumulate beneath a single bone (for example, the temporal squama) because the dura is fixed in the suture bounding it. The point of laceration is not usually difficult to locate at operation, for the blood is usually observed to be spurting from the defect in the vessel. At autopsy, however, this may be more difficult. The laceration is usually located where the fracture line crosses the meningeal artery or its branches. Unless this effusion of blood is promptly evacuated surgically, these lesions are almost invariably fatal.

Extradural "Hematoma".—A subacute or chronic state of extradural hemorrhage is extremely rare because of the tendency for these lesions to be fatal within a short time. However, one occasionally encounters a case in which the slow accumulation of blood with a slowly increasing intracranial pressure is compensated for in its evolution. This lesion is not a true hematoma because it is not an expanding lesion. The capsule is made up alone of connective tissue and there is no addition of free fluid because the lesion is not directly in contact with the arachnoidal space. In such cases the blood clot becomes inspissated, being dry and having a tendency to undergo fibrosis. If the patient should survive long enough, a deposit of calcium will be found about its margin. Ultimately new bone formation will appear about the margin of the "hematoma" where it lies adjacent to the inner surface of the skull.

Subdural Hemorrhage and Hematoma

A subdural hemorrhage is currently considered to be almost invariably traumatic. It was once thought that there is a special chronic encapsulated type of this lesion (recurrent subdural hematoma) which is the result of repeated hemorrhages of different etiology. Such lesions are actually quite rare. These cases of apparently repeated hemorrhages within the wall of the hematoma usually occur in alcoholics and are possibly the result of a series of alcoholic "binges".

Small subdural hemorrhages sometimes result from blood dyscrasias in infants, from thromboses of the intracranial venous channels incident to rupture of the cerebrocortical vessels, or from rupture through the arachnoid of hemorrhages primarily located within the brain itself. In these cases the etiology of subdural hemorrhage is therefore a simple matter because there is a history of an obviously primary source of bleeding in these cases.

It can now be accepted as fundamental that subdural hemorrhages are traumatic unless some other obvious cause can be demonstrated.

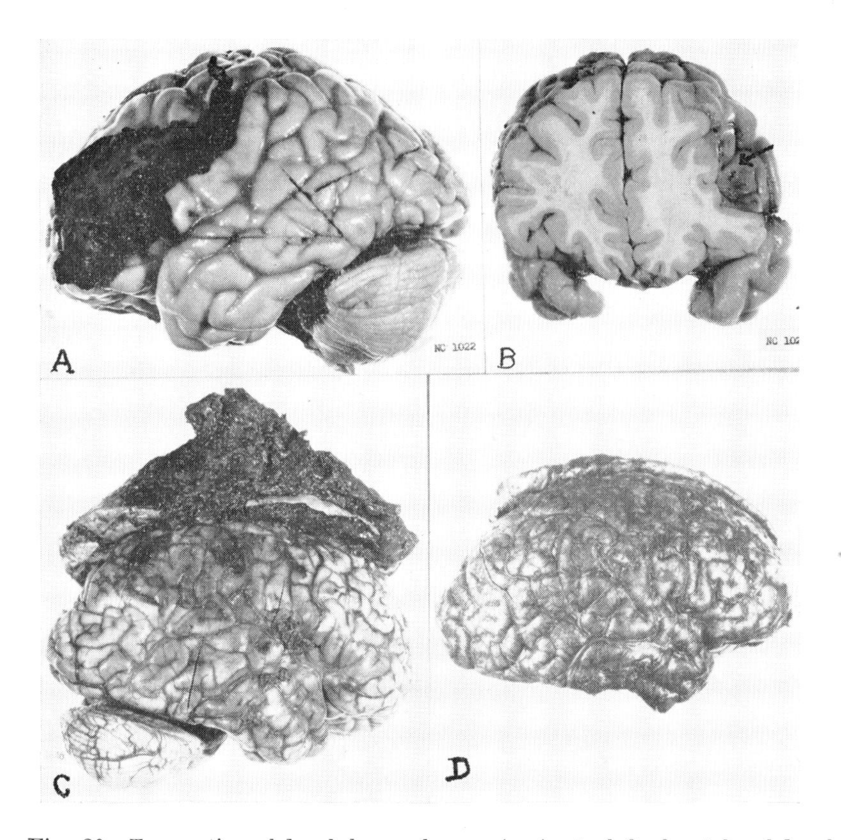

Fig. 20—Traumatic subdural hemorrhage. A. Acute left frontal subdural hemorrhage with localized compression of underlying brain (B). C. Acute subdural hemorrhage covering much of dorsolateral cortex of right cerebral hemisphere. D. Acute subdural hemorrhage in an alcoholic showing almost complete envelopment of right cerebral hemisphere, both dorsolateral and basal, by the liquid blood.

Mechanism of Bleeding.—Subdural hematoma is usually associated with other lesions resulting from Group C type of injuries (those sustained with the head in motion, resulting from traffic accidents or falls). When the moving head strikes in the frontal or occipital midline or close to it, the subdural effusion is usually bilateral. On the other hand, when the impact is sustained on one side of the head the lesion is more often unilateral and contrecoup. In the majority of instances, the bleeding is the result of tears where the superior cerebral veins enter the superior longitudinal sinus. These tears in turn are due to an excessive movement of the brain along the midline—an excessive movement beyond that permitted by the natural curves in the veins at this point. Occasionally, however, bleeding takes place along the course of one of these veins over the dorsolateral surface of the hemisphere (Rand, 1927) (1). In such instances the inner capsule of the hematoma is usually attached at this point. The amount of bleeding, the location and character, as well as the behavior of the subdural effusion of blood on the underlying cortex, is of significance in traumatic cases.

When the amount of blood is excessive and the subdural clot accumulates rapidly, the patient lapses into coma within a matter of 24 to 48 hours, when it is followed by fatal issue. If the bleeding is limited in amount, however, and accumulates slowly it may be controlled by the normal clotting mechanism. Under these circumstances the clot becomes progressively enveloped by an outer (subdural) and an inner (extra-arachnoidal) membrane to form a true subdural hematoma. This process will be discussed in detail in a subsequent section.

As far as its location is concerned, a subdural hematoma is usually located over the upper part of the cerebral hemispheres, falling short only by a centimeter or two of the superior longitudinal sinus. This interval is accounted for by the fact that the clot is held away from the midline by attachment of the veins to the dura mater. The clot may either lay forward over the frontal lobe or may be placed more posteriorly over the parieto-occipital region. At times a double clot united by a narrow isthmus may be found.[1] Under these circumstances there is formed a single or double saucer-like depression on the dorsolateral surface of the cortex. The thickness of these portions of the clot is dependent upon the rapidity of bleeding. It is thick if the bleeding is slow, thinner if rapid. The nature of the effusion within the ultimate capsule depends on the length of time

[1] The location of the clot either anteriorly or posteriorly or both gives rise to a variable electroencephalographic pattern during life (see Marsh, Hjartarson and Courville, 1949) (2).

since the onset of the hemorrhage (Fig. 21). A recent liquid clot tends to be widespread over a larger surface, extending even into the anterior and middle fossae of the skull. Under

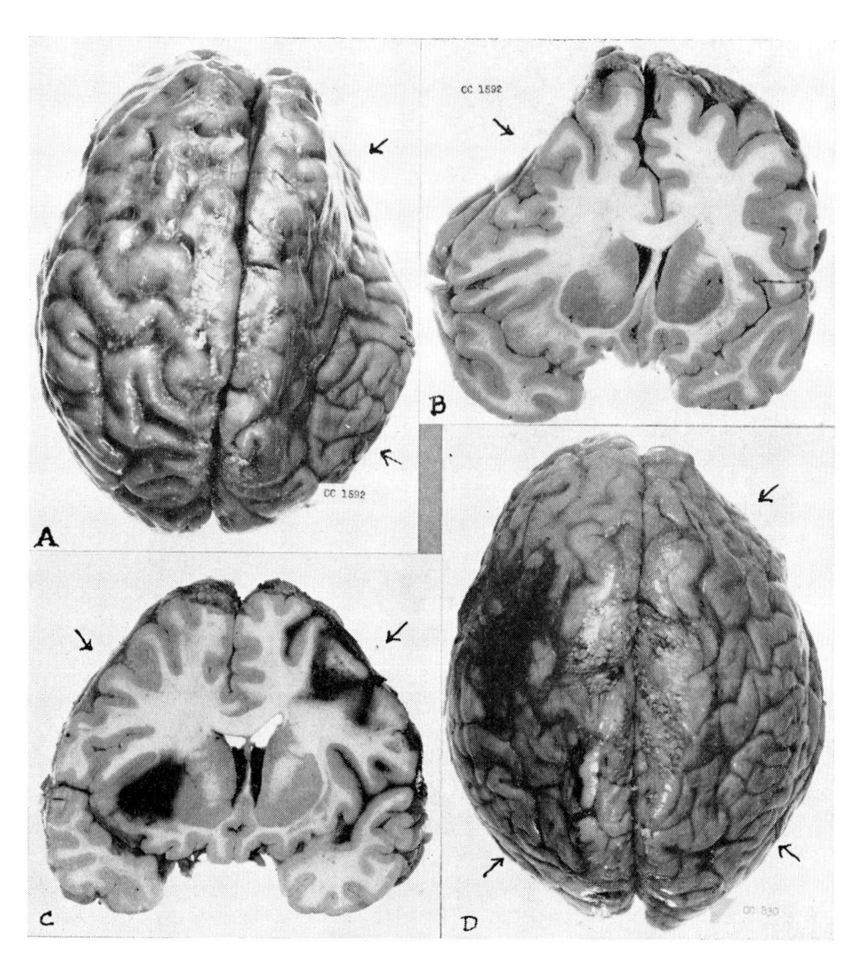

Fig. 21—Traumatic subdural hematoma showing compression of hemisphere by encapsulated lesions. A. Marked compression of the dorsolateral surface of the right cerebral hemisphere is also shown on cross section (B). C. Flattening of the dorsolateral surfaces of both hemispheres as well as an associated subarachnoid hemorrhage (D) on the left and an intracerebral hemorrhage on the right resulting from bilateral subdural hematomas. Hematomas themselves and covering dura have been removed.

these circumstances, the bleeding has usually occurred while the patient was under the influence of alcohol.[2]

The effects that the hemorrhagic effusion has on the underlying brain are characteristic. If the hematoma has been present for some time, there is a dark brown staining of the meninges beneath the hematoma incident to a breaking down of the erythrocytes. Externally, there is found a ridging of the underlying convolutions, giving them a triangular contour on cross section. It may also cause pressure on the underlying blood vessels with ultimate softening of the underlying brain tissue. More significant is the fact that pressure of the clot on the hemisphere as a whole tends to cause reduction in size of the corresponding lateral ventricle and a dislocation of the midline structures. This pressure also causes a herniation of the ipsilateral hippocampal uncus and cinguli gyrus, with subsequent pressure on the brain stem. These pressure manifestations further result in hemorrhages in the brain stem which constitute the terminal lesions under these circumstances.

The microscopic changes in the underlying cortex are variable, depending upon the age of the hematoma. In the early stages nothing significant can be seen; if a subsequent interference in the circulation of the cortex has taken place, status spongiosus or actual focal or laminar necrosis of the cortex will occur.

In acutely developing cases with rapid development of the hematoma and acute herniation of the uncinate and hippocampal gyri through the incisura, there may be an intermittent occlusion of the posterior cerebral artery with focal or extensive areas of red softening.

Bleeding in the brain stem is apparently the result of an overstretching of the long venous radicals draining the upper brain stem (midbrain and upper pons). The resulting hemorrhages are spotty, occurring either in the midline or on one or both sides. When severe, the effusions in the basilar pons

[2] The cause of excessive bleeding under the influence of acute alcoholism is not clear. Whether it is due to a breakdown of the clotting qualities of the blood or due to defect of the liver, or whether there is some influence of the alcohol itself on the clotting qualities has not been established.

and the midbrain may become confluent and the accumulated blood ultimately ruptures into the fourth ventricle. This is usually the last in a chain of reactions which ultimately results in the death of the injured patient.

Ultimate Residuals.—These are somewhat variable in extent, however there may be widespread finer changes in the superficial layers of the cortex in the form of focal softenings or laminar necrosis which ultimately result in atrophy, should the patient survive (Fig. 22). This situation is most likely seen in infants or in individuals who have had surgical intervention with drainage of the hematoma, but because of the long continued pressure do not fully recover. There may also be a softening of the cortex in the medial temporal, or temporo-occipital region. Small post-hemorrhagic cysts in the midbrain and upper pons may also be found.[3] All of these lesions are shown in the accompanying figure (Fig. 22).

Subdural Hematoma.[4]—The presence of a subdural hematoma, especially one occurring without a clear-cut history of cranial trauma, indicates the previous location of a smaller, often clinically unmarked, effusion of blood in the subdural space. The size of the hematoma is dependent upon the amount of blood lost at this time. The injury which causes this lesion is obviously much less severe than those resulting in acute or rapidly developing subdural hemorrhage. Clinically speaking, such injuries are entirely forgotten in approximately half of the cases. This smaller lesion permits a fairly active encapsulation by cells from the arachnoid on one hand and the under surface of the dura on the other.

[3] The location of these chronic lesions in the reticular formation at this level are undoubtedly responsible for the long continued coma and vegetative state such as occurs in occasional individuals who have failed to respond to surgical evacuation of the subdural blood clot (Courville and Amyes, 1952) (3).

[4] Subdural hematoma may occur also as a consequence of extensive compression of the fetal skull during birth. This results from an overlapping of the parietal bones with laceration of the superior cerebral veins of one or both sides. It may follow either difficult passage through a narrowed birth canal or excessive pressure by the obstetrical forceps. The lesion follows, therefore, a case of difficult delivery when after a few weeks or months a progressively enlarging head leads to the diagnosis of an internal hydrocephalus. This ordinarily does not become a forensic problem, hence does not need consideration at this point.

The "capsule" undergoes a progressive evolution leading to a thickening of this membrane. The external or subdural layer of the capsule developes fairly rapidly due to the elaboration of connective tissue elements with early formation of sinusoids. These sinusoids likewise soon make a functional connection with the blood vessels of the dura and develop a circulation of their own within the external layer of the capsule. On the other hand, the internal layer developes from a thin layer of fibrin which soon follows the develop-

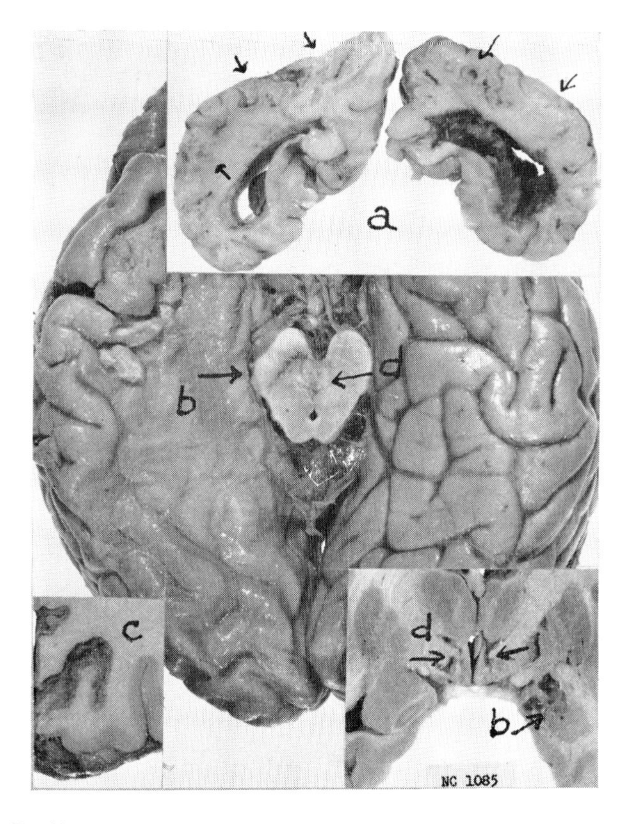

Fig. 22—Residual effects of compression and distortion by subdural hematoma. Photograph of base of brain shows softening of basilar temporal cortex by compression and occlusion of posterior cerebral artery (arrow) at (b) and central post-hemorrhagic cyst in the midbrain (d). Insets show (a) cortical and subcortical softening resulting from compression of bilateral subdural hematoma incident to birth injury, and (c) softening of temporal and occipital cortex.

ment of the blood clot. There often follows a liquification of the contents of the hematoma. This process results in an increased intracranial pressure which ultimately leads to the death of the patient if the hematoma is at all large, and its contents are not evacuated surgically. The stages in the development of the capsule of the hematoma betray the approximate age of the lesion.

An estimation of the age of the capsule is often of considerable value from a medicolegal viewpoint (Courville, 1957) (4). This can usually be estimated fairly closely, particularly within the first two or three weeks. The internal membrane or membrane adjacent to the arachnoid is first characterized by the formation of a thin layer of fibrin along the surface of the arachnoid. This appears within two or three days. In the following few days a single layer of flattened epithelioid type of cells will replace the fibrin, so that at the end of the first week the internal membrane can usually be seen in carefully selected microscopic sections. This membrane changes very slowly so that the only future alteration in it consists in the multiplication of cell layers.

The external layer lying subadjacent to the dura is first characterized by the presence of a zone of epithelioid cells (fibroblasts) which usually become obvious within five to seven days following the effusion of blood. This membrane thickens progressively over the next week until about the end of the second week, when vascular sinusoids become apparent. These become progressively more numerous and well developed until by the end of the third week a well defined zone can be seen. By this time vascular connections with the inner surface of the dura are also apparent. By the end of four weeks one can visualize a fairly well developed external layer of connective tissue whose elements infiltrate the blood within the hematoma. Compound granular corpuscles then begin to pick up the blood pigment from the degenerated erythrocytes. After one month the subdural membrane slowly thickens, but it is impossible to give any very accurate appreciation of the age of the hematoma after this point. However, the nature of this histological change is fairly consistent with the interval since the time of the injury. One must be careful about trying to estimate what this interval is in cases of an injury which has occurred at some unknown period in the past.

Subarachnoid Hemorrhage

Hemorrhage into the subarachnoid space is probably the most common traumatic intracranial lesion. It occurs in most instances of craniocerebral injury in which there has been a loss of consciousness of three hours or more, although exceptions to this rule may occur. It is particularly common in Group C cases (traffic accidents or falls). It is manifested clinically by the presence of uniformly bloody cerebrospinal fluid which tends to become xanthochromic as time passes. Opposed to this rather common post-traumatic effect there are many cases of spontaneous subarachnoid hemorrhages from other causes. The examples of subarachnoid hemorrhage that enter into consideration in cases of forensic autopsies may be divided into three groups. (1) *The basilar lesions,* usually very severe, involve the system of subarachnoid cisterns around the base of the brain and more or less completely fill these spaces. (2) A *dorsolateral group* of variable extent is usually found in the parietal region of one or both sides of the superior longitudinal sinus. (3) *Localized lesions* in variable locations envelope focal punctures, contusions, or lacerations, spreading out from the margin of such lesions into the regional subarachnoid space (Fig. 23). In the first of these groups, the hemorrhage is almost invariably spontaneous, while the second and third groups are usually traumatic. Only the second group is primary and incident to the force of injury, the lesion arising in a manner similar to subdural hemorrhage (laceration at the points of entrance of the superior cerebral or cerebellar veins into the dural sinuses). The third group is found around contusions or superficial wounds and is secondary to bleeding into the subarachnoid space about these lesions.

Basilar Subarachnoid Hemorrhage.—The essential feature of these basilar hemorrhages, in which the degree of the effusion appears to be responsible for the fatal issue, is their occupancy of the entire basilar cisternal system. The blood clot extends from about the optic nerves, anteriorly, to the lateral recesses and cisterna magna, posteriorly. It also

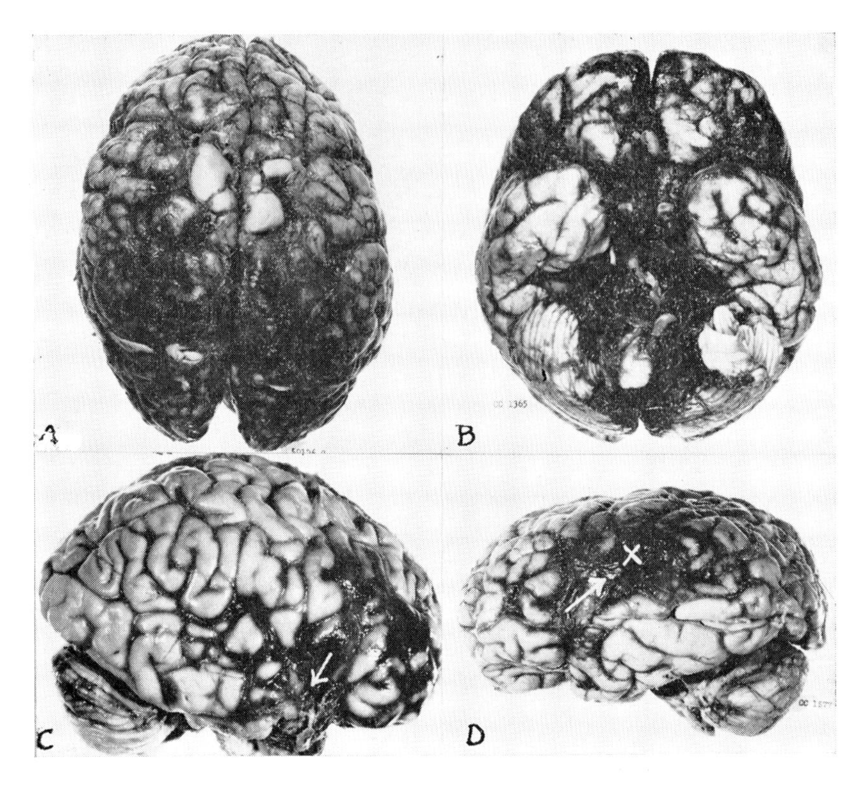

Fig. 23—Traumatic subarachnoid hemorrhage. A. Typical "primary" traumatic subarachnoid hemorrhage. B. Basilar subarachnoid hemorrhage from ruptured aneurysm for comparison. C. "Secondary" traumatic subarachnoid hemorrhage about a contusion. D. Gunshot wound of the brain (arrows).

spreads laterally into the sphenoidal cisterns, and, to variable degrees, onto the dorsolateral surface of the brain. The actual amount of blood clot in this system varies, but in instances of very short survival, the very excess of the effusion is of primary interest to the medical examiner. Under such circumstances, the cranial nerves and blood vessels in the vicinity are more or less completely obscured. The point of bleeding usually lies buried deep within the clot itself and, in the majority of cases, a ruptured aneurysmal dilatation can be found if carefully searched for. The bleeding point is discovered most easily if the body has not been embalmed prior to autopsy. But in spite of fixation, a gentle washing out of the clot from time to time in the course of exploration will usually disclose the arterial defect. Especially careful study should be given to the region of the anterior communicating artery, the first bifurcation of the middle cerebral artery, the two extremities of the tenuous posterior communicating artery, as well as the basilar artery where it divides into the two posterior cerebral arteries. Much more rarely is the aneurysm found over the basilar pons at the point of emergence of the posterior inferior cerebellar from one of the vertebral arteries.[5] In spite of the most careful search, however, in approximately 10 per cent of the cases the bleeding point cannot be discovered. In these cases what presumably happens is a rupture of a very tiny aneurysm whose thin sac is destroyed by the rapid effusion of blood. Nevertheless, a profuse basilar subarachnoid hemorrhage must be considered to be spontaneous under these circumstances and not an effect of trauma.

The aneurysm which is ruptured is usually unilocular but may be multilocular, and more than one of these lesions may be present. However, in the cases of multiple aneurysms, the one causing the fatal bleeding is usually easily identified.

Relation of Trauma to Rupture of Congenital Aneurysms and Spontaneous Basilar Subarachnoid Hemorrhage.—In any large series of Coroner's or Medical Examiner's autopsies, not infrequently one encounters a very severe basilar subarachnoid bleeding incident to a ruptured saccular aneurysm as the fatal issue. In not a few cases, there is a history of an antecedent traumatic episode, often with alleged blow to the head by a second party, when the question of homicide is raised. Under these circumstances the question arises whether trauma was actually responsible for the hemorrhage. This is particularly true where the sudden onset of symptoms occurs during or immediately after an altercation in which blows to the head had been presumably delivered. The situation is obviously important, for if the rupture occurred as an immediate consequence of a blow to the head, then the question of manslaughter is to be enter-

[5] A recent study by Dr. Abraham T. Lu (1961) of our laboratory indicates that saccular aneurysms may occasionally have a more peripheral location.

tained. On the other hand, if the rupture was spontaneous and purely incidental to the stressful situation, quite a different conclusion should be drawn.

In 1958 Newbarr and Courville (5) made a study of a series of cases in which this was the essential question. Criminal responsibility of the surviving party had to be decided. In order to establish trauma as the actual cause of rupture of a pre-existing aneurysm, the following postulates would have to be satisfied (Fig. 24). (1) The wall of the

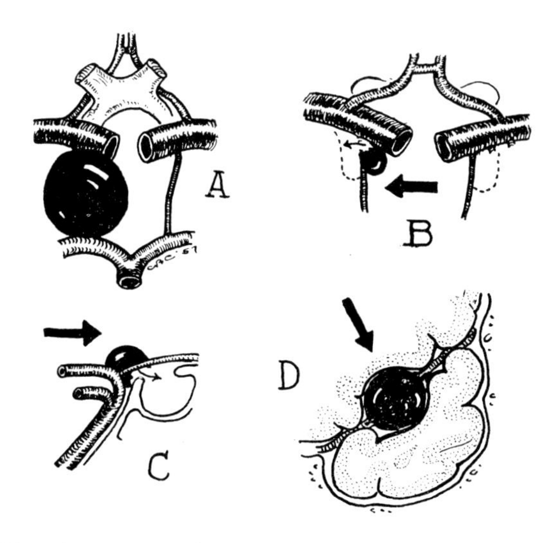

Fig. 24—Although rupture of most saccular aneurysms in presumed traumatic cases apparently result from transitory rise in blood pressure on an emotional basis, actual traumatic rupture may occur under certain circumstances, as suggested in these drawings: A. Rupture of thin-walled sac from excessive movement of the basal parts of the brain. B. and C. Thrust of aneurysmal sac against a bony prominence. D. Rupture of thin-walled sac between frontal and temporal lobes incident to movement of the brain in Group C cases. From Newbarr and Courville, J. Forensic Sc. (April) 1958.

aneurysm must be unusually thin, but one which had not been ruptured previously by the ordinary vicissitudes of life. (2) The degree of force applied to the head must have been sufficient to rupture such an aneurysm in accord with the concept of excessive movement of the brain. (3) The location of an aneurysm must be such as to make possible a direct application of force to its wall. (4) Other factors leading to rise of blood pressure, as physical or emotional stress, must have been of secondary significance. (5) The symptom of subarachnoid hemorrhage must immediately follow the cranial injury. (6) Symptoms and signs of bleeding in the living patient or when verified at autopsy must be in the regions where aneurysms are usually found (basilar cisterns). (7) The demonstration either by angiography in a surviving individual or at autopsy of bleeding from such an aneurysm not due to some other cause must be accomplished.

The chief arguments against true traumatic rupture of an aneurysm in most of this group of cases are based upon (1) the demonstration of unruptured saccular aneurysms in other individuals who have had previous severe injuries to the head. The author has observed this situation in more than one case where a severe craniocerebral injury has left unruptured such an aneurysm. This would indicate that ordinarily the walls of an aneurysm can withstand a rather severe degree of traumatic violence. (2) A study of a series of 6 cases showed that often there has been grave question whether or not the head has actually been injured, since there were no external marks such as contusions or lacerations of the scalp. (3) In suspected cases, the actual rupture of the aneurysm has ordinarily occurred after the alleged interval. Newbarr and Courville (5) concluded that the *possibility* of a rupture of an aneurysm on a traumatic basis must still be admitted, especially (a) if an aneurysm had a paper thin wall, (b) if the possibility exists of laceration of the aneurysmal wall by shearing stresses (as against a bony prominence), (c) if there exists the possibility of a large, thin-walled aneurysm between two opposing surfaces of the brain, as in the sylvian fissure, or (d) if the sac was obviously ruptured by puncture by some bony prominence (Fig. 24). The evidences in the cases which have been carefully investigated by the aforementioned authors seem to indicate that the essential factor in rupture under these circumstances is an elevation of blood pressure consequent to physical or emotional stress and not to trauma per se.

True traumatic subarachnoid hemorrhage does occur under circumstances in which the hemorrhage follows a well defined traumatic episode. This is most marked in instances in which the traumatic episode followed movement of the head with an impact against some quiescent object (Group C injuries). Even a simple analysis of focal post-traumatic lesion (puncture, contusion, or laceration) associated with subarachnoid hemorrhage tends to make this clear. Two types of traumatic subarachnoid hemorrhage have already been suggested: (1) A primary type, when subarachnoid hemorrhage is found in the upper and posterior part of the dorsolateral surface of the cerebral hemispheres on one or both sides, or (2) a secondary type, when subarachnoid hemorrhage envelopes other traumatic lesions of the cerebral cortex, such as punctures, stab or gunshot wounds, contusions or laceration. The first or primary type of subarachnoid hemorrhage is a result of movement of the brain, especially in the anteroposterior direction, such as in falls on the back of the head or the impact of the frontal region against some immobile or relatively immobile object, as in automobile accidents. As already noted, this is more likely to occur in traumatic lesions of Group C. These lesions occur much less likely in lateral impacts of the head, when the location of the hemorrhage is very likely to be contrecoup. The extent of the subarachnoid effusion is also less widespread. These bleedings are due to tears at the points of entrance of the superior cerebral veins into the superior longitudinal sinus.

In the second group the cause of subarachnoid hemorrhage is obvious. The contusion of the superficial surface of the brain permits bleeding from the surface vessels into the regional subarachnoid space. These may not only occur as the result of contusions of Group C but also of penetrating or puncture wounds (Fig. 23, C and D).

The location of these lesions of course is characteristic. Even when small and found in the upper parietal lobes they are important, if for no other reason, because of their significance in evaluating the traumatic mechanism. As the bleeding becomes more extensive they tend to extend forward and downward over the dorsolateral surface, until the entire hemisphere is affected. The amount of bleeding is therefore a rough index of the severity of the craniocerebral injury.

Intracerebral Hemorrhage

Because intracerebral hemorrhage is so often spontaneous, the fact that it may also be traumatic is often unknown or overlooked. This problem is complicated by the numerous known causes of spontaneous hemorrhage which are so often disclosed in medicolegal autopsies when the cause of death is not clear (Fig. 25). For instance, in a study of a large

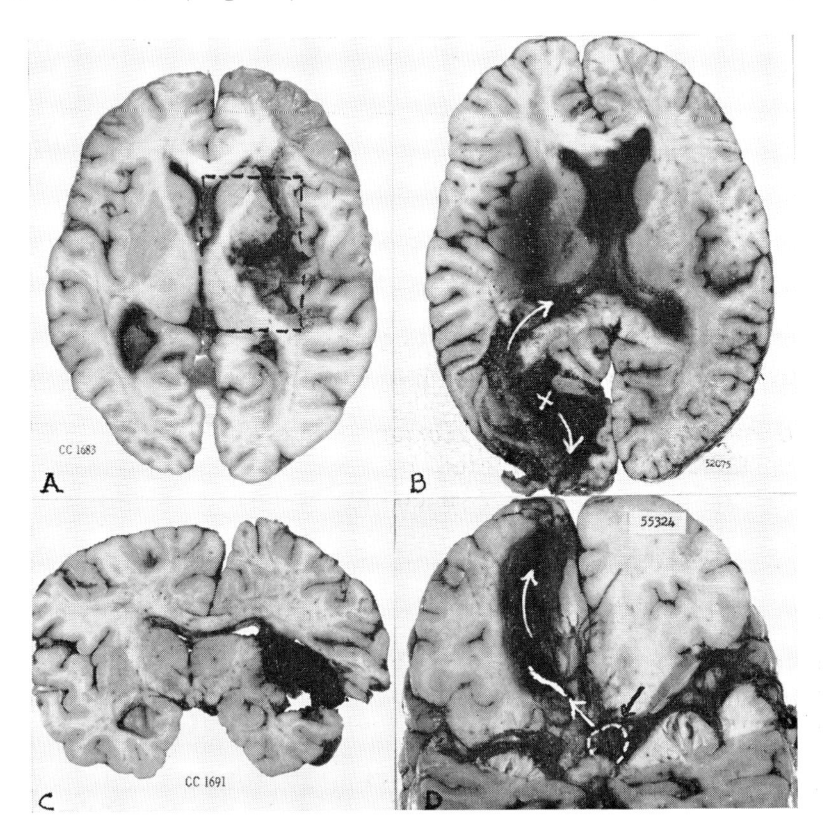

Fig. 25—Patterns of spontaneous (nontraumatic) intracerebral hemorrhage. A. Typical ganglionic hemorrhage consequent to arteriosclerosis and hypertension. B. Hemorrhage into the occipital lobe incident to rupture of an arterio-venous malformation with secondary ventricular effusion. C. Hemorrhage into temporal lobe and external capsule secondary to acute blood dyscrasia (leukemia). Similar lesions are produced by septic embolism. D. Hemorrhage into the frontal lobe from rupture of small saccular aneurysm of anterior communicating artery.

series of cases in the Los Angeles County Hospital (Courville, 1950) (6), 1487 out of 40,000 autopsies were accompanied by intracranial hemorrhage of arteriosclerotic and hypertensive origin. Embolism, brain damage from birth injury, ruptured aneurysms or vascular anomalies, blood dyscrasias, syphilis, tumors, eclampsia, uremia, thrombosis of the cerebral veins, meningitis, encephalitis, alcoholism, septicemia, and half a dozen other rare causes were also discovered as the cause of such hemorrhages. In an additional group of 91 cases of small focal hemorrhages within the brain in the form of petechiae, the apparent causes were pneumonia, arteriosclerosis and hypertension, arsphenamine poisoning, septicemia, meningitis, hemorrhagic encephalitis, polioencephalitis, uremia, diabetes mellitus, tuberculosis, pertussis and a number of other rarer causes.[6] The real medicolegal problem therefore lies in determining the cause of gross hemorrhage into the brain in individuals who have a history of a recent, fairly severe injury to the head, or have died under equivocal circumstances. This problem will now be considered.

Spontaneous Encephalic Hemorrhage.—The great majority of spontaneous encephalic hemorrhages of large size may be grouped into two categories on the basis of their location. In the first of these groups the effusion of blood is found in either the medial or lateral portions of the *ganglionic region* of the brain (Courville and Friedman, 1942) (7). Less often similar effusions are found in the brain stem or cerebellum. These effusions are most often the result of vascular disease (arteriosclerosis associated with hypertension, rarely syphilis). A second group of cases consists of gross hemorrhages into the *cerebral* or *cerebellar white matter,* therefore occupying a more peripheral location in the brain. Such lesions are due largely to rupture of aneurysms, vascular anomalies, blood dyscrasias and a few

[6] Scattered petechial foci in the white matter after cases of trauma usually follow fatal concussion so that this situation is not usually much of a problem when a severe and shocking degree of craniocerebral injury has been experienced (Courville, 1953) (8).

other rare causes. In either case the size of the resulting blood clot may vary between that of a small nut to that of the size of an apple. By progressive stages the typical "currant jelly" clot of the acute hemorrhage ultimately becomes a ragged, fibrous, brownish colored central mass. The once extensive, irregularly lacerated margin becomes smoothed off and contracted. Ultimately, only a small slit-like defect remains, with its margin stained with brownish-golden-orange to yellowish pigment. The cause of this group of lesions is usually made clear by a review of the clinical background as well as by the microscopic examination of sections from blocks taken from the margins of the hemorrhagic cavity. Arteriosclerotic or luetic changes in the walls of these vessels make clear the essential cause of the hemorrhage. This is also true in the case where one finds vascular anomalies adjacent to the wall of the clot, even though these anomalies which remain are small in size. Vessels loaded with immature leukocytes as well as perivascular accumulations or local areas of inflammatory cells also tell their own etiological story.

In addition to securing a clear-cut history of cranial trauma as well as the gross and microscopic findings of other traumatic lesions disclosed at autopsy, there are certain features of a true traumatic intracerebral hemorrhage which make the diagnosis unequivocal in most cases.

Traumatic Intracerebral Hemorrhage.—In a study on this phase of cranial traumatology made a number of years ago to determine the characteristics of such lesions (Courville and Blomquist, 1940) (9), it was found that such lesions are not particularly rare, especially as a result of traffic accidents or falls. As a matter of fact, hemorrhage within the cerebral hemisphere may follow craniocerebral injury of any of the mechanical groups. It may follow penetrating or perforating wounds including those produced by missiles (Abbott, 1961) (10) if any of the larger vessels are injured. More important because of their frequency, gross hemorrhages may follow severely depressed fractures, especially when the bone fragments have lacerated the dura and underlying brain (Fig. 26, A). If the patient survives, gross defects in the form of post-hemorrhagic brain cysts or pseudo-porencephalic cavities may be left as physical residuals (Fig. 26, B).

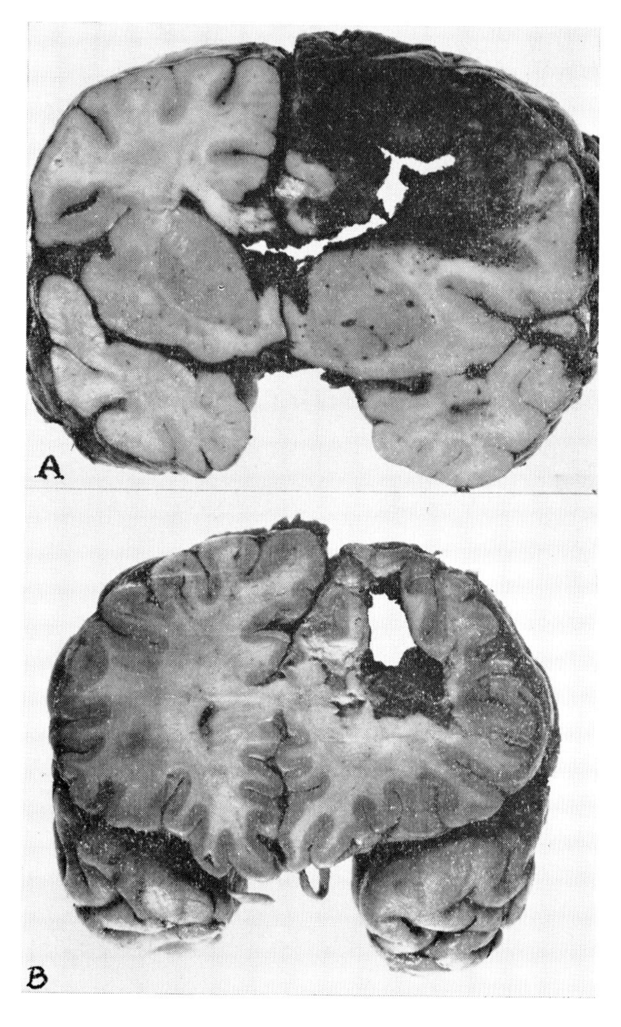

Fig. 26—Traumatic intracerebral hemorrhage incident to depressed skull fracture. A. Acute lesion. B. Residual cyst in old lesion.

Of particular interest because of their addition to the complexity of such cases is the discovery of such hemorrhages in brains injured by the coup-contrecoup mechanism (Group C). Such lesions correspond to the location of contusions with certain modifications (location in the temporo-occipital centrum, in the frontal centrum as *coup* lesions, or as isolated lesions in the basal ganglia). Two subgroups of the frontal and temporal lobes may be distinguished: (1) *primary lesions* within the lobe without any connection with a surface lesion (contusions or lacerations) and, (2) *secondary lesions* or internal effusions associated with severe contusions and lacerations and presumably an integral part of the same (Fig. 27).

In the frontal and temporal lobes, as well as in the basal ganglia, these traumatic intracerebral hemorrhages present a variety of patterns and occur in various sizes, depending upon the severity of the hemorrhages (Courville, 1962) (11). In the *frontal lobes* are found primary hemorrhages in the form of elongated clots whose lower ends point (in cross section) to the gyrus rectus, curvilinear lesions arching through the frontal centrum or circumscribed by it, and either small, smoothly contoured or large, irregular and often multilocular lesions which extend posteriorly into the basal ganglia. Secondary lesions as part of severe contusions or lacerations may involve the lateral, basal or (rarely) medial surfaces of the lobe. Bilateral lesions (symmetrical or asymmetrical) resulting from falls on the occiput are not uncommon.

In the *temporal lobes,* primary lesions may occur as circumscribed and deeply seated or larger and more irregular lesions tending to dissect posteriorly toward the occipital lobe or rupture externally through the dorsolateral cortex to produce a more or less severe subarachnoid and subdural hemorrhage. In other instances, an obliquely placed central hemorrhage may be found in the anterior part of the lobe. Larger effusions tend to be elongated, fusiform or diamond shaped clots, lying in the anterior-posterior axis of the lobe.

The relationship of this group of hemorrhages to the coup-contrecoup mechanism of injury is clearly pointed out by inspection of the location of a group of 50 consecutive cases as indicated on outlines of the cerebral hemispheres. Their similarity (other than the larger size of the individual le-

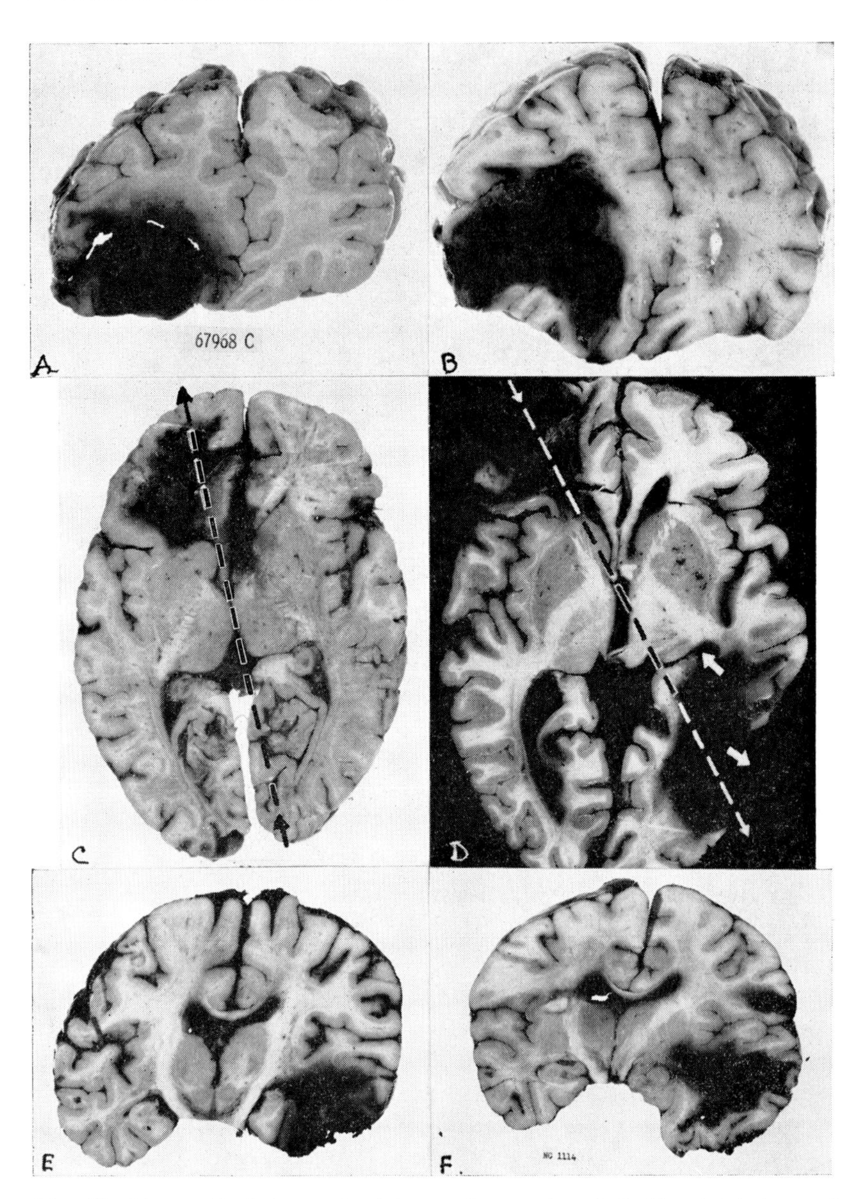

Fig. 27—Traumatic intracerebral hemorrhage. A and B. Frontal lesions of "secondary" (to contusions) and "primary" types. C. Gross contrecoup central "primary" hemorrhage with rupture into superior longitudinal fissure. D. Coup (secondary) frontal and contrecoup (primary) temporal hemorrhages showing mechanism of production (broken lines and arrows). E and F. "Secondary" (to contusions) and "primary" hemorrhages of the temporal lobe.

sions) to the pattern of a series of contusions (see study No. II) is quite remarkable (Fig. 28).

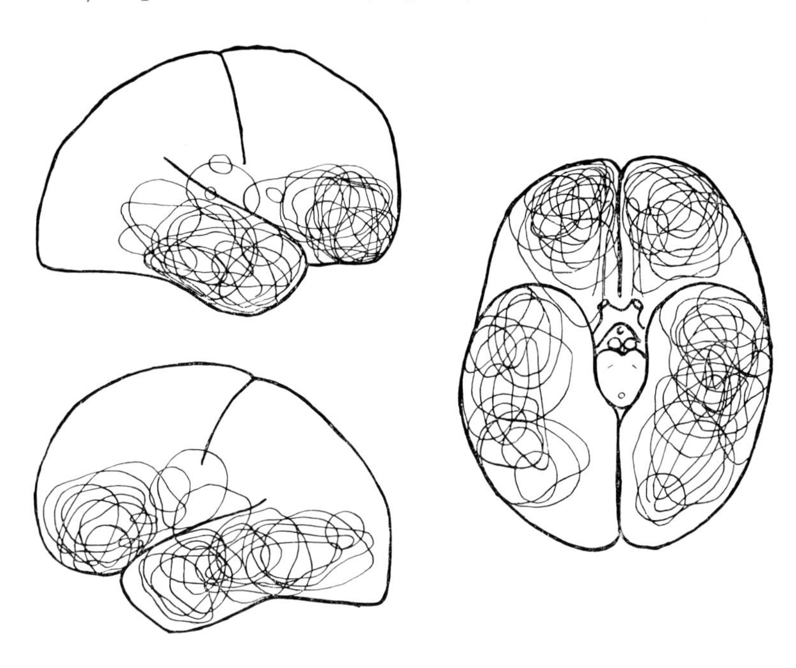

Fig. 28—Traumatic intracerebral hemorrhages in Group C cases. Location of hemorrhages in the brain in a consecutive series of 50 cases of Group C mechanism. The similarity of this pattern to the location of cortical contusions indicates their coup-contrecoup mechanism of production.

The occasional disclosure of what seems to be true traumatic hemorrhages on this basis in the basal ganglia creates one of the difficulties in differential diagnosis between ganglionic hemorrhages of spontaneous origin. Such a finding calls for critical analysis of the presumed traumatic episode as to its mechanism and severity, as well as its associated lesions. Attention to these details as well as an investigation of possible predisposing medical conditions and microscopic study of the regional tissues should make the differentiation clear.

The accompanying figure shows a variety of traumatic intracerebral hemorrhages and indicated mechanism of formation (Fig. 27). The lesson is clear. First of all it is necessary to recognize the possibility of traumatic intracerebral hemorrhage when the presence of associated traumatic lesions should make the nature of the hemorrhage quite certain. If there is any doubt, then the previous medical history of the individual for possible antecedent disease such as syphilis or hypertension and the findings of laboratory studies should be investigated to rule out all other causes.

Delayed Traumatic Apoplexy.—There has arisen what seems to be a clinical entity commonly designated as "delayed traumatic apoplexy", a term well known to experienced medico-legal examiners. The individual suffers a cranial injury of one of several mechanisms. After a somewhat variable but usually short period of time (from a few days to three weeks) the patient lapses into coma. This in itself suggests an "interval" hemorrhage but an extradural or subdural effusion of blood is usually suspected. Surgical exploration, however, discloses no blood in the subdural space, and unless the cerebral hemisphere is needled, the bleeding within its substance is often overlooked. These lesions are usually found in the same locations as other primary traumatic hemorrhages—the frontal, the temporal, or the temporo-occipital regions (Courville and Blomquist, 1940) (9). Oddly enough, these hemorrhages tend to occur in young or middle-aged adults rather than in elderly individuals, hence they are apparently not dependent upon a pre-existing arteriosclerosis and hypertension. The occurrence of various intervals between the traumatic episode and the onset of the "stroke" indicates that true traumatic apoplexy tends to occur in three weeks or less, usually within a few days. The reason for any interval between the two events is not fully understood, but preliminary softening of the surrounding tissue is presumed by some to permit rupture of a regional vessel. Nevertheless, the identity of such a lesion seems to be fairly well established.

The size of traumatic intracranial hemorrhages depends upon several possible factors. The severity of the injury is probably most important, but structural changes in the vessels, such as hypoplasia or anomaly, probably play an important role. Acute alcoholism at the time of the acute injury is also very important, as has been repeatedly emphasized in these studies. There are many injured individuals who die because of this attendant alcoholic state who might otherwise survive. Arteriosclerosis and hypertension oddly enough do not seem to be very important predisposing factors, nor have syphilitic disease or blood dyscrasias proved to be very significant. However, all possible secondary causes should be considered as possible contributing factors which may have some bearing on the ultimate conclusions regarding the matter of responsibility.

Intracerebral "Hematoma".—There occasionally arises a clinical state characterized by signs of progressively increasing intracranial pressure following a hemorrhage into the brain substance. In such cases, the hemorrhage may be either spontaneous or traumatic, although they seem to be more commonly traumatic. This is suggested by the location of such effusions in the proximity of the horns of the lateral ventricle. Following trauma to the head the patient does not fully recover but continues to suffer disturbing headaches. In time he also complains of blurred vision, becomes increasingly lethargic and may ultimately lapse into coma. The signs of unilateral motor disability with enlargement of the contralateral pupil tend to make the correct diagnosis very likely.

The exploring needle or trocar passed through a burr hole over the area of the brain showing evident cerebral dysrhythmia on the electroencephalogram usually results in an evacuation of fluid whose color and content varies with the age of the lesion. At first the fluid is frankly bloody or blood tinged and in which isolated bits of clot are present. Then the fluid becomes xanthochromic and a high protein content can be demonstrated. Release of this fluid, which is usually found to be under increased pressure, is usually followed by a dramatic relief of symptoms, although the hemiplegia which accompanies it usually persists.

The essential pathogenesis as described in another study (Courville, 1957) (4) lies in the proximity of the original hemorrhagic effusion to the lateral ventricle. The cavity is separated from the ventricle only by a thin pseudomembrane (made up of fibroblasts intermingled with glial elements) and the ependymal lining of the ventricle. This thin lamina of tissue acts as a semipermeable membrane, so that the ventricular fluid is drawn into the hemorrhagic cavity by osmosis, thereby diluting the content of the cavity. It is this steady accretion of fluid in the cyst which causes an increased intracranial pressure. Oddly enough, this type of lesion is seldom found at autopsy.

Hemorrhage into the Brain Stem.—These hemorrhages may be either *spontaneous* (arteriosclerosis and hypertension) or *traumatic* (usually associated with severe subdural hemorrhage or hematoma or severe contusion with secondary edema of the temporal lobe). The severity of the hemorrhage (more so in hypertensive disease) and pattern (multiple isolated hemorrhages which may become confluent in trauma) of the hemorrhage usually makes the situation clear (Fig. 29). Due attention to the lesion itself and accompanying phenomena helps establish the correct diagnosis.

Hemorrhage into the Cerebellum.—These are almost invariably spontaneous (arteriosclerosis and hypertension) although they may be traumatic in case of local missile wounds. Very rarely a spontaneous type of hemorrhage may be simulated by a traumatic one when a predisposing vascular

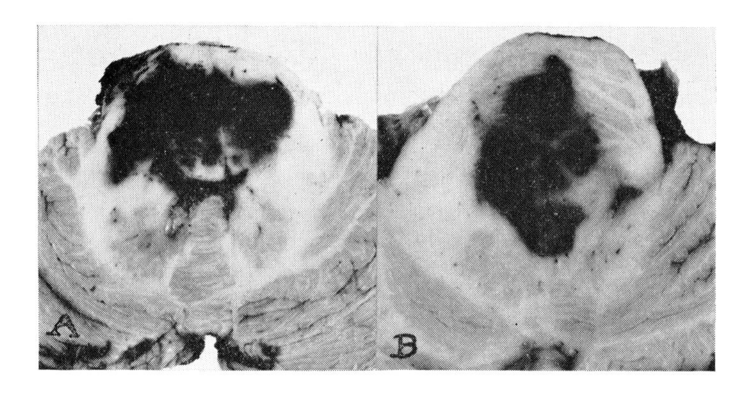

Fig. 29—Hemorrhages in the pons. Spontaneous (A) "versus traumatic" (B) patterns.

anomaly is present (Evans, Friedman, and Courville, 1940) (12) (Fig. 30).

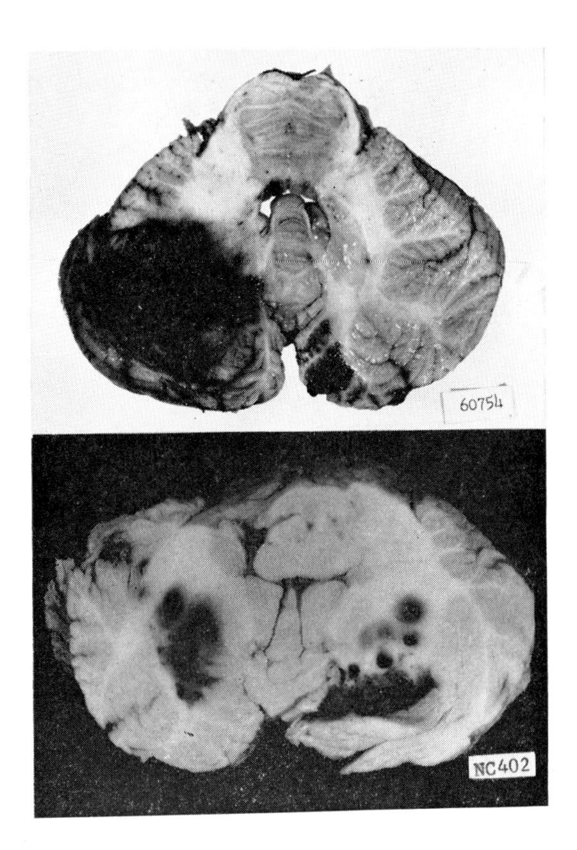

Fig. 30—Hemorrhages in the cerebellum. Spontaneous (A) versus traumatic (B) patterns.

Traumatic Intraventricular Hemorrhage

While not uncommon among effusions following trauma at birth, intraventricular hemorrhage is seldom significant. In adults, it usually follows gross hemorrhage into the cerebral centrum in blunt injuries or transventricular tracks in gunshot wounds. It is almost invariably a part of a fatal lesion complex and therefore not primarily significant per se.

Further Notes on Deep Traumatic Intracerebral Hemorrhages

Since this study was first published in the Journal of Forensic Sciences, three minor points regarding focal intracerebral hemorrhages after craniocerebral injury have come to the fore. In the first place a further word is advisable about the smaller effusions of the brain stem. Some years ago the writer was asked to present a brief survey on the effect of closed injuries on the midbrain and upper pons (Courville, 1945)(13). From the series of cases, which formed the basis of this study at that time, it was found that in most instances, hemorrhages in this part of the brain were secondary to dislocation of the midline of the brain as a result of the traumatic subdural hemorrhage (or hematoma) or severe contusion of the temporal lobe with secondary edema. Under these circumstances it was believed that such hemorrhages were due to stretching of the veins in this part of the brain stem. In the recent past, I have seen small hemorrhages in this region consequent to the direct impact of this portion of the head of a boxer against the lowermost rope of the ring in the course of a match. This case is still under study and it is hoped that a full discussion of this phenomenon will be published in the future.

Meanwhile, a further study of post-traumatic hemorrhages along the midline of the brain stem as found in the records of the Cajal Laboratory has been undertaken by a Dr. Juan Alberto Folle, of Montevideo, Uruguay. Because of the press of other matters, this contribution has not reached my desk, but when it does, it is hoped that further light will be shed on the mechanism of production of hemorrhages in this location.

Summary and Conclusion

The presence of gross effusion of blood in the intracranial space in case of death after trauma to the head always raises a single but important question—is the hemorrhage spontaneous or traumatic? From his knowledge of the manifold etiologic possibilities of such effusions the examiner is aware that it could be either. However, extradural hemorrhage is almost invariably traumatic. Subdural hemorrhage is very likely to be traumatic, except for occasional exceptions in infancy. Subarachnoid hemorrhage could also be either spontaneous or traumatic, but is much more often traumatic when the total factors in a series of cases are considered. Intraencephalic hemorrhage (including those of the brain stem and cerebellum) may also be spontaneous or traumatic but is statistically more commonly spontaneous (except for effusions in the brain stem); traumatic hemorrhage can usually be identified by its distinguishing characteristics and concomitant lesions.

The problem of causation in all of these cases of intraencephalic hemorrhage can usually be decided by a careful analysis of the antecedent history, particularly as to the severity, the mechanism, and the location of the effusion. A gross and microscopic study of other lesions of the brain further serve to make the situation clear. In most instances, there is little excuse for misinterpreting the cause of the bleeding in any given case, assuming that all of these precautions are taken.

REFERENCES

1. Rand, C. W.: Chronic Subdural Hematoma; Report of 7 Cases. Arch. Surg. 14:1136–1165 (June) 1927.
2. Courville, Cyril B., Marsh, C., and Hjartarson, D.: The Electroencephalogram Findings in Subdural Hemorrhage and Hematoma; Review of Literature and Report of Thirteen Cases. Bull. Los Angeles Neurol. Soc. 14:163–181 (Sept) 1948.
3. ———, and Amyes, E. W.: Late Residual Lesions of the Brain Consequent to Dural Hemorrhage. Report of 2 Cases with Old Brain Stem Lesions Verified at Autopsy. Bull. Los Angeles Neurol. Soc. 17:163–176 (Dec) 1952.
4. ———: Intracerebral Hematoma. Its Pathology and Pathogenesis. Arch. Neurol. & Psychiat. 77:464–472 (May) 1957.
5. Newbarr, F. D., and Courville, Cyril B.: Trauma as the Possible Significant Factor in the Rupture of Congenital Intracranial Aneurysms. J. Forensic Sc. 3:174–200 (Apr) 1958.
6. ———: The Mechanism of Coup-Contrecoup Injuries of the Brain; A Critical Review of Recent Experimental Studies in the Light of Clinical Observations. Bull. Los Angeles Neurol. Soc. 15:72–86 (June) 1950.
7. ———, and Friedman, A. P.: Hemorrhages into the Lateral Basal Ganglionic Region; Their Relationship to Recovery from Cerebral Apoplexy. Bull. Los Angeles Neurol. Soc. 7:137–149 (Sept) 1942.

8. ———: Commotio Cerebri: Cerebral Concussion and the Postconcussion Syndrome in Their Medical and Legal Aspects. Los Angeles, San Lucas Press, 1953.
9. ———, and Blomquist, O. A.: Traumatic Intracerebral Hemorrhage; with Particular Reference to Its Pathogenesis and Its Relation to "Delayed Traumatic Apoplexy." Arch. Surg. 41:1–28 (July) 1940.
10. Abbott, K. H.: Acute Missile Wounds of the Brain. An Atlas of Surgical Pathology. Bull. Los Angeles Neurol. Soc. 26:103–131 (Sept) 1961.
11. Courville, Cyril B.: Traumatic Intracerebral Hemorrhages. With Special Reference to the Mechanics of Their Production. Bull. Los Angeles Neurol. Soc. 27:22–38 (Mar) 1962.
12. Evans, H. S., Friedman, A. P., and Courville, C. B.: Calcification of Small Vessels of the Cerebellum. Bull. Los Angeles Neurol. Soc. 5:18–30 (Mar) 1940.
13. Courville, Cyril B.: Effects of Closed Injuries on the Midbrain and Upper Pons. Assoc. Res. Nerv. Ment. Dis., Proc. 1943. 24:131–150, 1945.

Chapter V. Complications of Cranial Fractures*

In a previous chapter (II. Traumatic Extracranial and Cranial Lesions) it was pointed out that in most instances, fractures of the cranium, especially the common linear variety, are of only incidental interest to the medical examiner. On the other hand, depressed fractures are often cause for concern because of damage to the underlying brain. One finds in a large series of autopsies on individuals who have had fatal craniocerebral injuries that complications of fractures are not particularly uncommon, although the brain is rarely directly or seriously damaged by them. Most complications of acute character are of interest to the clinician. Extradural and subdural hemorrhages which result from fractures of the skull concern the neurosurgeon and offer him favorable opportunity for saving patients' lives. Nevertheless, many of these acute lesions go undiscovered, perhaps because of the patient's rapidly downhill course or his failure to come under medical attention for diagnosis and treatment. It is vital, of course, that the medical examiner not only be aware of the nature of such complications, but also recognize their place in the complex end-results of craniocerebral injury. This article will therefore be dedicated to the discussion of these complications.

The variety of complications resulting from fractures may be outlined as follows:

---

* Complications of cranial fractures are likely to be found among cases of delayed effects of cranial injuries. These complications may be *structural,* as in the case of pyogenic infectious lesions, or assymptomatic disorders, such as convulsive attacks or psychic deteriorations. In the latter case, the aid of a clinician is often advisable in establishing a causal relationship between the original craniocerebral injury and the clinical residuals or the patient's demise.

1. *Laceration of the Meninges and Brain.*—Laceration of the brain may be simple, as a result of linear fracture, or complex, resulting from depressed fracture with indriven fragments of bone.

2. *Laceration of the Intracranial Blood Vessels.*—Blood vessels (the middle meningeal arteries and veins, more rarely the dural sinuses) may be lacerated occasionally or may be torn as a consequence of fragmentation of bone in depressed fractures. Lacerations of the larger carotid arteries as they enter the skull or pass along the sides of the sella turcica are of importance because of the occasional formation of an arteriovenous (carotid-cavernous) communication with the formation of "pulsating exophthalmos."

3. *Escape of Cerebrospinal Fluid.*—Cerebrospinal fluid may escape through the nasal passages (cerebrospinal rhinorrhea) or through the external auditory canal (cerebrospinal otorrhea). Less often, cerebrospinal fluid may leak directly through a laceration between the ventricle and the exterior of the head. This is particularly true in some cases of gunshot wounds of the temporal lobe, or compound comminuted fractures of the occipital region.

4. *Entrance of Air into the Intracranial Cavity.*—Air may collect in the subdural or subarachnoid spaces, within the substance of the brain (with formation of an air cyst), or in the ventricles to form an intracranial aerocele.

5. *Entrance of Pyogenic Bacteria.*—The invasion of pyogenic organisms, either through fractures involving the accessory nasal sinuses or the middle ear, less often through depressed fractures of the bone, frequently results in intracranial infectious lesions, such as (a) an extradural abscess, (b) a subdural abscess, (c) thrombosis of the dural sinuses, (d) pyogenic meningitis, or (e) an abscess of the brain.

6. *Escape of Brain Tissue.*—A large opening resulting from a compound comminuted depressed skull fracture often results in the escape of damaged brain tissue (a) as an acute process, (b) as a subacute process with formation of a cerebral hernia, or (c) as a delayed residual in the form of a fungus cerebri. In children, a linear fracture of the vault accompanied by increased intracranial pressure may result

in a traumatic meningocele, encephalocele, or hydroencephalocele.

7. *Further Injury to the Skull Itself.*—Traumatic lesions of the cranial vault may result in (a) the formation of sequestrum due to interference with the regional blood supply, (b) the development of an osteomyelitis through invasion of bacteria into the diploic spaces, or (c) local hypertrophy of bone in the form of hyperostosis.

Each of these several lesions will now be discussed in connection with the nature and location of traumatic bone lesions, usually fractures.

Laceration of the Brain

Lacerations of the brain incident to the various types of fractures may be either simple or complex. *Simple lacerations* are usually small, localized, and elongated, being the result of linear fractures. A linear fracture involving the bone forming the floor of the posterior fossae results in an elongated laceration, usually fairly superficial in degree, involving the basilar surface of the frontal or temporal lobe or the basilar surface of the cerebellum (Fig. 31, A). At times, such a linear fracture may extend onto the inferior portion of the dorsolateral surface of the cerebral hemisphere. Such superficial lesions form residual scars, very much like contusions of the brain, although they are usually complicated by the presence of more compound granular corpuscles and the formation of a complex connective tissue-glial scar. Such a scar tends to become adherent to the regional dura, although this adhesion seldom affects the normal functioning of the brain. More extensive simple lacerations follow the long horizontal linear fractures which involve the crown of the cranial vault. Because of their more severe effects, such fractures are not usually survived.

Complex lacerations of the brain are the usual result of larger compound comminuted depressed fractures with indriven bony fragments. These foci of laceration may be fairly large when the cranial injury is the result of impact of a large object striking with considerable force. Smaller foci of this type of damage may also be found in gunshot wounds accompanied by indriven fragments of bone and/or foreign bodies (Fig. 31, B). A complex laceration is usually greater in extent and deeper, and consists of a mixture of grossly softened brain tissue and blood clots. A complex connective tissue-glial scar is formed if the softened brain tissue is left in place. A central focus of connective tissue is formed and becomes attached to the regional blood vessels of both the brain tissue and the dura, or scalp. These vessels exert a "pull" on the regional brain with its sensitive nerve cells. The significance of this "pull" on the surrounding brain tissue (which is presumed to be the cause of traumatic convulsive seizures) is attributed to Foerster and Penfield (1930) (1). If the area is debrided surgically, the wound in the brain heals more quickly because the scar is much simpler, resembling that resulting from a small superficial contusion. It is a local anisomorphic scar, and becomes continuous in the adjacent white matter of the involved gyrus as an isomorphic scar.[1]

A high percentage of these lesions result in traumatic convulsive seizures with localizing phenomenon pointing to the region of the scar (Rand and Courville, 1932) (2).

Laceration of the Intracranial Blood Vessels

Even a laceration incident to a linear fracture, appropriately placed, may be responsible for an interruption of blood vessels, particularly the anterior, middle, or posterior meningeal arteries and their venae comites. This complication more commonly involves the middle meningeal artery, less commonly the anterior meningeal vessels, and least commonly the posterior meningeal artery. Tears of these vessels may occur when fractures pass through their grooves on the interior surface of the skull. In case of the middle meningeal arteries, however, such tears are most common in fractures passing through the base of the middle fossa, or across the vascular tunnel at the tip of the sylvian ridge. Such fractures

[1] An anisomorphic scar is one in which the glial elements are distributed in the form of a netlike meshwork, while an isomorphic scar is one resulting from a progressive loss of the myelinated nerve sheaths, permitting the remaining glial fibers to assume a parallel arrangement.

often result in severe degrees of extradural hemorrhage. These hemorrhages may be of either rapid or slow evolution depending upon the size of the vessel lacerated, the degree of blood pressure, and perhaps other limiting factors. These hemorrhages are usually limited by their dural attachment to the bone in which they groove; therefore, intracranial pressure may evolve rapidly as the blood accumulates beneath this membrane lining the particular bone. On an average, the accumulation is sufficient to give rise to serious intracranial pressure within a period of 24 to 48 hours. This results in a progressive lethargy deepening to coma, as well as the production of localizing symptoms. Occasionally, the blood clot may be small and result in a more chronic "extradural hematoma."

Less often do such fractures result in subdural hematoma, which more often arises from laceration of the terminal portions of the superficial cerebral or cerebellar arteries.

Occasionally, a depressed fracture over the dural sinuses may result in laceration of the sinuses, permitting an extradural accumulation of blood. When located over the superior longitudinal sinus, blood may appear beneath the scalp or even pour through a laceration of the scalp to the exterior. Such hemorrhages, of course, are more common in cases of gunshot wound than in depressed fractures of other causes (Abbott, 1961) (3).

As a rule, such extravasations are dealt with surgically, so that it is on rather rare occasion that the medical examiner has opportunity to inspect such lesions.

Tears in the Carotid Artery by Transverse Linear Fracture through the Sella Turcica.—A well-known post-traumatic lesion described as "pulsating exophthalmos" results from a transverse linear fracture extending into the base of the skull, passing through the floor of the sella turcica. It is recognized that such a fracture at times produces a tear in the wall of the carotid artery within the cavernous sinus. This produces an arteriovenous fistula which results in a typical pathological complex with characteristic clinical symptoms. On the side of the lesion, the eye becomes increasingly prominent, the vessels in the region become congested, and the mucous membranes of the eye become edematous and protrude through the eyelids to form what has commonly been known as "pulsating exophthalmos." The pulsation of the eye, of course, is incident to the arterial "beat" transmitted through the collection of venous blood in the cavernous sinus. A second feature of unusual interest, from the standpoint of the patient, is the presence of a blowing, whistling, murmur, incident to the escape of the column of blood from the artery into the cavernous sinus.

The pathological picture of this lesion is also of special interest, since it is followed early by engorgement and tortuosity of the regional veins draining into the cavernous sinus, but ultimately may disappear after spontaneous occlusion of the carotid cavernous fistula or ligation of the carotid artery (Fig. 32, A). Such vascular lesions, even though fairly large, are not fully appreciated at autopsy by the medical examiner because they are found adjacent to the sella turcica or are obscured by the overhanging sphenoidal ridge (Fig. 32, B). If one cares to pursue the course of the lesion by opening the roof of the orbit, the marked congestion of the contained veins associated with more or less edema of the tissues of the orbit will be seen to account for the exophthalmos. Relatively little change is found, however, in the veins draining into the cavernous sinus from the brain (mainly the superficial and deep middle cerebral veins). However, such an enlargement may occur.[2]

Traumatic Saccular Aneurysms.—Regional formation of saccular aneurysms has been considered by some to be a result of trauma to the carotid artery, however this has never been verified. It is very unlikely that the so-called congenital or saccular aneurysms ever have this origin, as has been pointed out in the third chapter. It is quite possible, however, that trauma may rupture a pre-existing aneurysm of this type, thereby causing an arteriovenous communication.

Traumatic dissecting aneurysms of the internal carotid artery have been reported (Dratz and Woodhall, 1947) (4).

---

[2] An arteriogram performed during life gives some interesting impressions as to the altered circulation causing the pulsating exophthalmos. Not only can one see the dilated orbital veins, but also engorged veins of the face which ultimately become apparent clinically under these circumstances. In addition, the intracranial venous channels appear to be dilated.

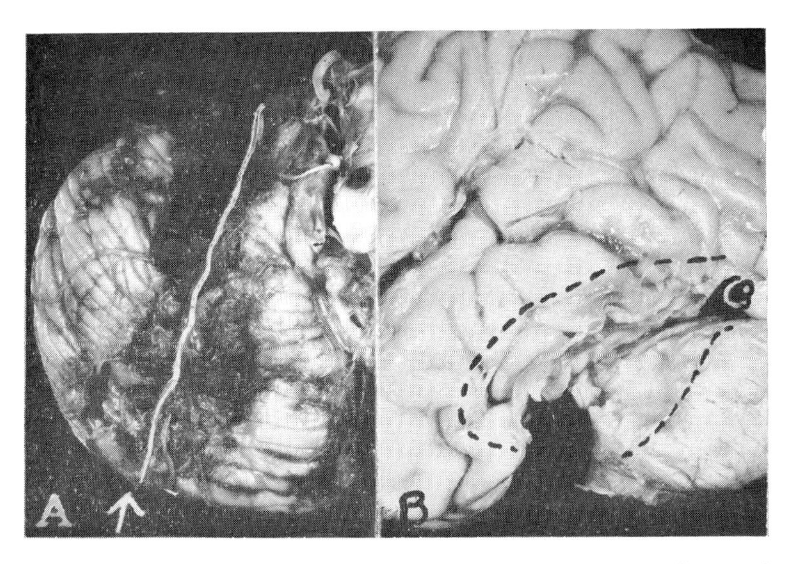

Fig. 31—Laceration of the brain. A. Simple laceration of basilar surface of right cerebellar hemisphere incident to linear fracture of occipital bone. B. Complex laceration of left temporal lobe and cerebellum incident to previous missile wound.

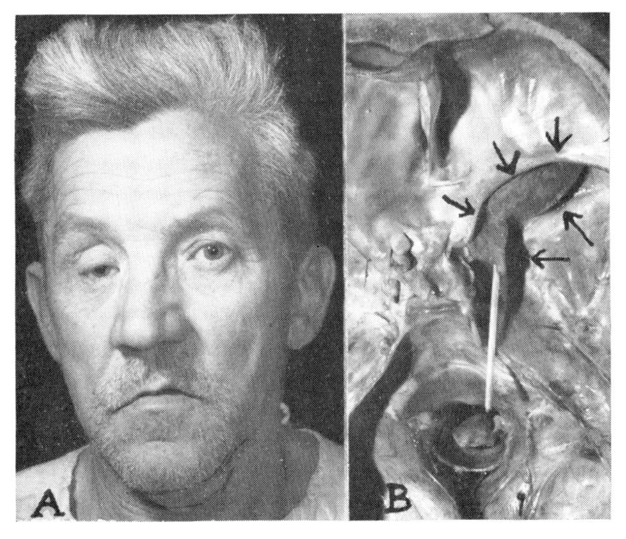

Fig. 32—Traumatic carotid-cavernous fistula. A. Late residual (enophthalmos) of a one-time pulsating exophthalmos. This was evidently a spontaneous cure. B. Huge enlargement of the cavernous sinus.

It is doubtful, however, that such a lesion can be accounted for by the presence of a fracture. The writer has described this compound type of lesion from a gunshot wound of the orbit; however, it was the missile rather than a fracture which was responsible for the lesion (Courville, 1960) (5).

Escape of Cerebrospinal Fluid to the Exterior

Cerebrospinal fluid may escape to the exterior of the skull in blunt injuries with fracture through the frontal sinus or the external auditory canal, and occasionally in cases of severe depressed fractures of the occipital bone or penetrating severe depressed fractures of the occipital or temporal bones. When the cerebrospinal fluid escapes through the nose it is designated clinically as "cerebrospinal rhinorrhea." As a rule, this fluid appears as a clear or slightly blood-stained fluid having the cellular and chemical constituents of cerebrospinal fluid. This fluid escapes through the cranial vault by way of a linear or depressed fracture involving the nasal sinus, less through a fracture involving the wall of the ethmoid or sphenoid sinuses.

The escape of the fluid usually occurs in a gush when the patient bends forward. In such a situation, escape of the fluid is accompanied by an inrush of air. An intracranial aerocele is usually formed by this progressive replacement of fluid by air. A "trapdoor" mechanism often follows a small opening in the bone covered by a flap of dura between episodes of evacuation of fluid. The direct communication between the intracranial space, subarachnoid space, and the sinuses may also result in infectious sinusitis, and in turn meningitis, subdural abscess, or even abscess of the brain. Such lesions may complicate an intracranial aerocele.

When the fracture results in a communication between the mastoid cells, the middle ear, or the eustachian tube and the intracranial space, the cerebrospinal fluid may escape into the throat or external auditory canal. The causative linear fractures in this region are more difficult to determine by roentgenograms, but if pictures are taken in several positions their presence may sometimes be demonstrated. As in the case of rhinorrhea, cerebrospinal otorrhea may result in intracranial infections, particularly in suppurative meningitis. Of the two locations, cerebrospinal otorrhea indicates the more serious lesion, because the basal location of the causative fracture has a close proximity to the structures of the brain stem. It also heals slowly, if at all.

The escape of cerebrospinal fluid from gunshot wounds of the temporal lobe or depressed compound comminuted fractures of the occipital bone is much more rare. In the former, the penetrating wound, incident to passage of a missile, extends vertically into the middle fossa at the base of the skull. Although it is complicated, intracranial aerocele may still result. In the case of the latter, the cerebrospinal fluid may flow directly to the exterior through a gross traumatic communication between the posterior horn of the lateral ventricle, through a laceration of the overlying soft tissues and skin. The latter two types of lesions almost invariably follow gunshot wounds, particularly in time of war, although occipital lesions may result from compound comminuted depressed fractures with laceration of the underlying brain.

Traumatic Intracranial Aerocele.—As was pointed out, the escape of cerebrospinal fluid, especially through the frontal sinus and upper nasal air passages, is frequently associated with the entrance of air into the intracranial spaces. This avenue of escape may entail a trapdoor mechanism, placed between a lacerated dura and a small traumatic aperture in the bone. The escape of fluid is usually facilitated when the patient tips his head forward, coughs, or sneezes, and is often followed by a sudden entrance of a volume of air into the intracranial space. This situation has been well described by Walter Dandy (1926) (6). The air may remain in the subdural space, or it may enter and follow along the subarachnoid space (with appearance simulating that of a surgically produced pneumoencephalogram). It may force its way into a defect in the brain by way of a pocket formed by laceration of the inferior surface of the frontal lobe. The air seems to spread the walls of this linear defect to form a pocket by compression of the lacerated tissues. It then dissects its way along the fibers of the forceps major toward the anterior horn of the lateral ventricle. Under these circumstances, what is known as an "air cyst" is formed. As this "air cyst" increases in size, it may actually tear its way into the anterior horn of the ventricle, when a simple roentgenogram of the skull will disclose air in this cavity. Of course, the steps in the process of passage of air into the ventricular cavities will not be detected by the medical examiner as he performs the necropsy on the injured individual. All he may find is a slitlike cavity within the medial portion of the frontal lobe, which he may mistake for a posthemorrhagic cyst. In case of doubt, the true nature of such a cavity is made clear by the characteristic pseudoepithelial appearance of its walls (Courville, 1943) (7).

A traumatic communication between the external auditory canal and the posterior or medial fossa results in the entrance of air, as a rule, into the subarachnoid space only, although a true traumatic ventriculogram is also possible.

The entrance of air into the posterior horn of the lateral ventricle by way of a compound comminuted depressed fracture of the occipital region usually results in a traumatic ventriculogram, there being a direct communication via the damaged brain between the scalp laceration and the ventricular cavities.

All three of these types of lesions (Fig. 33) have been described in another connection (Courville, 1943) (7), to which the reader is referred for further details.

Traumatic Infectious Lesions of the Intracranial Space

The presence of a fracture through either the accessory nasal sinuses or the internal ear (mastoid area) always constitutes a potential atrium for the invasion of pathogenic organisms. At the present time, however, the danger of intracranial invasion of bacteria has been greatly minimized by the use of antibiotic substances following cranial injuries complicated by leakage of cerebrospinal fluid. In former times, however, this danger was not only potential, but actual. Many patients have died of pyogenic meningitis resulting from this type of fracture. It is important to recognize that while the invasion of infectious material may follow immediately after the fracture has occurred, in cases of fractures in the region of the ear in particular, trauma may only set the stage for the subsequent development of an infectious process (Nager, 1930) (8). Thus, a delay, often involving a period of weeks, months, or even years, may follow the occurrence of such a fracture before meningitis may ensue.[3]

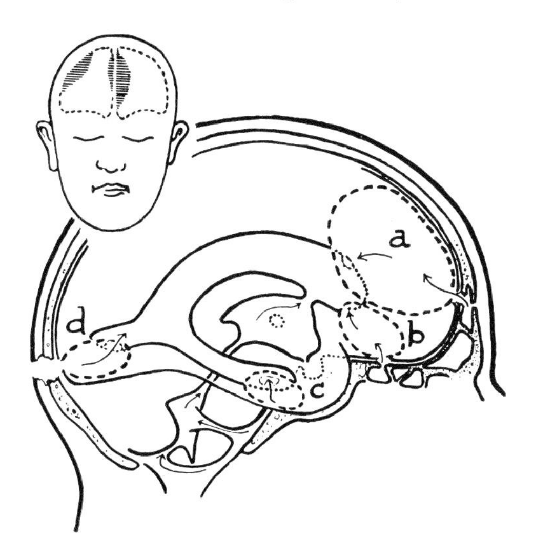

Fig. 33—Traumatic pneumocephalus. Indicating mechanism of formation. a. Air cyst formed by communication between frontal sinus and anterior contusion of frontal lobe. b. Air cyst formed by communication between ethmoid sinus and subfrontal contusion. c. Spontaneous ventriculogram resulting from penetrating wound of middle fossa of skull. d. Same, resulting from compound fracture of occipital region with laceration of underlying brain. (Courville, Fig. 132, Pathology of the Central Nervous System, ed 4, Pacific Press Publishing Assn., Mountain View, California, 1950.)

---

[3] It is also important to remember that trauma to the region of the sinuses or the mastoid *without fracture* may result in a traumatic sinusitis or mastoiditis. Thus, the actual intracranial invasion may develop under circumstances of a blunt injury, yet be truly traumatic. The writer has examined the brain in a case of traumatic mastoiditis without fracture which ultimately resulted in the formation of a typical temporal lobe abscess. The laborer sustained his injury by a fall from a ladder while picking fruit. He was just as entitled to compensation as one whose fall had produced a fracture with direct invasion of organisms. It has been pointed out by some observers (i. e., Nager, 1930) (8) that delayed meningitis, particularly after fractures passing through the petrous portion of the temporal bone, may develop after months and years have passed. The writer has seen a case with fracture

An intracranial lesion incident to the invasion of pyogenic organisms may be in the form of a local extradural abscess (usually of not great significance unless the dura is also torn), a subdural abscess, thrombosis of the dural sinus, septic meningitis, and abscess of the brain in various locations.

Extradural Abscess.—These occur but rarely and are usually not of importance clinically. They are ordinarily small and lay outside the dura along the line of the fracture, such as in the vicinity of a sinus or about the petrous bone. These lesions may be found at the time of operation for other traumatic lesions (such as repair to stop cerebrospinal rhinorrhea or an aerocele).

The relatively rare extradural abscess secondary to a focal lesion of the cranial vault, known eponymically as Pott's "puffy tumor," may be of greater significance. If such a lesion continues to develop, other and more serious complications may follow. Extradural abscess secondary to osteomyelitis of the skull may at times become quite extensive, although here, again, the extradural reaction is usually limited to the area of the bony infection.

Subdural Abscess.—This is likewise a rare lesion and usually follows an implantation of infectious material into the subdural space through a compound fracture of the bone, as is the consequence of a gunshot or stab wound. This lesion may also be due to an extension of an infection from cellulitis of the scalp of traumatic etiology (Fig. 34, A). It may develop as a very focal lesion at the point of exit of cerebrospinal fluid and ingress of air by way of a fracture through the posterior wall of the frontal sinus. It may likewise be secondary to traumatic frontal sinusitis or traumatic otitis media, even though a fracture per se may not be present. Spontaneous rupture of a traumatic cerebral or cerebellar abscess may also be a possible cause of this lesion. In spite of these many possibilities, subdural abscess is a lesion that rarely concerns

---

through the cribriform plate in which a fatal meningitis developed after an interval of ten years. Moreover, in these days of antibiotics, episodes of meningitis may repeatedly recur at intervals, unless the traumatic opening through the bone is repaired by dural transplants. The writer has seen three episodes of meningitis in a young man, each time relieved by antibiotics, before the dural-bone opening was finally occluded at operation.

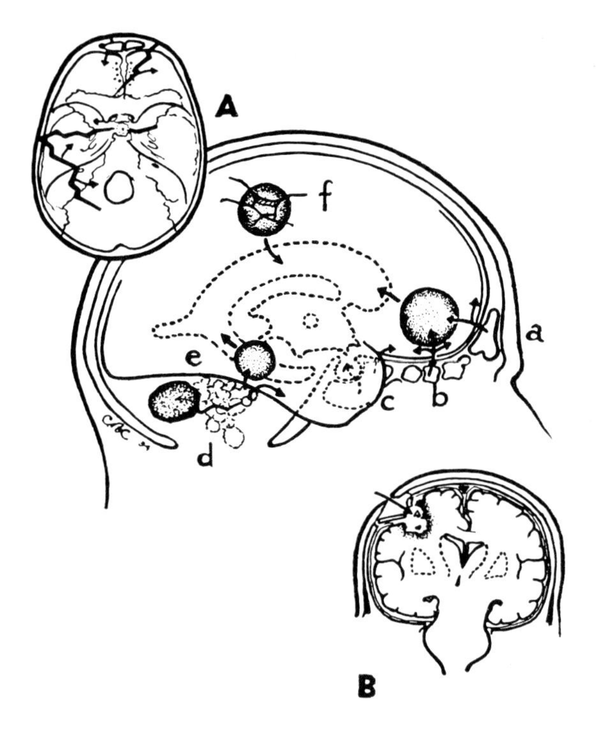

Fig. 34—Traumatic brain abscess. Diagram showing regions of entrance of infectious material to form brain abscess. A. Frontal lobe from fractures through frontal sinus (a) or at the base (b and c). Fractures through auriculomastoid region causing abscess of the cerebellum (d) or temporal lobe. Abscesses of the dorsolateral region of the brain following local compound comminuted depressed skull fractures (f). See also inset B. (Courville, Fig. 131, Pathology of the Central Nervous System, ed 4, Pacific Press Publishing Assn., Mountain View, California, 1950.)

the medical examiner. Fig. 35, A shows an example of subdural abscess.

Thrombosis of the Dural Sinuses.—Traumatic thrombosis of the dural sinuses is a lesion which must be extremely rare, one which has not come to the personal attention of the writer. It would most likely follow a penetrating wound involving such a sinus directly, or as incident to a depressed fracture. Secondary infection of the soft tissues of the scalp might extend into the partially occluded sinus and result in a septic thrombosis of a dural channel. It might also follow a traumatic mastoiditis (lateral sinus) or traumatic frontal sinusitis (superior longitudinal sinus).

Purulent meningitis.—On the other hand, purulent meningitis is still not too rare a development of ingression of infectious material through a cranial fracture. While this may be due to a penetrating gunshot or stab wound, septic meningitis is more likely the result of a linear fracture through the accessory nasal sinuses or the petrous bone. This condition may be classified as *primary,* due to direct extension of infection through the fracture, or *secondary,* incident to the spread of some focus of infection, which in turn has been due to trauma (Courville and Platner, 1938) (9). Primary purulent meningitis may follow fractures through the sinuses (especially the frontal sinus), the auditory canal, depressed fractures of the cranial vault, or penetrating wounds (Fig. 35, B). Secondary meningitis more likely follows sinusitis or otitis media, which may be traumatic but unaccompanied by fracture. Blunt injuries of the scalp and skull may cause cellulitis, from which meningitis may subsequently develop. A subpericranial abscess or osteomyelitis of the skull are causes of less frequency, particularly since the antibiotic era has been introduced.

The pathology, either gross or microscopic, of traumatic meningitis has no particular characteristics which distinguish it from meningitis of other types, unless perchance the brain has also been injured at the same time.

Traumatic Abscess of the Brain.—This is not at present a common complication of injury to the head. Even in the recent past such lesions were relatively rare because cranial wounds that were obviously depressed or penetrating were ordinarily carefully explored and any infectious material removed at the time of operation. Such lesions are extremely rare, particularly since antibiotics have been introduced in the therapy of inflammatory conditions. The writer has seen very few in the past two decades, and these have invariably been exposed at operation rather than at autopsy. However, the possibility still exists that an abscess may follow a direct implantation of infectious material within the brain, as in the case of missile wounds or compound fractures of the skull (Fig. 35, C). Abscesses may result from traumatic atria (fractures) between the intracranial space and actually infected areas, such as the nasal sinuses, or potentially infected areas, such as the middle ear. Post-traumatic infections of the mastoid or frontal sinuses favored by, or actually produced as a result of trauma, may in turn cause abscess following invasion of the usual channel of infection into the brain. Traumatic abscesses of the brain may therefore be classified from the standpoint of location into two groups: (1) those following depressed fractures of the cranial vault, and (2) those adjacent to the

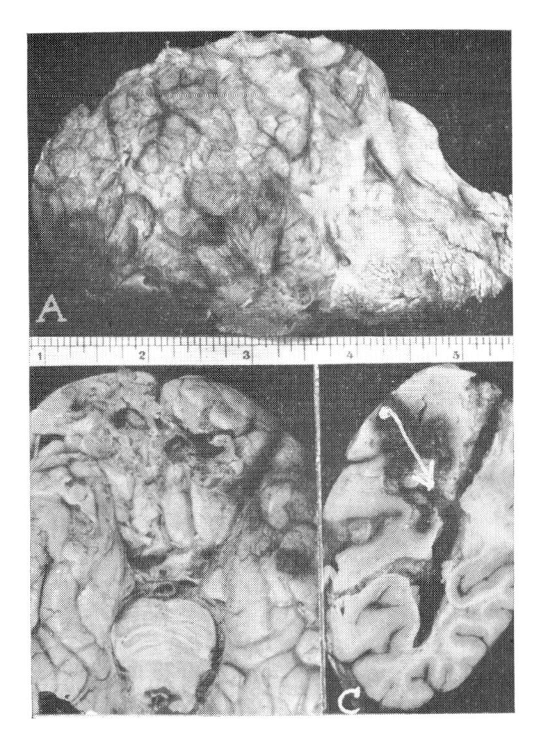

Fig. 35—Traumatic infectious lesions of the intracranial space. A. Subdural abscess. B. Evidences of meningitis associated with old subfrontal contusion. C. Acute brain abscess with spread in brain of infectious process.

accessory nasal sinuses, middle ear, or mastoid. The most common are those following depressed fractures with indriven dirt, foreign material (such as fragments of a cap or hair), or infectious organisms carried in with a missile or other penetrating object. The presence of infection in these cases often provokes the development of a heavy capsule which makes surgical drainage more successful than in abscesses of other types. However, acute nonencapsulated abscesses do occur. In the writer's experience, most abscesses have been correctly diagnosed and successfully operated upon with recovery of the patients.

Abscesses of the brain following bullet wounds usually result in a different pattern. One may find these abscesses deep within the brain tissue along the track of the missile, sometimes forming a chain of lesions, with one or more of them attached to a linear scar. The deep location of the abscesses and their complex structure creates a somewhat more difficult situation as far as surgical cure is concerned.

Escape of Brain Tissue through Traumatic Defect in the Skull

The escape of brain tissue through a traumatic defect in the skull is not ordinarily looked upon as a complication of fracture per se. This is because such a lesion is more or less incidental to a depressed fracture and acute laceration of the brain, with edema of the surrounding material favoring the escape of macerated nervous tissue to the exterior. For example, it is not too rare to find macerated brain tissue on primary dressings after a patient with severe cranial injury has been admitted to the hospital for definitive care. This situation also may be encountered in a medicolegal autopsy if the body has been brought directly to the morgue. The escaped tissue is usually very much traumatized and mingled with blood, foreign bodies, and fragments of bone.

Traumatic hernia cerebri is a result of a more severe degree of edema of the brain tissue beneath a recent traumatic defect in the cranial vault. This lesion usually follows a depressed skull fracture with extensive loss of bony fragments. A superficial contusion of the brain, perhaps abetted by the presence of local hemorrhage, causes swelling of the underlying brain, which protrudes progressively from the cranial defect (Fig. 36, A). The swelling may be so extensive as to produce further laceration of the protruding tissue by the sharp margins of the bony defect. With the recession of the edema, the herniated tissue gradually recedes. A scar forms which tends to be adherent to the regional dura. Such lesions are quite rare, at least in modern practice.

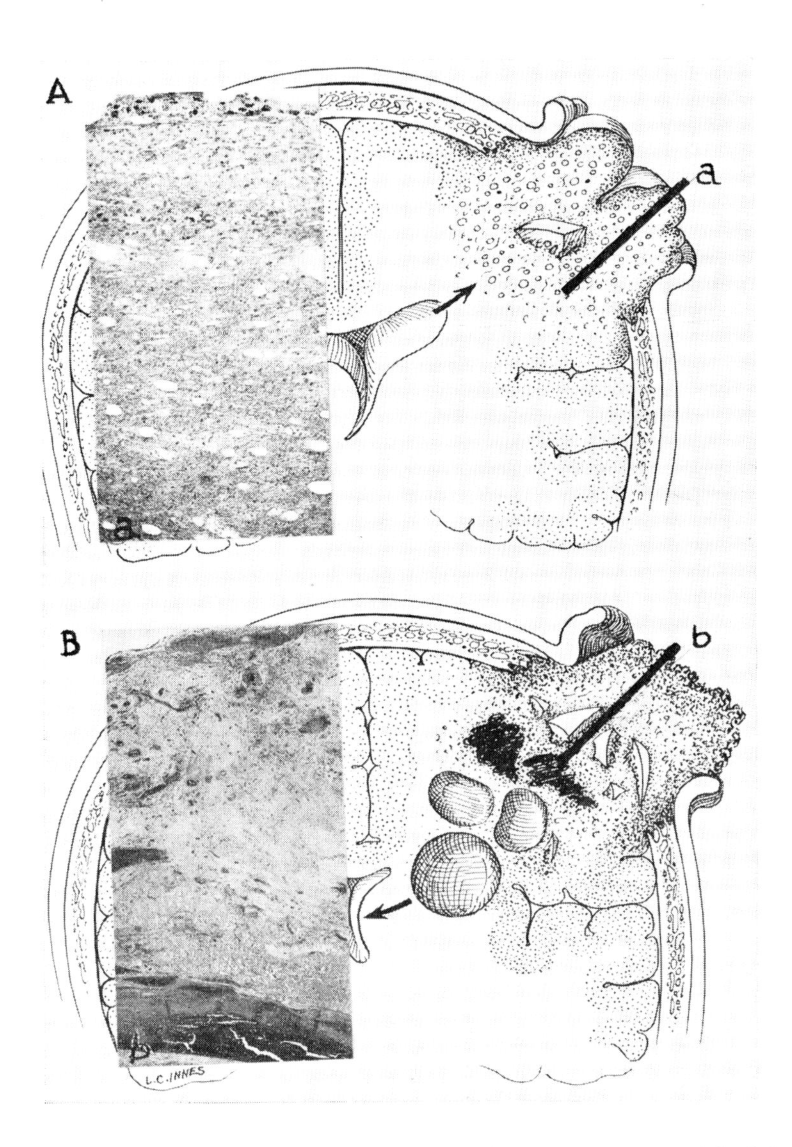

Fig. 36—Traumatic protrusions of the brain through a cranial defect. A. Hernia cerebri, showing its composition of edematous brain tissue. Inset a, showing microscopic section through a hernia cerebri. B. Fungus cerebri, showing underlying abscesses of the brain. Inset b, showing microscopic section through a fungus cerebri.

A number of years ago the writer had occasion to study a boy who had a severe craniocerebral injury with a depressed fracture of the left temporal region. His post-traumatic clinical course was rather stormy; the traumatized brain tended to protrude to the point at which some of the cortex and subcortical tissues were lost. However, the acute lesion ultimately became quiescent and it was thought that the patient was recovering. The child died, however, of an acute complication, and an opportunity to study the focal lesion was thereby offered. The lesion then consisted of a rather firm covering scar with deformation of the surrounding brain and a "wandering" of the ventricle toward the cranial defect.

Fungus Cerebri.—This is a lesion somewhat different in its gross and histological details. It too follows a gross compound comminuted fracture of the skull. It is particularly well known to army surgeons as a consequence of missile wounds with indriven foreign material, as well as fragments of bone. A cerebral fungus develops progressively after a variable interval following wounding of the individual. It is a progressive lesion, whose exposed superficial surface is soon surmounted by a layer of granulation tissue intermingled with pus. The lesion tends to protrude more and more until actual evulsion of the degenerated tissue takes place. In the past, efforts have been made to resect repeatedly this degenerated tissue, until a considerable amount of the brain tissue has been lost. The point of greatest significance, which was demonstrated years ago and rediscovered recently (Richland and Courville, 1951; Courville et al., 1956) (10, 11), is that a cerebral fungus never forms unless an abscess is localized deep within the brain. Expansion of this infectious lesion constitutes the essential mechanism for the progressive herniation of the mass. It is therefore made up of a complex tissue matrix of brain tissue and scar together with one or more abscess cavities with heavy connective tissue capsules, secondary vascular softening, and secondary deformation of the ventricular system (Fig. 36, B). Since this lesion is in most cases a military one, it is very unlikely that the medical examiner will have to deal with this problem. Should this come to hand, however, it will profit him to consult the references cited for further details.

Traumatic Cephaloceles.—These rare lesions usually develop in children who have sustained a vertical linear fracture of the parietal and temporal bones (Brooks and Olsen, 1936) (12). With increasing intracranial pressure, the fracture is progressively widened until the underlying brain tissue begins to herniate through enlarged bony defect. The lateral ventricle likewise undergoes enlargement, sufficient at times to become a part of the herniation (*traumatic hydroencephalocele*). These lesions are rarely fatal, hence do not ordinarily come to the attention of the medical examiner.

Traumatic Porencephaly.—This lesion may be described in this connection as a *late residual* of loss of cerebral tissue through a traumatic cranial defect.[4] The original cranial lesion again consists of a compound comminuted and depressed fracture. The sharply edged depressed bone fragments lacerate the underlying brain. The macerated tissues are intermingled with blood clot which assists in the process. This necrotic material escapes through the original traumatic defect or is gradually softened and absorbed by the natural phagocytizing processes of repair. There ultimately remains a defect in the superficial part of the brain, whose size corresponds closely with the cranial lesion producing it (Fig. 37).

Evolution of the Original Bony Lesion

It is of rare occurrence that the primary traumatic lesions of the skull undergo any subsequent changes to which attention should be called. Perhaps the most important of these changes are (1) necrosis of bone of the cranial vault resulting from an interference with the regional blood supply, and (2) osteomyelitis due to invasion of the diploic spaces by pyogenic bacteria. *Necrosis of the bone* most often follows avulsion of the scalp, especially when associated with fragmentation of bone. This necrosis seems to follow an interruption of the

---

[4] This type of "brain cyst" can also result from the rupture to the surface of a traumatic intracerebral hemorrhage. See chapter on traumatic intracerebral hemorrhages (Chapter IV).

nutrient arteries derived from the dura. It was also formerly reported in cases of tangential sabre cuts or other incised wounds with more or less detachment of the scalp from the bony fragments of the cranial vault.

Osteomyelitis of the skull usually follows an infection of the scalp in compound comminuted depressed fractures (Adelstein and Courville, 1933) (13). The bone fragments are usually bathed in the purulent exudate and gradually are eroded and broken down to form sequestrum, to be eliminated from the wound (Fig. 38). Occasionally, osteomyelitis may follow

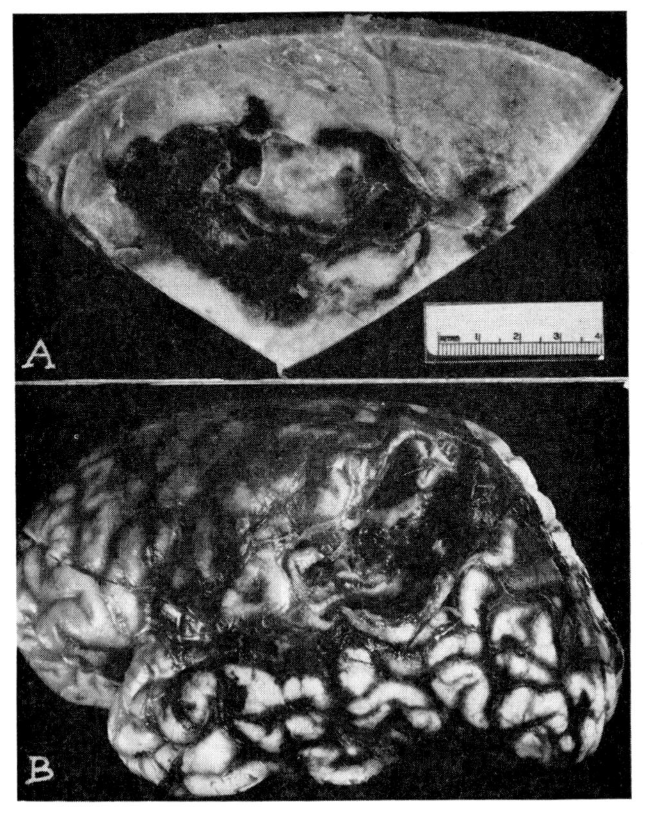

Fig. 37—Traumatic porencephaly. A. Old healed depressed skull fracture, the cause of brain damage in B. B. Irregular deep defect in brain produced by laceration of bone fragments. Recent subarachnoid hemorrhage due to second fatal injury.

abrasions of bone in which street dirt has been ground into the opened diploe. Such eventualities are now extremely rare, thanks to antibiotics.

Perhaps even more rare is *hyperostosis* following traumatic lesions of the cranium or *healed traumatic osteomyelitis,* as is sometimes noted in prehistoric skulls, i. e., of the Incas, in whom osteomyelitis was apparently fairly common.

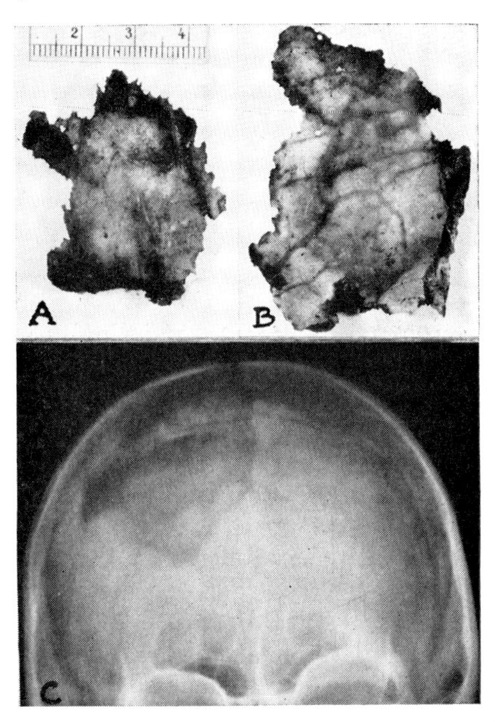

Fig. 38—Traumatic osteomyelitis of the skull. A and B. Sequestra with eroded margins from extensive area of osteomyelitis following comminuted fracture of skull. C. Roentgenogram showing necrotizing bone fragments in large defect in cranial vault.

Nonvisible Cracks in the Cranial Basis

It has already been suggested that "hair line" fractures may occur in the rather brittle bone forming the internal wall of the accessory nasal sinuses or of the tegmen tympani or mastoid cells. In the later situation, not only is such a fracture possible but it is also less likely to heal. The forensic surgeon should not overlook the possibility of such a cause in a cryptic septic meninges whose fracture may not be any more apparent at autopsy than on X-ray studies made during life. This is particularly true if the injury which caused the fracture had taken place many months or years before the onset of the meningitis. Under these circumstances a true traumatic infectious lesion may be considered purely a spontaneous lesion and its relationship to a previous injury overlooked. When this is in doubt, any previous cranial injury should be analyzed to determine whether or not the mechanism of a fracture might not be forthcoming.

It would seem that it should be possible in some manner to demonstrate the avenue by which the infection has gained entrance to the intracranial space. This is a vital link in the chain of invasion. The steps in establishing this link are to determine the viability of the extracranial infectious focus (sinus or mastoid cell infection), the presence of the avenue of invasion through the bony wall, and finally a corresponding focus of infection in the dura and leptomeninges. This may involve the medieval method of applying a dye of some sort to show up a "hair line" crack not otherwise visible. Fortunately this complex effort is not often necessary, but if this sort of a situation is to be really demonstrable, it may take this amount of attention to details.

Another approach to the problem may involve the development of microroentgenology. If it is suspected that the invasion of infection has resulted from an old fracture through a petrous bone, careful removal of the bone in question and a microroentgenological study, perhaps in stereo, may be able to demonstrate a thin fracture line. This would have to be preceded by critical study of clinical history of the injury in order to establish the correct approach to the region in question.

Summary

This study constitutes a brief survey of the many and varied types of complications of fractures of the skull, acute and chronic, which occasionally demand careful medicolegal evaluation. As a rule, these complications do not require critical study, since by their very nature, the mechanism of their formation is quite clear. The importance of understanding these complications is that first of all, they should not be mistaken for nontraumatic lesions, which is rarely the case. Secondly, they should not be confused with other traumatic lesions and thereby cause misunderstanding of their true causative mechanism (i. e., a laceration of the superficial tissues of the brain may be confused with a contrecoup contusion). Residuals of such complications are not likely to be found in great numbers except in cities where large numbers of traumatic lesions are exposed for evaluation in the course of time. Nevertheless, in any community, the medical examiner may be suddenly confronted with such a lesion, even though they be rare. For this reason such a survey calling attention to all these complications has seemed to be worthwhile.

REFERENCES

1. Foerster, O., and Penfield, W.: Structural Basis of Traumatic Epilepsy and Results of Radical Operation. Brain 53:99–119 (July) 1930.
2. Rand, Carl W., and Courville, Cyril B.: Histologic Changes in the Brain in Cases of Fatal Injury to the Head. IV. Reaction of the Classic Neuroglia. Arch. Neurol. & Psychiat. 27:1342–1379 (June) 1932.
3. Abbott, Kenneth H.: Acute Missile Wounds of the Brain. An Atlas of Surgical Pathology. Bull. Los Angeles Neurol. Soc. 26:103–131 (Sept) 1961.
4. Dratz, H. M., and Woodhall, B.: Traumatic Dissecting Aneurysm of Left Internal Carotid, Anterior Cerebral and Middle Cerebral Arteries. J. Neuropath. & Exper. Neurol. 6:286–291 (July) 1947.
5. Courville, Cyril B.: Traumatic Aneurysm of an Intracranial Artery. Description of Lesion Incident to a Shotgun Wound of the Skull and Brain. Bull. Los Angeles Neurol. Soc. 25:48–54 (Mar) 1960.
6. Dandy, Walter E.: Pneumocephalus, Intracranial Pneumatocele or Aerocele. Arch. Surg. 12:949 (May) 1926.
7. Courville, Cyril B.: Traumatic Intracranial Aerocele; Some Comments on Its Pathology Based on a Review of the Literature and a Study of Three Autopsied Cases. Bull. Los Angeles Neurol. Soc. 8:97–117 (Dec) 1943.
8. Nager, F. R.: Ueber Spätmeningitis nach Labyrenth-fraktur. Acta Otolaryng. 14:127–134, 1930.
9. Courville, Cyril B., and Platner, C. D.: The Etiology of Traumatic Meningitis; A Survey of Ninety Cases Verified at Autopsy. Bull. Los Angeles Neurol. Soc. 3:150–168 (Dec) 1938.
10. Richland, K. J., and Courville, Cyril B.: Fungus Cerebri. Report of a Case with a Brief Review of Its History, Pathogenesis and Pathology. Bull. Los Angeles Neurol. Soc. 16:267–291 (Sept) 1951.

11. Courville, Cyril B., Moyar, J. B., Eberlin, E. W., and Haymaker, Webb: Fungus Cerebri as a Complication of Missile Wounds of the Brain. Some Comments on Its History and Pathogenesis with Report of Case. Military Medicine 118:473–487 (May) 1956.
12. Brooks, M. B., and Olsen, C. W.: Traumatic Cephalhydrocele. Bull. Los Angeles Neurol. Soc. 1:127–131 (Sept) 1936.
13. Adelstein, Leo J., and Courville, Cyril B.: Traumatic Osteomyelitis of the Cranial Vault. Arch. Surg. 26:539–569 (Apr) 1933.

Chapter VI. Trauma to the Spine and Spinal Cord and Its Medicolegal Significance*

Injuries to the spine and spinal cord have recently become of considerable interest from a medicolegal viewpoint. While undoubtedly such injuries have been observed since prehistoric times, it has only been with the advent of rapid transportation and modern warfare that the importance of such injuries has been particularly emphasized. Arrowheads lodged in the vertebrae of skeletons found in both Europe and America indicated that such injuries occurred in warfare among the indigenous peoples of prehistoric times. As far as the medical literature is concerned, injuries of the spinal cord have been reported chiefly in the literature of the latter half of the eighteenth century and the entire nineteenth century. Military surgeons of the nineteenth century also reported injuries to the spinal cord, resulting from gunshot wounds. Extensive volumes on missile injuries call attention to the American Civil War and gunshot wounds of a century ago.

From a medicolegal viewpoint, however, interest in injuries to the spinal cord was aroused in the latter decades of the nineteenth century, when Erichsen (1882) (1) began to write on a peculiar clinical entity which he called "concussion of the spine." Such injuries were so common among the numerous railroad accidents of that era that the lesion came to be known as "railway spine," or Erichsen's disease. The introduction of the automobile and the increase in industrial activity have resulted in a greatly increased frequency of spinal injuries.

---

* Unfortunately, most problems involving forensic lesions of the spinal cord are not exposed at autopsy. Therefore the structural changes in the spinal cord are not well evaluated. A critical study on groups of these lesions are very much in order.

One must recognize that when dealing with a case involving an industrial accident or an injury from an automobile collision (question of compensation) the medical examiner does not prove to be so helpful as he does in cases of craniocerebral injury. The reason for this, of course, is that aside from an extremely severe injury with fracture-dislocation of the spine and resultant cord crush, there is usually little evidence as to the nature or the significance of the spinal injury. However, there are cases in which alleged injury of the spine is accompanied with clinical symptoms of disease of nontraumatic etiology. In such a case, the medicolegal autopsy makes clear that some other cause produced the crippling manifestations attributed to trauma. In an extensive middle ground, in which less severe whiplash injuries of the cervical spine or industrial flexion-twisting injuries result in herniation of the nucleus pulposus, the etiological diagnosis cannot wait for autopsy. For the most part, of course, flexion-extension injuries do not damage the cord; they rarely result in extrusion of the nucleus pulposus, and only occasionally compression of a nerve root. The use of the electromyogram and of the opaque myelogram makes it fairly simple to arrive at a diagnosis in a case of such injury. Herniation of the nucleus pulposus in the lower spine, which results in a fairly typical nerve root compression syndrome, is usually made clear by the same methods. Hence, the medicolegal examination rarely discloses either of these lesions.

Nevertheless, it is necessary for us to consider traumatic lesions of the spine and spinal cord in order to complete our survey of trauma in medicolegal cases. It is desirable to open this discussion with presentation of a selected group of 79 autopsied cases of both clearcut and assumed injuries of the spine. The details of these cases are made clear in the accompanying table (Table I). From these cases we shall be able to make certain conclusions which will be of value in forensic medicine. In the first place, there is a great difference between the gross traumatic lesions of the spine verified roentgenographically (especially when associated with paraplegia below the level of injury) and the second group of alleged injuries of the spine of minor degree in which the disease of the cord, manifested by a variety of clinical syndromes, seems to be completely unrelated to the alleged injury. Such injuries as flexion-extension (whiplash) injuries and herniation of the nucleus pulposus comprise a third group of lesions, which are usually easily diagnosed. A comprehensive discussion of traumatic injuries of the spine and spinal cord can therefore be divided into three parts: (1) gross traumatic lesions of the spine and spinal cord, (2) nontraumatic cord lesions found in cases of alleged injury, and (3)

Table I

Necropsy Examination on Actual or Presumed Injuries to the Spine

1. Whiplash injuries without cord damage	8 cases
2. Minimal uncertain trauma with minor cord changes (unproven)	2 cases
3. Alleged "back injuries" with nontraumatic spinal cord disease	12 cases
4. Penetrating injuries	
a. Gunshot wounds	6 cases
b. Stab wound	1 case
5. Fracture-dislocation of spine with or without injuries of the spinal cord	
a. Cord crush	32 casse
b. Cord contusion	5 cases
c. Hematomyelia *	6 cases
d. Extradural hematomyelia	1 case
e. Herniated nucleus pulposus	1 case
f. Without any cord damage	4 cases
g. With chiropractic manipulation	1 case
TOTAL NUMBER IN SERIES	79 cases

minimal lesions of the spinal cord and nerve roots following minor functional injuries of the spine. Before we become too deeply involved in these divisions, it is advisable to consider the applied anatomy of the spine, the different types of spinal injury and the mechanisms involved.

The Anatomy and Nature of Traumatic Lesions of the Spine and the Mechanism of Their Production

Although both the brain and spinal cord compose the central nervous system, the traumatic lesions of these portions are

* In 1 case of old hematomyelia the traumatic etiology was uncertain.

remarkably different in nature and severity. This is due to the nature of their bony investments and the distribution of the functional divisions of the two organs.

Applied Anatomy of the Spine—The spine is a flexible, curved column of flattened bony segments separated from each other by a fibrocartilaginous pad and bound together by a pattern of firm ligaments. The individual bones are smallest in the cervical region and largest in the lumbar region. The individual bones are made up of a body, two lateral pedicles, and laminae with a posterior arch and process. This column describes three curves when viewed laterally—anterior curves in the cervical and lumbar regions and a posterior curve in the dorsal section. The weight of the trunk is supported by the bodies and articular surfaces. The extent of flexion and extension of the spine is greatest in the cervical region and least in the lumbar. Spinal rotation is relatively slight in the cervical region, somewhat more free in the upper dorsal region, but diminished to almost zero in the lumbar region.

The anatomical characteristics of the individual vertebrae and the arrangements of their articular surfaces contribute to dislocations and fractures of the spine as a whole. The relation of the spinal cord to the vertebrae, lying as it does in the spinal canal interposed between the vertebral bodies anteriorly, the articular surface of the pedicles laterally, and the spinous process of the neural arch posteriorly, also accounts for the various types of injury to the cord and its emergent nerve roots.

Traumatic Lesions of the Spine—The several portions of the spine may be dislocated, fractured or penetrated by foreign bodies. *Dislocation* is determined largely by the arrangement of the articular facets. In the cervical region, these facets slope downward and backward, hence dislocation in this region occurs when the upper portion of the cervical spine is pressed forward, lying anterior to the lower portion. Dislocation is usually unilateral, unless fracture of one or both pedicles has occurred. Luxation usually affects the fourth, fifth, and sixth cervical vertebrae.

The atlas may also be dislocated, either anteriorly or posteriorly, by rupture of the transverse ligament, fracture of the odontoid process, or slipping of the process beneath this ligament.

Fracture is frequently associated with luxation, especially in the lower cervical region. The spinous and articular processes may also be broken and pushed inward into the spinal canal to injure the spinal cord. The bodies of the vertebrae (especially the dorsal and lumbar) and their intervening disks may be compressed, crushed, or fragmented, with variable degrees of injury to the spinal cord. Even though dislocated, the vertebrae are rarely fixed in their new position, as in the case of the fracture-dislocations of the lower cervical spine.

Clinical localization of the lesions in injuries of the spine and spinal cord is determined not only by examination of the spinous processes externally, but also by checking the clinical symptoms referable to the spinal cord itself. This is especially true of *penetrating injuries,* such as stab or gunshot wounds, which may be entirely or partially segmental.

As in our cases of craniocerebral injuries, we shall briefly discuss the *mechanism* of spinal cord injuries. It is obvious that damage to the cord may result from a variety of mechanisms. Collapse of a vertebra incident to tuberculous or malignant disease may result in mechanical pressure, with distortion of the cord and nerve roots. In such an instance, only a failure of spinal support would be seen. We are more concerned, however, with the lesions in the first group, true traumatic injuries. They may be divided into three subgroups: (1) *Crushing injuries* result from falls from a height, striking a beam transversely, or being pinned beneath some collapsing structure or an overturned automobile. (2) *Fracture-dislocation* of the spine may result in damage to the spinal cord by compression of the cord by the vertebrae. This may be either (a) *cervical,* when an individual dives or falls on the head with severe flexion of the lower cervical or upper thoracic spine, or (b) *dorsal,* resulting from falling objects or heavy weights compressing the upper spine and causing a fracture-dislocation of the lower dorsal vertebrae. Jefferson (1927) (2) has designated the first as the civilian group and the second as the industrial group. (3) *Penetrating wounds* of the spine usually result from (a) stab wounds or (b) gunshot wounds. It is now important to demonstrate that these mechanisms may produce a variety of lesions of the spinal cord, many of which follow a more typical pattern. These mechanisms, illustrated in the accompanying figure (Fig. 39), also produce certain syndromes which can be briefly discussed with respect to their inherent pathology.

Clinical Symptom Complexes and Their Pathological Counterparts

A group of symptom complexes which result from injuries of the spinal cord and which are fairly characteristic of certain cases will now be briefly described.

Spinal Concussion—Concussion of the spinal cord following blunt trauma has been compared to cerebral concussion following mild injuries of the head. There are certain differences, however, which should be stressed. In the first place, it apparently takes a much more severe blunt injury to produce concussion of the spine than it does to produce concussion of the brain. This is most likely to occur when a patient has been injured by a fall, or has been struck in the dorsal region of the spine by an automobile. The patient is immediately paralyzed below the level of the injury (Clevenger, 1889) (3). This is associated with loss of sensation in the lower extremities. As a rule, a loss of control of the urinary and rectal sphincters is also present. These symptoms are usually short lived and the patient soon regains function in all areas.

Spinal concussion also differs from cerebral concussion in that it apparently is not a purely functional disorder. This is suggested in the first place by the location of the functional disturbances in the cord, which may extend some distance above and below the immediate point of contact. It is theoretically presumed that these more distant manifestations are the result of the impact on the cerebrospinal column, with a reverberation up and down the spinal canal. It has been presumed that local edema, small hemorrhages, and laceration of the cord may be found in the vicinity of the impact. Those who have described the pathology of such lesions state that anemic softening, focal hemorrhage, alterations in the nerve cells and nerve fibers, and hemorrhage into the subarachnoid space, as well as trauma to the regional nerve roots may be found. When physical changes have taken place, of course, one would expect to find phagocytosis of degenerated tissue and, in the late stage, resultant glial proliferation, as has been described by Davison (1945) (4). The author has not had an opportunity to see these changes in any of his cases. He has, however, found local edema, which is probably an early stage of the same process.

Traumatic Hematomyelia—In flexion injuries of the spine which are not accompanied by gross dislocation or fracture, focal damage to the spinal cord may be found. This lesion does not involve the complete cord. Rather, there is found within the spinal cord a hemorrhagic softening of the enclosed gray matter, observed only on cross or horizontal section. It is thus supposed that the internal gray matter, being softer than the enveloping white fibers, is more easily damaged. At the point of injury an extensive destruction of gray matter occurs while the outer portion of the white matter is preserved. Above or below the point of impact the gray matter is less extensively damaged. This peculiar pattern results in a fusiform cavitation of the center of the cord. Microscopic examination of these sections discloses the injured gray matter to have undergone softening intermingled with hemorrhage. The nerve cells and fibers in the damaged area are totally or subtotally destroyed, the intervening substance being involved as well.

Not all lesions of this type are immediately fatal. As time goes on, the degenerated tissue is broken down, there is an accumulation of compound granular corpuscles transformed from the regional microglia (Bailey, 1961) (5), the degenerated tissue is phagocytized and removed, with ultimate formation of a peripheral glial scar surrounding a central cystic cavity. This scar is of the anisomorphic variety. Its constituent astrocytes ultimately become hyalinized, a pseudomembrane is formed around the cavity and the structural changes in the lesion become more or less stablilized. There results, therefore, a residual multilocular, irregularly shaped cavitation whose walls stain orange-yellow (Fig. 40).[1] The

[1] The writer (Courville, 1937) (6) has shown that this tendency for more extensive destruction of the interior of the cord than of the external white matter is the rule in injuries of this sort. Only focal lesions result in this

patient may survive such a lesion for a considerable length of time (Elsberg, 1919) (7).

Contusion of the Cord—A simple contusion of the cord is a rather uncommon lesion, as will be observed by reference to Table I. Of 5 suggestive cases studied in this laboratory, only one would strictly qualify for designation as a contusion. This was due to a depression of only a small portion of the overlying lamina. A contusion may be a more external wound of the cord, involving only the immediate portion of the cord which is compressed by bone. Such a lesion would be manifested clinically by symptoms from the portion of the cord actually compressed by the bone, a nonfatal condition. This lesion would later become adherent to the overlying leptomeninges and a meningeal-spinal scar of varying depth and extent would be formed.

Contusion-Compression of the Cord (Cord Crush)—Severe fracture-dislocation of the spine, whether cervical or thoracic, as a rule results in contusion-compression of the cord (Fig. 41). This lesion is much less common in the lumbar regions, where the vertebrae are not easily dislocated. Crushing of the cord is not necessarily a fatal lesion, although many individuals do die within a few days or a week after injury to the cervical cord because of interference with the elimination of heat from the body or the development of pulmonary or other complications. The extent and location of cord crush varies remarkably (Fig. 42). In some patients the lesion is quite marked, being only a simple transverse or slightly oblique defect in the cord. If the injury has occurred at some interval prior to the patient's demise, above and below the defect the cord will be well preserved and may be flexed at this level, indicating only a small transverse defect in the cord. In other instances the softened area of the cord may be fairly extensive, corresponding to the extent of compression by depressed bone. In such cases it is quite obvious that the spinal damage is extremely severe. At first the tissue may be stained by infiltration of hemorrhage. As time goes on, this pigment becomes brown, then orange, then yellow, and

---

typical fusiform lesion. Under other circumstances, one finds that the gray matter of the cord has undergone severe damage above and below the immediate area of impact and depressed section of the spine.

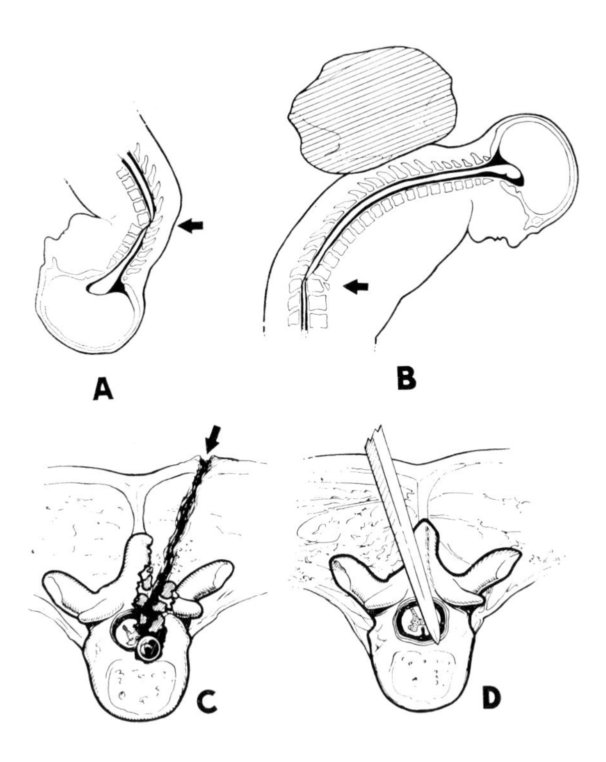

Fig. 39—Mechanisms of spinal fractures. A. Acute flexion injury of cervical spine (fall on head) with fracture-dislocation and cord crush. B. Acute flexion injury by crushing weight on shoulders with fracture-dislocation of lower thoracic vertebrae and cord crush. C. Penetrating missile wound of spine, with injury to spinal cord. D. Stab wound of spinal cord.

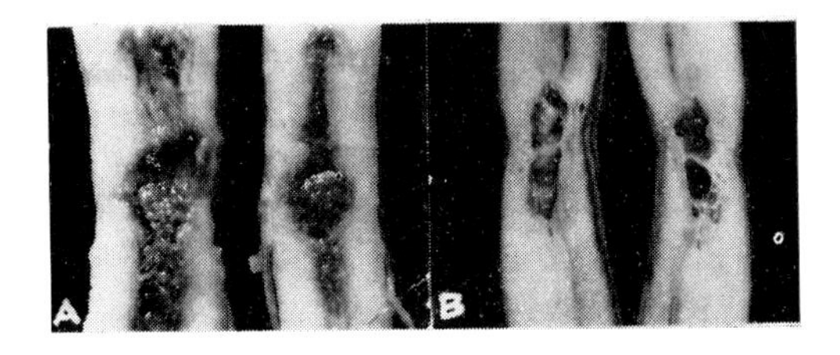

Fig. 40—Traumatic hematomyelia. A. Recent lesion. B. Chronic residual cyst. Note tendency to fusiform shape of lesions involving predominantly central gray matter.

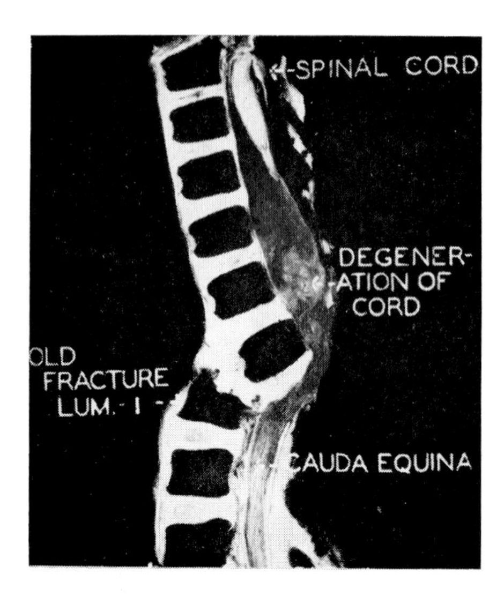

Fig. 41—Fracture-dislocation of spine with compression of spinal cord.

finally fades out entirely. The covering leptomeninges may also be stained in this way. Ultimately, with thickening and increasing opacity of the meninges, an adhesive leptomeningeal scar enveloping the area of cord crush develops.

Histology of Cord Crush—The immediate effect of cord crush essentially consists of damage to the tissue of the spinal cord intermingled with a moderate degree of hemorrhage. Edema and acutely swollen oligodendroglia soon develop in the immediate area of injury (Bailey, 1961) (5). In the first few hours, there becomes evident an infiltration of hemorrhagic pigment into the regional nerve cells, especially those of the anterior horn. The microglia show early swelling and the formation of vacuoles in their substance. The nerve fibers begin to show a breakdown in their myelin, with irregularities in the contour of the myelin sheaths. This, of course, is followed by fragmentation, and ultimately by segments of the myelin sheaths, the formation of myelin balls and myelophages. In sections stained by Cajal's reduced silver technique, the earliest changes seen in the axis cylinders are swelling and varicosity, particularly in the region adjacent to their interruption (Bailey, 1959) (8). This is followed by a breaking down of the axis cylinders in more distal segments, with ultimate disappearance of these elements. The proximal segment of the interrupted fiber also undergoes fragmentation for a short distance. Here end-bulbs are formed (Bailey, 1960) (9). These changes in the nerve fibers are coincident with a rapid loss of tigroid material. Adjacent to the wound, the nerve cells undergo severe change, which varies in proportion to their proximity of the injury itself (Bailey, 1943) (10). Subsequently, the compound granular corpuscles pick up the debris of the nervous elements and carry it away through the regional blood vessels. These macrophages remain until all the decadent material is removed. Ultimately, a typical anisomorphic glial scar with a proliferation of astrocytes develops in the region of the defect (Bailey, 1961) (11). The final picture, therefore, is a replacement gliosis with the altered remains of both parenchymatous and interstitial elements. These changes are seen in the accompanying figure (Fig. 43).

Penetrating Injuries

In this series of cases, we have relatively few penetrating injuries, although such injuries are not at all uncommon. The injuries in which there were medicolegal questions were relatively few in number. There were six gunshot wounds of the spinal cord and only one stab wound.

The degree and location of destruction in *gunshot wounds* are quite variable (Thorburn and Richardson, 1919) (12). It is a matter of chance where a bullet lodges, and the extent of damage is dependent upon the points of entrance and exit and the injury to the spinal cord between the two openings. Most of our cases have been acute wounds, and hemorrhage and laceration have been characteristic (Fig. 44). However, in one case of an old lesion, a certain amount of repair had been attempted, in the form of a glial scar lying in the site of the injury. To completely evaluate such wounds, it is worthwhile to take sections of the spinal cord at regular intervals between the point of entrance of the missile and its exit. By reproducing these sections, even when stained routinely, one can reconstruct in a series of drawings the area

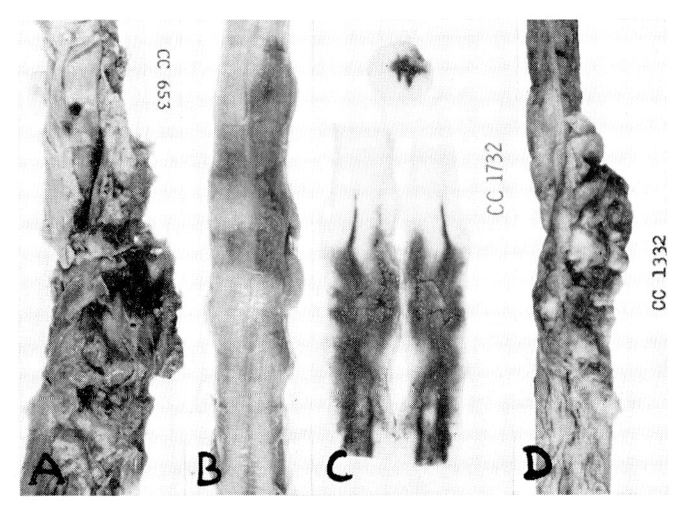

Fig. 42—Acute lesions of cord crush. A. Death in *ca* 48 hours after auto collision with fracture of lower cervical spine. B and C. Death 5 days after fracture of cervical spine; patient struck in back of head and neck by heavy lid while cleaning tank. D. Death in 4 hours after injury while water skiing; fracture of 7th cervical spine.

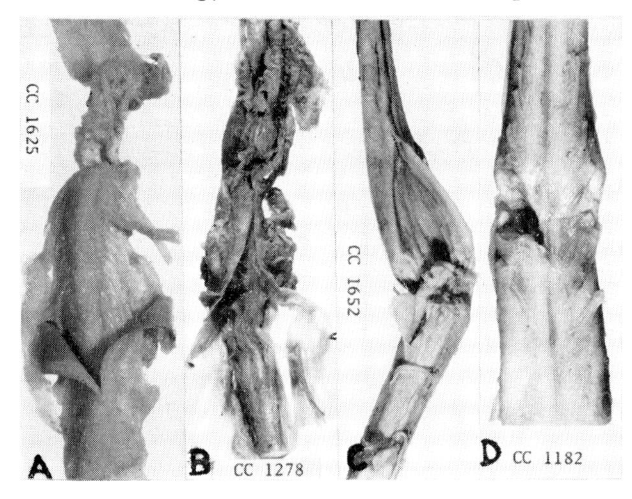

Fig. 43—Subacute and chronic residual cord lesions incident to fracture of the spine. A. Fracture-dislocation of lower cervical spine in auto collision. Survival *ca* 2 months. B. Fracture lower cervical spine with cord crush after automobile collision. Survival for 3 weeks. C. Focal crushing of cord from transitory dislocation of lower cervical cord; quadriplegia after fall from swing. Survival period 7 years, 10 months. D. Complete cord crush lower cervical cord after automobile accident. Survival for 3 weeks.

of damage and thereby give a visual explanation of the neurological symptoms resulting from the injury.

A most unusual case which has come to our attention is that of an individual with a gunshot wound of the abdomen, with profuse hemorrhage into that cavity, as well as hemorrhage into the subarachnoid space of the spinal cord. The connection between the two effusions could not be made out.

In our one verified example of a *stab wound* of the spinal cord, evidence of transection was still quite clear after a survival period of 6 months (Fig. 45, A). A 22-year-old Mexican woman was stabbed in the back while dancing. She immediately became completely paralyzed and fell to the floor. Below the level of the injury all sensation was lost. Death came from a bulbar palsy. At autopsy, the wound in the spinal cord was seen to be practically complete. This was verified by microscopic section (Fig. 45, B). Such injuries are, of course, quite rare (Rand and Patterson, 1929) (13).

Actual Findings in the Spinal Cord in Cases of Alleged "Back Injury"—In this segment of neuropathology one can learn a great deal about what is often assumed from a simple "back injury" which is not followed by any immediate, well-defined manifestations, and the relatively long interval between the time of the injury and the postmortem examination.

In a series of cases in which individuals gave a history of "back injury," the following lesions were actually discovered by gross and microscopic examination: (1) thrombosis of the anterior spinal artery, (2) softening of the spinal cord on the basis of arteriosclerotic thrombosis, (3) compression of the spinal cord by metastatic carcinoma of the lumbar spine, (4) amyotrophic lateral sclerosis (2 cases), (5) necrotizing myelitis, (6) tabes dorsalis, (7) hematomyelia due to vascular anomaly (questionably traumatic in 1 case), (8) mild compression of the spinal cord by a cotton pledget after surgery, and (9) a meningioma (alleged to be due to a lumbar puncture 10 years before).

The presence of such lesions in a series of forensic cases which were ultimately recognized as being of some nontraumatic etiology points out the rather loose ideas regarding trauma as a cause of spinal cord disease. Were one to be slip-shod in his interpretation, he might perhaps assign one of these cases demonstrated to be amyotrophic lateral sclerosis to trauma

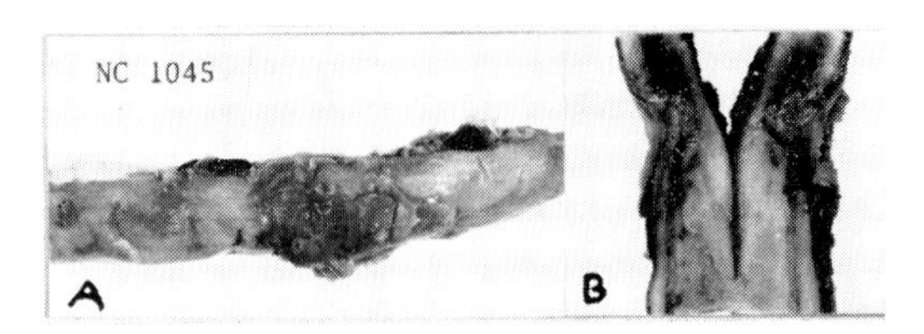

Fig. 44—Gunshot wound of spinal cord. A. Bruise of cord by impact of missile. B. Vertical section of cord showing point of impact of missile and consequent hemorrhage into spinal cord. Survival period 6 weeks.

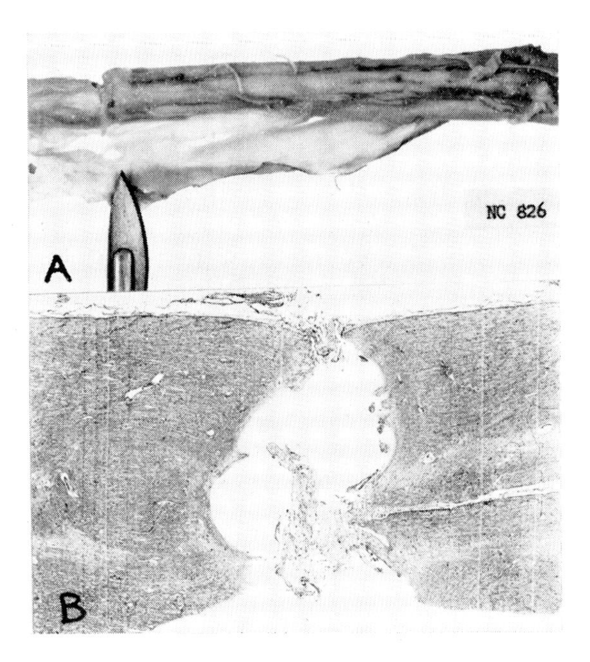

Fig. 45—Stab wound of spinal cord in a young woman. Assaulted by jealous lover while dancing; immediate quadriplegia. Survival period 6 months. A. Photograph showing almost total section of cord. B. Low-power photomicrograph showing same defect.

to the cervical spine, since it is true that a few cases of this disease are credited to such an injury. Furthermore, some cases of tabes dorsalis have supposedly been activated by a local injury to the back, although in many such cases the likelihood of pure coincidence must be acknowledged. In one of the two cases of hematomyelia due to the presence of a vascular anomaly, the possibility of traumatic rupture was considered. However, there are no cases in the medicolegal literature known to the writer in which there was a clear relationship of trauma to rupture of such a vascular anomaly. In one instance, an absolutely normal spinal cord was found, although it was alleged that the patient developed spinal symptoms after an injury.

Miscellaneous Problems

There are always a few cases in any extensive series such as this in which some aberrant factors are to be explained. For example, there were 8 cases of whiplash injury without any evidence of cord damage, the examinations simply being done to disprove the presence of such injuries. There were also two cases in which seemingly minor injury of the spinal cord was followed by symptoms of atypical pattern. Possibly, these two cases may have represented "cord concussion", although history was inadequate to prove this point.

There were 4 cases of fracture-dislocation of the spinal cord, without any injury to the cord itself, illustrating that once in a while severe injuries of the spine with automatic separation of the lamina may spare the cord from damage.

It is also of interest that in one instance a vigorous chiropractic manipulation resulted in physical damage to the spinal cord.

In two cases, investigation of the spinal cord after alleged injury disclosed a herniated nucleus pulposus, a lesion much more likely to be exposed by a neurosurgeon than by a medical examiner.

Additional Notes on Effects of Physical Agents

In addition to the immediate and direct action of heat on the tissues of the nervous system, there must also be considered certain remote effects of severe external burns on the body. These effects are not always to be registered in changes in the nervous tissue but are presumed to be due to the action on the body of shock, renal dysfunction or central influences on the automatic components of the brain stem. These later symptoms resemble an encephalopathy with signs of striatal manifestation (athetosis, tremors) as well as the cortex (convulsive disorders, psychic manifestations). The associated structural changes consist of hyperemia, punctate hemorrhages, and edema. As late residuals central demyelination and gliosis may occur. An anoxic mechanism has been charged as the cause of these changes but this is problematical (Globus and Bender) (15).

Nervous Tissue Damage by Electrical Current.—The actual effects of transmission of electrical current on nervous tissues depends upon the amount of current and the duration of its application. This would indicate whether the exposed tissue was involved by high, medium or low voltage. Direct exposure to high voltage may show charring on or near the surface, hemorrhage or necrosis. With exposure to lower voltage, the tissue appears swollen and marked by petechiae; microscopically the tissue is edemous and marked by small perivascular hemorrhages. The nerve cells have undergone variable degrees of pyknosis or severe nerve cell change leading to ghost cell formations. Still lesser injury from lower voltage (electroshock therapy) may leave no changes at all. Alpers (1946) (16) found cloudy swelling of cortical nerve cells, oligodendrocytosis with acute swelling and widening of the pericellular and perivascular spaces. However, the writer has not observed such changes in two cases of fatal issue from electroshock therapy.

Changes in Brain Tissue from Ultrasound.—No fatal cases of ultrasound administered to the brain of man have been studied in our laboratory. In animals, Lynn and Putnam (1946) (17) found changes in the skin and soft tissues of the scalp but no significant alterations in bone and meninges. The cerebral tissues show alterations suggestive of mechanical laceration of the tissues in the form of focal necrosis with central disintegration enveloped by a zone of vascular proliferation with infiltration of red cells from vascular rupture. This area is surrounded by a zone of gliosis.

Summary

The most severe injuries of the spinal cord result from grossly evident fracture-dislocations of the spine, which occur most often in the lower cervical and lower dorsal segments of the spinal column. Most fracture-dislocations in the cervical region are the result of a fall on the flexed neck, while in the lower thoracic region they usually result from the impact of a heavy weight on the shoulders, transverse injury to the spine by a fall, or compression in an automobile accident. These lesions are associated with crushing of the cord, usually with complete transection resulting in permanent paraplegia. Penetrating injuries of the spine, with an acute onset of symptoms localized at the level of injury, may be due to stab or gunshot wounds. In such instances, the obvious relationship between the injury of the cord and the traumatic episode leaves little reason for doubting their etiology.

In minor injuries without symptoms or clean-cut neurological manifestations, any connection between the traumatic episode and the disease of the patient is most doubtful. When a subsequent, latent syndrome develops and simulates a known medical complex, such as that produced by posterolateral sclerosis, amyotrophic lateral sclerosis, tabes dorsalis, or delayed sensory dissociation (question of syringomyelia), it must be considered as a purely medical problem, not as a consequence of injury. When such complexes are encountered clinically, grave doubts of any traumatic etiology should be entertained.

Flexion-extension (whiplash) injuries of the cervical spine almost never produce cord damage, although occasionally they may injure the local nerve roots or cause herniation of the nucleus pulposus in this region.

A twisting-flexion injury of the lower back may produce an extrusion of a herniated disk, which is usually demonstrated by electromyography or opaque myelography as a typical localized and usually lateralized root compression syndrome. Since this is not ordinarily a fatal injury, the resultant lesion is not likely to be uncovered in a medicolegal examination.

Two rather characteristic clinical syndromes from traumatic injuries of the cord merit brief mention. A penetrating injury, particularly a stab wound, tends to produce signs of an atypical or typical hemisection of the cord (Brown-Sequard's syndrome). Dissociation of pain and temperature from tactical sensation, without associated paraplegia may also follow a blunt injury to the back of the neck because of a hematomyelia of the cord, although such a lesion can be simulated by a spontaneous (nontraumatic) rupture of a vascular anomaly.

Trauma may accentuate certain medical diseases, such as tabes dorsalis, amyotrophic lateral sclerosis, multiple sclerosis, and tuberculous meningitis from Pott's disease. In these cases, the cause and effect relationship must be clearly established before one is entitled to attribute the cord changes to trauma.

REFERENCES

1. Erichsen, J. E.: Concussion of the Spine, ed 2. New York: Burmingham & Co., 1882.
2. Jefferson, G.: Fractures of First Cervical Vertebra. Brit. M. J. 2:153–157 (July 30) 1927.
3. Clevenger, S. V.: Spinal Concussion. Philadelphia: F. A. Davis, 1889.
4. Davison, C.: Pathology of Spinal Cord as Result of Trauma. A. Research Nerv. & Ment. Dis., Proc. (1943) 24:151–187, 1945.
5. Bailey, Frank W.: Histological Changes in the Spinal Cord of Man in Cases of Fatal Injury. V. Alterations in the Oligodendroglia and Microglia. Bull. Los Angeles Neurol. Soc. 26:172–185 (Dec) 1961.
6. Courville, Cyril B.: Pathology of the Central Nervous System. Mountain View, Cal.: Pacific Press Pub. Ass'n., 1937, pp 234–240.
7. Elsberg, C. A.: On Some Lesions Observed in Operations for Old Injuries to Spinal Cord with Remarks as to Treatment. Ann. Surg. 69:239–244 (Mar) 1919.
8. Bailey, Frank W.: Histological Changes in the Spinal Cord of Man in Cases of Fatal Injury. II. Alterations in the Neurocytons. Bull. Los Angeles Neurol. Soc. 24:204–213 (Dec) 1959.
9. ———: III. Alterations in the Nerve Fibers. Ibid. 25:147–160 (Sept) 1960.
10. ———: Nuclear Changes in the Anterior Horn Cells Following Local Injury to the Spinal Cord. Ibid. 8:129–136 (Dec) 1943.
11. ———: Histological Changes in the Spinal Cord of Man in Cases of Fatal Injury. IV. Alterations in the Classical Neuroglia. Ibid. 26:32–40 (Mar) 1961.
12. Thorburn, W., and Richardson, G.: The Pathology of Gunshot Wounds of the Spine and Spinal Cord. Brit. J. Surg. 6:481–496 (Apr) 1919.
13. Rand, C. W., and Patterson, G. H.: Stab Wounds of Spinal Cord: Report of 7 Cases. Surg. Gynec. & Obst. 48:652–661 (May) 1929.
14. Courville, Cyril B.: Trauma to the Central Nervous System and Its Envelopes, in Tice's Practice of Medicine. Hagerstown, Md.: W. F. Prior Co., Vol 10, 1950, pp 139–221.
15. Globus, J. H., and Bender, M. B.: Disseminated Toxic, Degenerative Encephalopathy (Disseminatory Sclerosis Demyelination) Secondary to Extensive and Severe Burns. J. Nerv. & Ment. Dis. 83:518, 1936.
16. Alpers, B. J.: The Brain Changes Associated with Electroshock Treatment: A Critical Review. Journal Lancet. 66:363, 1946.
17. Lynn, J. G. and Putnam, T. J.: Histology of Cerebral Lesions Produced by Focused Ultrasound, Am. J. Path. 20:637, 1944.

Chapter VII. Changes in the Brain Incident to Extreme Variations in Temperature, Barometric Pressure, Electrical Current, and X-Radiation*

Thus far in these studies, "trauma" or "injury" to the brain has been applied to the mechanical effects of force. Because the term "injury" has also been used to include structural damage from other types of physical factors, a separate study of these will be included. Such changes as are produced by extreme temperature, altered barometric pressure, electricity, and x-radiation will be discussed since they are sometimes encountered in medicolegal problems. Elevated barometric pressure (or air embolism) and lowered barometric pressure (or cerebral anoxia) will be discussed more completely in a later chapter. The characteristic structural changes produced in the brain by x-radiation will be given attention in this chapter. Electricity, which so often produces disappointing changes in the brain, will also be included for the sake of completeness.

Cerebral Changes from Extreme Variations in Temperature

A human being whose brain has been exposed to extreme degrees of temperature rarely survives to tell the story. When death occurs from such exposure, there is usually little doubt as to the cause of the patient's demise.

---

* The cases in this chapter describing lesions due to physical agents other than trauma are relatively rare, but are here included for sake of completeness. References are added which will be a source of help to pathologists seeking to learn more about individual problems.

When the brain is exposed to extreme cold, the intracranial fluids become crystallized, as do the body fluids in general. Apparently no residual changes occur in the brain if an individual recovers from the effects of exposure to cold, unless some intercurrent factor, such as shock or pneumonia, complicates the case.[1]

When the head is directly exposed to fire, death usually occurs from the general effects of burning, such as shock and hemorrhage, before the heat can pass through the skull to leave any characteristic marks upon the brain. Less extreme degrees of elevated temperature, however, do leave some residuals which merit brief attention.[2]

Heatstroke, Sunstroke.—Exposure of the human being to extreme solar heat, with direct exposure of the unprotected head or under conditions of high humidity, results grossly in congestion of the brain. Even the small pial vessels become crowded with red cells. Especially in cases of sunstroke, the brain appears small and dehydrated. In proportion to the degree of congestion, patchy subarachnoid hemorrhages occur over the dorsolateral surface of the brain; rarely hemorrhages

---

[1] Four persons succumbed as a result of severe hypothermia (8° to 12°C) while having cardiac surgery. Terminal symptoms referable to the brain stem were reported by Egerton et al. (1). Cortical ischemia, degeneration of cells of the basal ganglia, loss of Purkinje cells and changes in the myelin sheaths, as well as gross stasis and focal hemorrhages have been described in nine other fatal cases (2). Mateva, cited by Egerton et al. (1) in 11 individuals dying after exposure to cold found similar changes. Cellular changes are attributed to cerebral anoxia.

[2] In one questionable case of this sort studied in this laboratory, an infant was put into his crib at night wrapped in an electric blanket. He was found dead the following morning. Congestion was the only change visible in the brain. It was uncertain whether death was due to accidental electrocution or to long continued excessive temperature.

In another case, an elderly woman was found dead, with one side of her head exposed to the heat of a lamp. The brain on the exposed side was grossly congested, and microscopic examination showed that the regional cortical tissues were edematous, with widened perivascular and pericellular spaces. The nerve cells on that side stained poorly.

Minimal congestion and mild edema were found in the brains of two patients (even though the bodies had been embalmed) whose deaths were ascribed to heat exhaustion from working in the desert during the summer.

occur within the nervous tissues. Histologically, the congestion is very evident. It is greater in the cortex than in the white matter, although the large veins in the basal ganglia and choroid plexus also appear distended with dark blood. If the hyperemia persists for any length of time, signs of edema appear. The perivascular and pericellular spaces become distended with fluid. Perivascular, ring, or ball-shaped hemorrhages may also appear. Changes in the nerve cells are nonspecific and usually consist of acute swelling. Minimal changes occur in the nerve fibers. Insofar as the other elements are concerned, only the oligodendroglia are altered. They show acute swelling.

Undoubtedly, some residuals occur to account for chronic headaches and neurasthenic manifestations. Chronic thickening of the leptomeninges, especially about the pacchionian granulations, associated with unusual fullness of the larger external cerebral veins has been described in necropsies of sunstroke cases. Unfortunately, no cases with residuals of certain identification have been seen.

Exposure to Extremes of Barometric Pressure

There is considerable doubt whether extremely high or low barometric pressure produces specific alterations in the brain, either grossly or microscopically. The effects of *increased barometric pressure* are usually noted under circumstances of immersion in deep water (divers), which results in the release of nitrogen from the blood with lodgement of gas emboli in the brain. The effects of air or gas embolism are much like the effects of embolism of other types, with localized cerebral manifestations if the individual survives sufficiently long. These emboli are fatal when numerous and death comes before grossly evident softening occurs. Congestion and patches of subarachnoid hemorrhage may be seen externally. Punctate hemorrhages are at times observed microscopically, associated with small infarcts. Of the 5 cases of air embolism recorded in the necropsy files of the Los Angeles County Hospital, none were due to prolonged or excessive immersion. In 3 cases of air embolism seen in the Coroner's service, no bubbles of air were found in the superficial arteries of the brain.

The effects of *lowered barometric pressure* of serious degree are at present observed only in high altitude flyers whose supplies of oxygen have been interrupted. In these instances, the effects on the brain are manifested by an anoxic state. These effects, both acute and chronic, were reported by Titrud and Haymaker in 1947 (1), who found typical anoxic alterations in the brain. These changes will be described extensively in a subsequent chapter on asphyxia.

Effects of X-Radiation on the Brain

Damage to the tissues of the central nervous system can occur (1) by excessive exposure to x-rays (of the fetus or the adult) in the course of diagnostic procedures or treatment, or (2) by exposure to ionic radiation via certain metals or the explosion of an atomic (or hydrogen) bomb. Exposure to radioactive materials usually presents no medicolegal problem, except under industrial circumstances. A brief survey, however, of the chronological developments in the brain after such exposure will be made. The changes which occur in the first situation will be discussed more fully.

Effects of Atomic Radiation on the Brain.—The effects of atomic radiation on the brains of 49 casualties of the bombing attack on Hiroshima and Nagasaki were studied by Shiraki, et al., in 1958 (2). Forty-seven of these patients survived from 16 to 69 days. Two others lived approximately 4 and 6 years. Mental and neurological disturbances developed but the precise cause could not be determined.

Scattered perivascular hemorrhages of the brain were of a high incidence. Glial changes (glial nodules, reactive gliosis, enlargement of the astrocytic nuclei, deposition of lipochrome pigment in the glia of the globus pallidus), alterations in the nerve cells (globus pallidus, substantia nigra, and motor nuclei of the cranial nerves), and changes in the blood vessels, as well as increased vascular permiability were also observed. There was some question whether these changes were a reflection of the attendant anemia or the hypoxia.

Exposure of Fetal Brain to X-Radiation.—Damage to the nervous tissues which results from exposure to x-rays is usually consequent to excessive radiation treatment. Occasionally the abdomen of a pregnant woman is accidentally overexposed and the brain of the fetus seriously affected. A case was re-

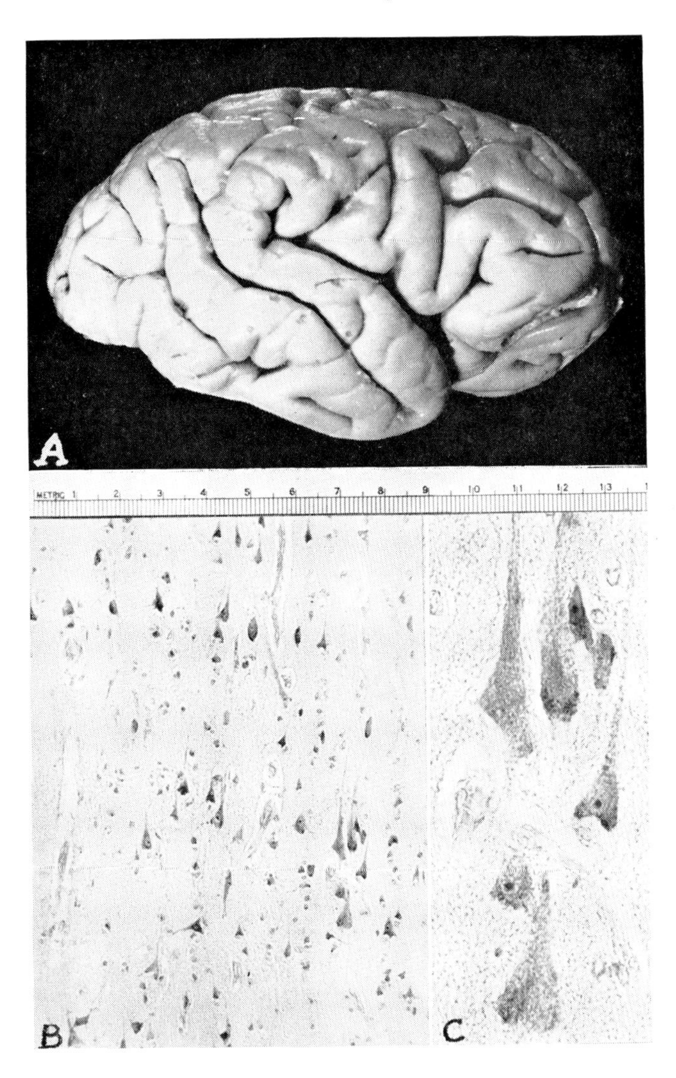

Fig. 46—A. Simple convolutional pattern in brain of microcephalic idiot after radiation of abdomen of mother to induce abortion. B. Dropping out of cortical nerve cells (frontal lobe). Nissl preparation X 150. C. Changes in remaining cellular elements. Nissl preparation X 500.

ported by Courville and Edmondson in 1958 (5) in which deliberate exposure of the fetus produced serious results.

A pregnant woman was subjected to a course of radiation to produce a therapeutic abortion which was recommended because of tuberculosis of the sacroiliac joint. The treatment failed to produce an abortion, however, and a diminutive baby, weighing only 2¾ pounds, was delivered by Caesarean section after the eighth month of pregnancy. The child, who developed slowly mentally and physically, proved to be a microcephalic dwarf. She died at the age of 13 years from an otitic osteomyelitis of the skull. The brain was very small and had an embryonic pattern of convolutions (Fig. 46, A). Microscopically, there was a marked reduction in the cortical nerve cells, especially of the frontal lobes, with deterioration of those which remained (Fig. 46, B).

The typical clinical pattern of microcephalic idiocy seen in this child is an obvious effect of x-radiation in utero. In 1938 Johnson (6) reported another similar example of this which was also verified at autopsy.

Results of Overexposure of the Mature Brain to X-Radiation.—The changes produced in the adult brain by excessive exposure to x-radiation were described by Courville and Myers in 1958 (7). A 15-year-old boy, along with a younger brother, was given an overdosage of x-radiation during treatment of ringworm of the scalp. The brain was later studied and characteristic changes were seen. Scarred areas were present in the cortex of the parietal regions, with extensive spotty softening of the white matter in the postcentral parietal and occipital regions (Fig. 47, A and B). Closer inspection revealed that the foci of softening enveloped small blood vessels (Fig. 48, C and D). An advanced degree of demyelinization and necrosis extended from the centrum to the cortex. Areas of gliosis, necrosis, and liquefaction occupied the centrum. The only intactly myelinated fibers were in the periphery beneath the cortex. Small perivascular cysts represented the liquefaction. Scattered foci of hemorrhage were seen. In the posterior portion of the cerebral hemispheres, focal cortical hemorrhages, focal red cortical softening, edema, and abscesses were found.

Microscopically, the changes in the cortex varied with the proximity to the area of advanced necrosis. In the anterior portion of the brain the small blood vessels were mildly congested, but the cortex was essentially unaltered. Some of the

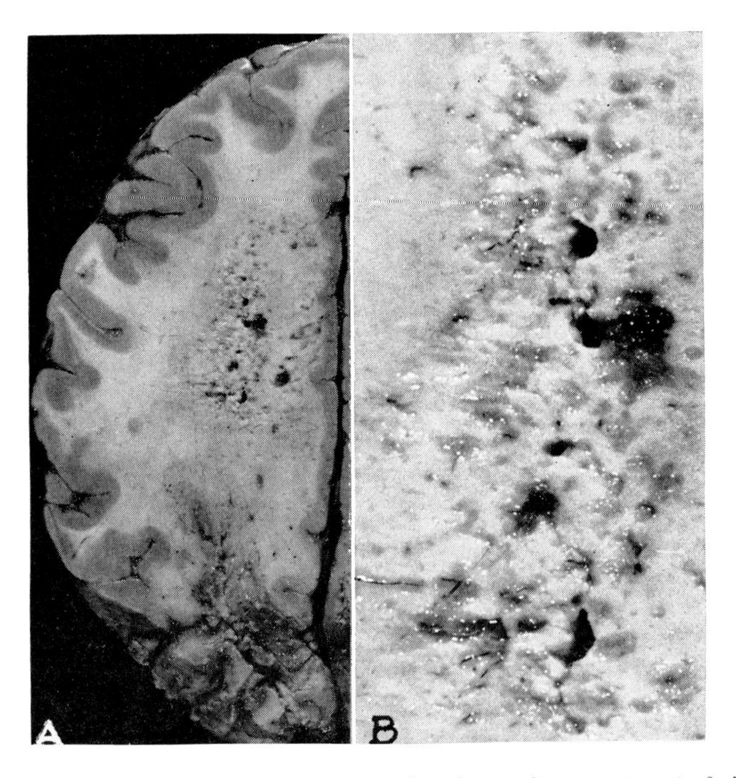

Fig. 47—Brain damage from x-radiation. Overdosage from treatment of ringworm of scalp. A. Softening and demyelinization of cerebral white matter. B. Enlarged view showing nature of central necrosis.

large nerve cells showed loss of tigroid granulation and accumulation of lipoid globules in the cytoplasm. Near the areas of necrosis focal cortical hemorrhages were found, and in some regions there was endothelial proliferation. The areas of cortex over the necrotic foci were largely devoid of nerve cells and were occupied by newly formed blood vessels. In the white matter, all stages of demyelination, gliosis, and necrosis were found (Fig. 48, A and B).

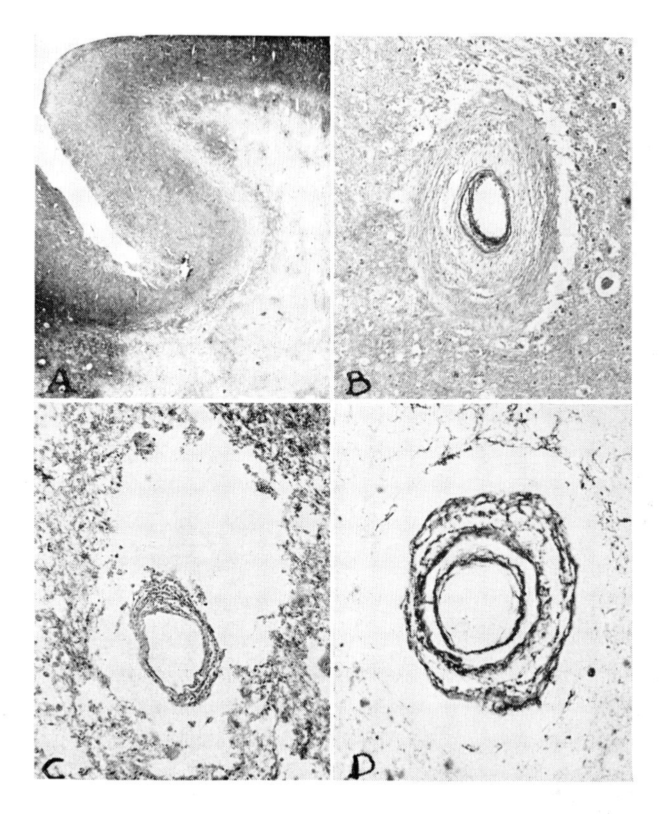

Fig. 48—Photomicrographs showing pathogenesis of demyelinization. A. Low power view indicating sharp demarcation of central damage. Myelin sheath stain X 3. B. Demyelinization about thick-walled arteriole. H & E X 70. C. Necrosis about degenerated blood vessel. Phosphotungstic acid-hematoxylin X 65. D. Changes in damaged vessel (multiple lamination of reticulin). Perdrau X 350.

The Perdrau method of staining the reticulin showed that the walls of the blood vessels were split into laminae or net-like patterns in which lymphocytes, leucocytes, red cells, collections of fat droplets, and macrophages were entangled.

From the thickening of the walls of the blood vessels and occlusion of their lumens by various materials, it was concluded that, while direct damage by x-rays could occur, in most instances regressive changes resulted from an interference with the local circulation.

A review of the literature disclosed a number of typical cases in which gross damage to the brain was found (Fischer and Holfelder, 1930; Markiewicz, 1935; Windholz, 1937; Marburg, Rezek, and Fleming, 1945; Pennybacker and Russell, 1948; Zeman, 1949; and Denny-Brown and Foley, 1953) (8–14).

Effect of Radiation Therapy for Intracranial Tumors.—A less serious type of injury to the brain results from deliberate radiation of a tumor of the brain.[3] This situation has been described by a number of observers (Freid and Davidoff, 1951; Greenfield and Stark, 1948; Horrax, et al., 1955; Horrax, 1958; Ingraham, et al., 1948; Malamud, et al., 1954; and Pennybacker and Russell, 1948) (15–21).

Only one case in which this therapeutic radiation resulted in obvious damage has been seen in this laboratory.

A 49-year-old Negro woman had failing vision which proved to be due to a bitemporal hemianopia. The presence of an enlarged sella turcica without any conspicuous changes indicative of hypereosinophilia led to the diagnosis of a chromophobe adenoma of the pituitary. The patient refused the recommendation of surgical removal of the lesion, so x-ray treatment was suggested and was accepted by the patient.

The patient was given a million units of radiation over a period of 3 years. She died at the age of 58 in another hospital and the brain was brought to the Cajal Laboratory for study.

The brain was rather small. In the region of the optic chiasm and posterior to it was a partially collapsed, membranous capsule containing some soft yellowish tissue, evidently the remains of the adenoma. The lower dorsolateral aspect of the right frontal lobe was depressed, suggesting the presence of a cystic cavity. On cross section through the frontal lobes, just anterior to the splenium of the corpus callosum, a smoothly walled cyst measuring 3 cm. by 2.4 cm. was found (Fig. 49, A). The cortex above the cyst was yellowish colored, but otherwise normal in appearance. The ependyma of the lateral and third ventricles was also yellowed.

---

[3] The spinal cord may also be damaged by radiation. This most often happens in treatment for a malignancy of the spine or spinal cord. The cord first undergoes swelling and then deterioration in the area in which the radiation is administered.

A heavy connective tissue capsule, partially hyalinized, could be seen microscopically in the remains of the adenoma, which seemed to be a compact granular structure. A mass of calcium was deposited in the wall of the cyst. A glial scar occupied the entire lower frontal centrum (Fig. 49, B). Swol-

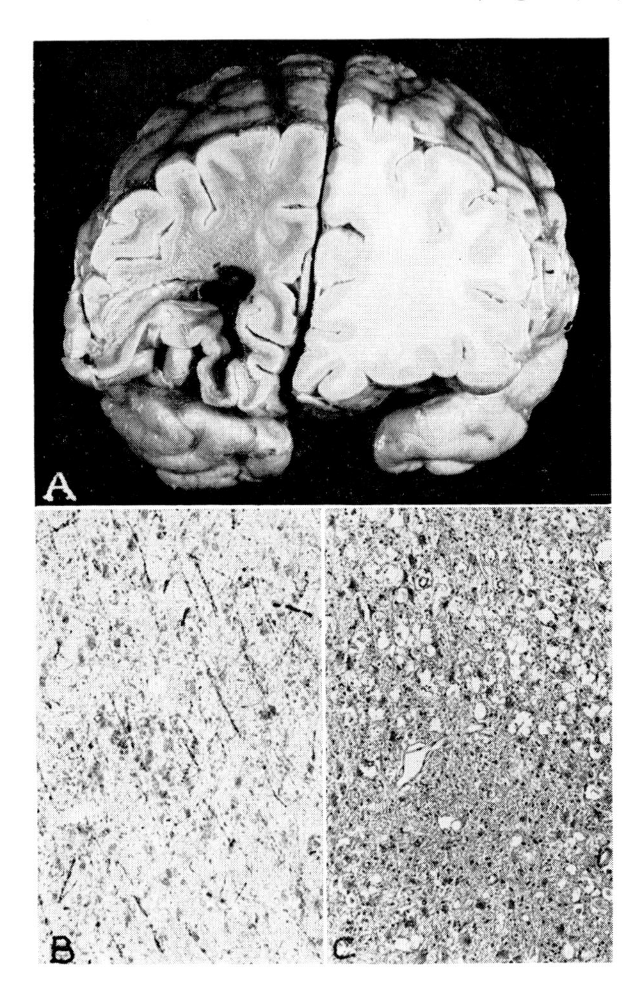

Fig. 49—A. Demyelination of white matter of right frontal lobe after several courses of x-radiation for chromophobe adenoma of pituitary with million volt x-ray machine associated with necrotic cyst. B. Photomicrograph showing almost total loss of myelinated nerve fibers in white matter. Myelin sheath stain X 75. C. Secondary gliosis of demyelinated centrum. H & E X 75.

len, hyalinized astrocytes were embedded in the interstices of the stroma. The walls of the blood vessels in this area were thickened and infiltrated by round cells, and the tissue was marked by hemorrhagic infiltration. Many fat laden macrophages were demonstrated by scarlet red preparations (Fig. 49, C).

Although the changes in the brain were not as severe as those in the case reported by Courville and Myers in 1958 (7), it seems clear that the demyelination and necrosis of the white matter of the frontal lobe were the result of excessive therapeutic radiation to the pituitary adenoma. They apparently resulted from thickening of the blood vessels and alteration of the circulation caused by the radiation. This process was clearly reflected in the altered tissues of the brain.

Effects of Ionizing Radiation.—The brains of two individuals exposed to radioactive substances have been studied. One was the brain of a Negro man of 26 years who had served as a shipping clerk handling radioactive material for a period of three months. He was found dead one morning in bed. Examination revealed congestion and nonspecific cell changes suggestive of toxic (alcoholic or barbiturate) reaction, but nothing of a chronic nature to suggest exposure to radioactive material.

The second was the brain of a 35-year-old Caucasian man who worked on the atom bomb during the war with an unknown amount of exposure to radiation. He experienced no known effects of this exposure during his life. He died from rupture of a gastric ulcer. The brain was somewhat atrophic for a man of his age, but this change was thought to be the result of chronic alcoholism.

Effects of Electric Current on the Central Nervous System

The medical literature is devoid of satisfactory information on the structural effects of electricity on the brain and spinal cord. There seems to be no report of a case in which the electric current entered the cranium and passed out of the body by way of the extremities. In very severe cases of electric shock, instantaneous death is usually presumed to be due to central respiratory paralysis or ventricular fibrillation, which leave no marks on the brain. These usually occur when an individual is struck by lightning, accidentally electrocuted, or legally executed. In the brains of 3 cases of death from electrocution which were studied in the Cajal Laboratory, neither gross nor microscopic changes were evident to account for sudden death. Changes are also lacking in cases of so-called delayed, interrupted, or late death from electrocution (Jaffe, 1928) (20). When death occurs from complications of electrocution, the abnormalities in the brain are usually due to secondary effects, such as hemorrhage, embolism, or infection. In some cases of electrocution, death seems to be due to some pre-existent conditon, such as coronary disease.

Hassin (1933, 1937) (21, 22) stated, however, that visible changes sometimes occur in the central nervous system as a result of accidental or legal electrocution. He has postulated that such changes are produced by a mechanism comparable to that of concussion, with minute tears, fissures and areolar fragmentation of the nervous tissues being followed by edema, enlargement of the perivascular and pericellular spaces, with swelling and tigrolysis of the ganglion cells and acute swelling of the oligodendroglia. The various tunics of the arterial walls are supposedly torn by the effects of the electrical current. These observations have not been confirmed.

Electroshock therapy has not been known to produce any demonstrable changes in the brain.

Accidental electrical shock by passage of current through the extremities and spinal cord can produce local burns of the skin at the points of entrance and exit. Paralytic phenomena indicate considerable dysfunction of the peripheral nerves, which may be of variable severity, as indicated by the electromyographic findings. No cases representative of this have been studied at postmortem in this laboratory, so the evolution of structural changes, if they do occur, cannot be described. From the clinical descriptions of the victims of such accidents, it is almost certain that some degree of parenchymatous damage with residual scarring does take place. In an experiment conducted on this problem in 1932, Langworthy and Kouwenhoven (23) found that the spinal cords were unusually soft, with lesions consisting of broken nerve fibers, necrotic debris, fat laden macrophages, and red cells occupying the posterior columns of the cord. Langworthy (1932)

(24) was also able to produce cavitations of the cord by low voltage electrical current. Little is known about the structural changes in the brain, but it is presumed that any changes may be predisposed by arteriosclerotic vascular disease.

Traumatic Intracranial Complications of Injuries to the Cervical Spinal Canal

I

Too little is known of traumatic lesions of the spine which are capable of producing minor temporary lesions of the cervical spinal cord. This is particularly true of injuries of the cervical segments which are so exposed to such injuries. A recent case studied by the writer presented a typical Brown-Sequard syndrome which suggested an intraspinal tumor. The patient had sustained cervical spinal injury years before which almost had been forgotten as a possible source of trouble. The lesion turned out to be a herniated nucleus pulposus which had become calcified and fixed in place. It was removed with great difficulty by a double operation by both a posterior and anterior approach. Another group of cervical cord lesions resulted from dislocation of the disk occurring from chiropractic adjustments. One takes occasion to wonder how common such lesions may be.

Still another cluster of potential lesions arise from injuries to the intraspinal portion of the vertebral arteries which give rise to embolic localization within the basilar artery.

Even structural injuries to the bones of the cervical spine may be overlooked in poor positioning on the X-ray table. A recent case of fracture had been overlooked, the patient's complaints of persistent pain and stiffness being explained away as malingering.

Summary

There is little to report concerning the effects of physical agents such as heat, cold and altered barometric pressure. Elevated barometric pressure does sometimes cause gas embolism of the brain, and lowered barometric pressure may cause cerebral anoxia, but otherwise changes in the brain after exposure to these elements usually consists of congestion and focal hemorrhage.

X-rays and ionizing radiation, however, produce alterations in the brain. Depending upon the amount of exposure to x-radiation, the changes vary in degree, mechanism and location. Exposure of an embryo to radiation results in retardation of the morphogenesis of the brain. If an overdosage of radiation is directed at the mature brain, extensive demyelination or necrosis results, which appears to be secondary to thickening of the walls of the blood vessels. If the radiation is sharply focused, damage to the overlying cortex may also occur. Central gliosis with regional demyelination may follow radiotherapy directed to the brain for intracranial, cranial, or pericranial neoplasms.

There is much uncertainty as to the effect on the brain of electrical currents especially those of high voltage. No characteristic pattern has been demonstrated in the central nervous system of man, even in cases of electrocution or in instances of severe electric burns associated with peripheral nerve injury. Severe electrical injuries, especially those of the peripheral nerves, should be studied more critically until this information becomes established.

REFERENCES

1. Egerton, Nancy, Egerton, W. S., and Kay, J. H.: Neurologic Changes Following Profound Hypothermia. Ann. Surg. 157:366–374 (Mar) 1963.
2. Bjork, V. O., and Hultquist, G.: Brain Damage in Children after Deep Hypothermia for Open Heart Surgery. Thorax 15:284, 1960.
3. Titrud, L. A., and Haymaker, W.: Cerebral Anoxia from High Altitude Asphyxiation. Clinicopathologic Study of Two Fatal Cases with Unusually Long Survival and Clinical Report of Nonfatal Case. Arch. Neurol. & Psychiat. 57:397–416 (Apr) 1947.
4. Shiraki, H., Matsuoka, S., Takeya, S., Koyano, K., Araki, M., Uchimura, Y., Miyake, M., Tamagawa, C., Amano, S., Ayres, W. W., and Haymaker, W.: Effects of Atomic Radiation on the Brain in Man. A Study of the Forty-nine Hiroshima and Nagasaki Casualties. J. Neuropath. and Exper. Neurol. 27:79–137 (Jan) 1958.
5. Courville, Cyril B., and Edmondson, H. A.: Mental Deficiency from Intrauterine Exposure to Radiation. Bull. Los Angeles Neurol. Soc. 23:11–20 (Jan) 1958.
6. Johnson, F. E.: Injury of the Child by Roentgen Ray During Pregnancy. J. Ped. 13:894–901 (Dec) 1938.

7. Courville, Cyril B., and Myers, R. O.: Process of Demyelination in the Central Nervous System. II. Mechanism of Demyelination and Necrosis of the Cerebral Centrum Incident to X-Radiation. J. Neuropath. and Exper. Neurol. 17:158–173 (Jan) 1958.
8. Fischer, A. W., and Holfelder, H.: Lokales Amyloid im Gehirn. Eine Spätfolge von Röntgenbestrahlungen. Deutsche Ztschr. f. Chir. 227:475–483, 1930.
9. Markiewicz, T.: Über Spätschadigungen des menschlichen Gehirns durch Röntgenstrahlen. Ztschr. f. d. ges. Neurol. u. Psychiat. 152:548–568, 1935.
10. Windholz, F.: Zur Kenntnis der Blutgefässveränderungen im Röntgenbestrahlten Gewebe. Strahlentherapie 59:662–670, 1937.
11. Marburg, O., Rezek, P. R., and Fleming, R. M.: Changes After Treatment of an Unprotected Brain with Large Doses of Roentgen Radiation. Am. J. Roentgenol. 53:171–178 (Feb) 1945.
12. Pennybacker, J., and Russell, D. S.: Necrosis of the Brain Due to Radiation Therapy; Clinical and Pathological Observations. J. Neurol., Neurosurg., and Psychiat. 11:183–198 (Aug) 1948.
13. Zeman, W.: Zur Frage der Röntgenstrahlenwirkung am tumorkranken Gehirn. Arch. Psychiat. 182:713–730, 1949.
14. Denny-Brown, D., and Foley, J. M.: Clinicopathological Conference. Radiation Necrosis of Right Hemisphere in Hodgkin's Granuloma of Meninges with Epilepsy. Neurol. 3:615–629 (Aug) 1953.
15. Freid, J. R., and Davidoff, L. M.: Roentgen Therapy of Primary Neoplasms of Brain. Radiology 57:25–36 (July) 1951.
16. Greenfield, M. M., and Stark, F. M.: Post-Irradiation Neuropathy. Am. J. Roentgenol. 60:617–622 (Nov) 1948.
17. Horrax, G., Smedal, M. I., Trump, J. G., Granke, R. C., and Wright, K. A.: Present Day Treatment of Pituitary Adenomas. Surgery Versus X-Ray Therapy. New England J. Med. 252:524–526 (Nov) 1955.
18. Horrax, G.: Treatment of Pituitary Adenomas. Surgery Versus Radiation. Arch. Neurol. and Psychiat. 79:1–6 (Jan) 1958.
19. Ingraham, F. D., Bailey, O. T., and Barker, W. F.: Medulloblastoma Cerebelli; Diagnosis, Treatment and Survivals with a Report of Fifty-six Cases. New England J. Med. 238:171–174 (Feb 5) 1948.
20. Malamud, N., Boldrey, E. B., Welch, W. K., and Fadell, E. J.: Necrosis of Brain and Spinal Cord Following X-Ray Therapy. J. Neurosurg. 11:353–362 (July) 1954.
21. Pennybacker, J., and Russell, D. S.: Necrosis of Brain Due to Radiation Therapy; Clinical and Pathological Observations. J. Neurol., Neurosurg., and Psychiat. 11:183–198 (Aug) 1948.
22. Jaffe, H. R.: Electropathology: Review of Pathologic Changes Produced by Electric Currents. Arch. Path. 5:837–870 (May) 1928.
23. Hassin, G. B.: Changes in Brain in Legal Electrocution. Arch. Neurol. and Psychiat. 30:1046–1060 (Nov) 1933.
24. ——————: Changes in Brain in Accidental Electrocution. J. Nerv. and Ment. Dis. 86:668–673 (Dec) 1937.

25. Langworthy, O. R., and Kouwenhoven, W. B.: Injuries Produced by Contact with Electric Circuits. Am. J. Hyg. 16.625–666 (Nov) 1932.
26. ——————————: Necrosis of Spinal Cord Produced by Electrical Injuries. Bull. Johns Hopkins Hosp. 51:210–216 (Oct) 1932.

Chapter VIII. The Mechanism and Structural Effects of Poisons Upon the Brain*

In order to make a proper forensic evaluation of the structural effects of toxic agents in the central nervous system, the mechanisms of their production must be understood. Drugs and poisons produce their ill effects on the brain through alterations of structure or function. This chapter will be concerned with the *structural* changes which occur in the central nervous system consequent to poisoning. The forensic pathologist should not forget, however, that these *physical* alterations are invariably accompanied by complex *chemical* changes which contribute to the intercurrent *physiological* processes which account for symptoms during life.

A brief analysis will first be made of the ways in which noxious agents may affect the nervous tissues. These agents will then be classified on the basis of their common methods of attack and, finally, the pattern and sequence of formation of the resultant lesion will be discussed.

The effects of poisonous substances on the tissues of the nervous system are often difficult to ascertain. In many cases of acute fatal poisoning, although death is actually due to the effects of the toxic agent on the central nervous system, no demonstrable changes are found in the tissues on gross or

---

* In order for poisons to exert their noxious effect upon the brain, they must gain entrance to the cerebral circulation, either through the gastrointestinal tract by ingestion, or the respiratory tract by inhalation. Occasionally the brain may be indirectly affected through action of the original poison on the liver or kidneys. This process usually produces an *interim* poison of a metabolic nature.

microscopic examination. In many instances, the ultimate structural changes in the brain are produced so indirectly that they can only be explained as the result of secondary or even tertiary processes. Evaluation of these effects is further complicated because different types of poisons may result in lesions which are similar grossly or microscopically. It is the purpose of this chapter on the effects of poisons on the nervous system to re-emphasize and elaborate upon the known lesions, and to investigate the less certain mechanisms involved. These poisons will be dealt with in groups which are related in both mechanisms and effects.

A poison is any substance which, by its deleterious action on the nervous system, seriously impairs health or results in death. Certain drugs and anesthetic agents must be considered as poisons when taken in excess. Poisoning may be accidental, suicidal, or homicidal. Accidental poisoning may result from an error in medical treatment, from mistaken ingestion of a poisonous substance in the home, or from hazardous employment. Whatever the circumstances under which it occurs, the possibility of poisoning in any case makes it one of medicolegal concern, and demands a special type of examination.

Poisons in General

There are many kinds of poisons and they affect the human organism in a variety of ways. Poisons may be classified, on the basis of their effects, as (1) those which act locally (the irritant and corrosive poisons), and (2) those which act generally (the systemic poisons). *Irritants* (oxalic acid, arsenic compounds, phosphorus) exert their undesirable affects on the skin or mucous membranes with resultant inflammation. *Corrosives* (the mineral acids, caustic alkalies, and certain mineral substances), when taken in concentrated form, destroy the tissues with which they come in contact. Most irritant or corrosive poisons also exert a systemic effect after absorption. *Systemic poisons* act upon the viscera, including the tissues of the nervous system, usually without any localized effect. The systemic poisons which affect the central nervous system include many vegetable substances and most drugs. Noxious gases may have either local or general effects, while most food poisons are constitutional in action. These systemic poisons affect the liver, the kidneys, the heart, and the nervous system. In some instances, however, certain organs seem to bear the brunt of their action. This study will be concerned with agents which influence adversely the function of the nervous system. These may be direct and selective or indirect and incidental.

Predisposing Factors—The action on the body of a poison depends upon several factors. A personal idiosyncrasy (inherited or acquired) to the action of the poison may be present, such as tolerance to a noxious agent after repeated use. The age of the individual influences the outcome of the poisoning; children are generally more susceptible than adults. The effects of poisoning are often exaggerated in the presence of disease. The amount of poison taken, the form of the poison (solid or liquid), and the mode of administration (intravenous administration always results in a more acute and profound action) also determine how great the effect of the poison will be. The influence of these various factors will be discussed in connection with the groups and individual types of poisons.

Mechanisms of Central Poisonings

Poisons which affect the nervous system may produce their deleterious effects by a variety of mechanisms, either direct or indirect (Fig. 50). The mode of entrance to the body and the primary and secondary effects of the poison may differ greatly. It is most unusual for a poison to have only a direct and immediate effect on the brain. As a rule, other reactions are interposed. Most common, of course, are reactions in the skin or the mucous membranes of the mouth, respiratory or gastrointestinal tract. With some poisons, alterations in the lungs (irritant gases), the stomach (corrosive poisons), the kidneys and the liver (systemic poisons), or the blood stream (carbon monoxide) constitute the primary response.

The specific nature of a poison and its concentration in the tissues determines *direct* central involvement. Precursor (phenol poisoning with gastrointestinal changes) or coincidental effects (lead poisoning with changes in the blood) on

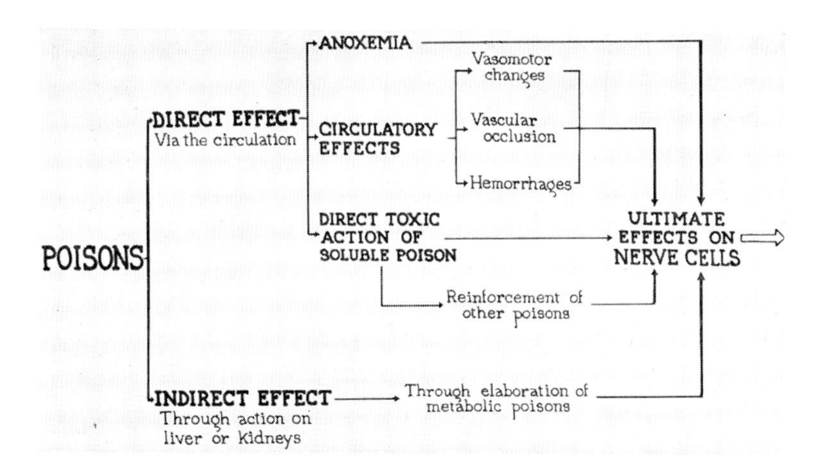

Fig. 50—Routes through which poisons affect the central nervous system.

organs or tissues which sometimes occur should not obscure the fact that the poison is also exerting a direct and primary effect on the nervous system.

Indirect effects of poisonous substances are seen with the asphyxiant gases (Courville and Myers, 1954) (1), when the cerebral effects are purely anoxic. The anoxia is produced by inhalation of toxic concentrations of the asphyxiant gas. Another mechanism of indirect action of poisons on the brain is seen when a poison acts primarily on the kidneys or liver. Severe phenol poisoning, for example, results in extreme damage to the kidneys, with typical cerebral symptoms of uremia.

Pathogenesis of Nervous Lesions

In many cases of poisoning, it is not possible to distinguish between the effects of one process and another. The pathogenesis of the lesions are varied and at times manifold, even though the lesions themselves may be uniform.

Direct structural and cellular changes in the tissues of the nervous system are accounted for by (1) the specific action of the poison on the parenchymatous elements, (2) through the action of anoxemia on these elements, or (3) by certain disturbances in the circulation.

Specific Action—The specific action of poisons on the individual nerve cells varies from one noxious substance to another. Certain drugs apparently act upon the synapses (Fig. 51). The organic solvents act upon the lipoids in the sheath of the cell. Other substances act upon the constituents of the cytoplasm, either by altering their physical qualities (wood alcohol) or by interfering with their metabolic functions (arsenicals). Some poisons act directly on the nucleus, either specifically or together with other cellular alterations (the alcohols). Very little information is available about this phase of the action of poisons.

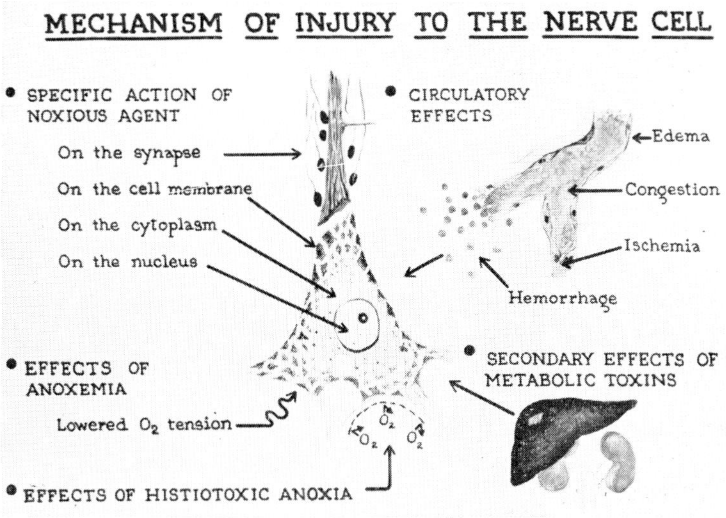

Fig. 51—Mechanism of injury to individual cellular elements of the nervous tissues.

Anoxemia—Anoxemia produces damage to the nervous system through circulatory disturbances and through often lethal cellular changes. Congestion incident to cerebral anoxia cannot be distinguished grossly from that incident to other causes. It is believed that significant architectural changes result from some secondary circulatory change, usually manifest by congestion, which acts through the vasomotor system. When this is due to an asphyxiant gas, the etiology is usually known and the problem of pathological diagnosis does not arise. If the victim survives the poisoning for a week or more, the anoxemia results in gross softening of the cortex and basal ganglia or characteristic architectural changes (focal cell loss or necrosis, laminar or subtotal necrosis) in the cortex. When delayed death occurs due to certain heavy metals (lead, manganese, nickel), some metalloids (phosphorus, arsenic, phosgene, hydrocyanic acid), and some of the asphyxiant gases (particularly carbon monoxide), the gross softening in the cortex-subcortex or centrum is best accounted for on the basis of a disturbed circulation.

Anoxemia presumably acts directly on the individual nerve cells by slowing down their internal respiration, hence affecting their vital metabolic functions. Certain metabolites, notably glucose and catalyzers such as thiamin, are intimately involved in this process (Courville, 1954) (2).

Circulatory Disturbances—Circulatory changes may be an integral part of anoxemia or a direct component of the noxious process. Determination of the correct etiology is therefore difficult. The congestion, edema, and ischemia which are particularly evident in heatstroke are direct effects of a noxious process. When direct circulatory changes occur after acute intoxication, gross examination of the brain reveals leptomeningeal congestion, with accentuation of the small pial blood vessels. At times focal hemorrhages resulting from the congestion may be seen. When the brain is sectioned, the cerebral gray matter is found to be grayish blue.

Congestion is most characteristically found in heatstroke or sunstroke, or in poisoning with the alcohols (methyl alcohol), tetra-ethyl lead, manganese, vanadium, barium, arsenic, hydrocyanic acid, the aliphatic esters, certain organic solvents, and the asphyxiant gases. Small hemorrhages are also found in poisoning with manganese, mercury, phosphorus, tin, phosgene or nitric acid.

Edema of the brain appears after acute congestion, although it is not an invariable consequence. The superficial vessels are not prominent; the convolutions of the dorsolateral surface of the cerebral hemispheres are flattened, with a corresponding narrowing of the intervening sulci. The cerebral substance seems somewhat doughy to palpation. When sectioned, the gray matter appears pallid, the white matter swollen, and the subarachnoid and ventricular system reduced in size. Edema is most characteristically seen in acute intoxication with lead, nickel carbonyl, manganese, the arsenicals, phosgene, fluorine, hydrocyanic acid, and the alcohols (notably methyl and ethyl).

The *indirect action* of poisons is typically seen through damage to the kidneys or liver, with nervous symptoms arising through injury to these organs.

The following outline indicates the mode by which noxious substances affect individual elements of the nervous system.

I. Direct Action of Poisons on the Nervous Parenchyma
   A. Action on Nerve Cells
      1. Cerebral and cerebellar cortex
         a. Exhaustion of cells—strychnine, tetanus
         b. Functional depression—general anesthetic agents such as ether
         c. Specific toxic effect—lead
         d. Asphyxial action—nitrous oxide, carbon monoxide, ethyl alcohol, cyanides
      2. Brain stem
         a. Extraocular nuclei—botulism
         b. Respiratory and cardiac centers—barbiturates, narcotics, asphyxiant gases
      3. Lower motor neurons—strychnine, tetanus
      4. Fundus oculi—methyl alcohol, nicotine
   B. Action on Nerve Fibers
      1. Central white matter (only through circulatory and vascular disturbances)—nitrous oxide, carbon monoxide, cyanides
      2. Optic nerve—arsenic, phosgene
      3. Peripheral nerves
         a. Toxic action—lead, arsenic, alcohol
         b. Asphyxial action—carbon monoxide

II. Indirect Action of Poisons on the Nervous Parenchyma
   A. Through Secondary Toxins
      1. Damage to kidneys—arsenic
      2. Damage to liver—lead, copper
   B. Through Circulatory Effects
      1. Severe edema—arsenic, ether, alcohol
      2. Congestion—lead, arsenic, carbon monoxide, the alcohols, benzol, opiates

3. Petechial and gross hemorrhages—mercury, arsenic, salvarsan, carbon monoxide, nitrous oxide, alcohols, opiates
4. Ischemia—carbon monoxide, lead, salvarsan
5. Endothelial changes
   a. Acute degeneration—arsenic
   b. Proliferation—lead, chenopodium, alcohol, asphyxiants

Many of these poisons produce their effects through more than one mechanism. Because of complex clinical manifestations and structural changes it is difficult to identify the noxious agent solely on the basis of alterations in the brain. Other evidence is necessary in establishing the precise poison involved. In forensic practice, it is essential to determine the source of the poison (i. e., the discovery of a container), whether there has been any local action of the poison on the skin or mucous membranes, and what indirect toxic effects it has had on the kidneys and liver. Most important is the recovery and identification of the poison from the contents of the gastrointestinal tract, the blood, or the tissues of the brain.

Selective Susceptibility of Individual Structures and Cellular Elements

Regardless of the mechanism by which a noxious agent acts upon the nervous system, it is clear that in some cases the substance has a specific affect on certain nerve cells or structures. These localized responses to poisons may be readily distinguished from the general effects on the cerebral cortex, which result in mental confusion, delirium, or stupor.

One of the most typical and well defined of these specific effects is manifested by certain heavy metals (lead) and metalloids (arsenic) on the peripheral nerves. In the case of heavy metals, the severity of damage to the nerves is determined by the amount of activity in the affected part. Carbon monoxide, carbon disulfide, thallium and gasoline may also produce typical peripheral neuropathy. The production of cranial palsies in gasoline poisoning is particularly noteworthy. The effect of methyl alcohol, trichlorethylene, nicotine and thallium on the nerve cells of the retina and fibers of the optic nerves is constant and not dependent upon any local functional state.

The cerebral cortex is very commonly affected by organic solvents.[1] The effect on the cortical nerve cells of asphyxiant gases such as carbon monoxide and nitrous oxide, metals such as lead, mercury, manganese, thallium, zinc, vanadium and antimony, the alcohols, some halogens (bromine), and some chemical compounds such as carbon disulfide and the halogenated hydrocarbons (von Oetingen, 1940) (3) is well known.

The cerebral centrum may be affected acutely by congestion and hemorrhage or as a chronic degenerative process. Petechial hemorrhages are an acute effect of exposure to the asphyxiant gases, phosphorus, mercury, arsenic (particularly of the organic compounds), nickel carbonyl, and the cyanides. Chronic degenerative changes in the centrum are found as residuals of chronic intoxication with the cyanides, carbon monoxide, nitrous oxide, and carbon disulphide.

The specific action which some noxious substances (the asphyxiant gases and certain metals and metalloids, particularly arsenic, manganese, and possibly magnesium and thallium) have on certain portions of the extrapyramidal system (globus pallidus) seems predisposed by peculiarities of the vascular pattern which render the structure more vulnerable to anoxia. A typical parkinsonism syndrome occurs after poisoning with carbon monoxide and manganese. The occurrence of tremors after poisoning with DDT suggests either striatal or cerebellar involvement, although neither animal nor human experimentation has disclosed any commensurate changes in these structures. It must be concluded, therefore,

[1] It is inadequate to discuss the effects of noxious substances on the cerebral cortex as a whole. Critical study of the clinical manifestations, particularly the chronic ones, of such poisons as the mercury compounds, manganese, thallium, selenium, carbon disulfide, and gasoline and allied solvents, has made it clear that these various substances produce specific effects on certain regions of the cortex. This is indicated especially by the early appearance of fear and anxiety in selenium poisoning (? temporal lobe), the intellectual perversions and defects in poisoning with mercury and carbon disulfide (? frontal lobe), the early convulsive seizures in manganese poisoning (? central cortex), and the excitement, hyperkinesis, and hysterical laughter (? subfrontal cortex) seen in other poisonings.

that clinical symptoms indicating disturbed function need not be accompanied by regional histological alterations.

The cerebellum is less often specifically altered by noxious substances, although it is frequently involved in the general toxic effects. This is indicated by the common occurrence of vertigo and ataxia after acute intoxication, especially with the alcohols. There is some evidence to suggest that this organ is damaged more severely by such substances as carbon disulfide, tetra-ethyl lead, mercury, thallium, and possibly cadmium.

The cardiac and respiratory centers are predominantly affected by the cyanides and asphyxiant gases. Depression of these centers is generally rapid and fatal if exposure is severe. Less often, fluorine, benzene, carbonyl sulfide, and possibly selenium, depress these vital centers.

The localization of effects of noxious substances is illustrated in Figure 52.

As for the specific action of poisons on the spinal cord, there is little to be said. It is recognized that severe lead

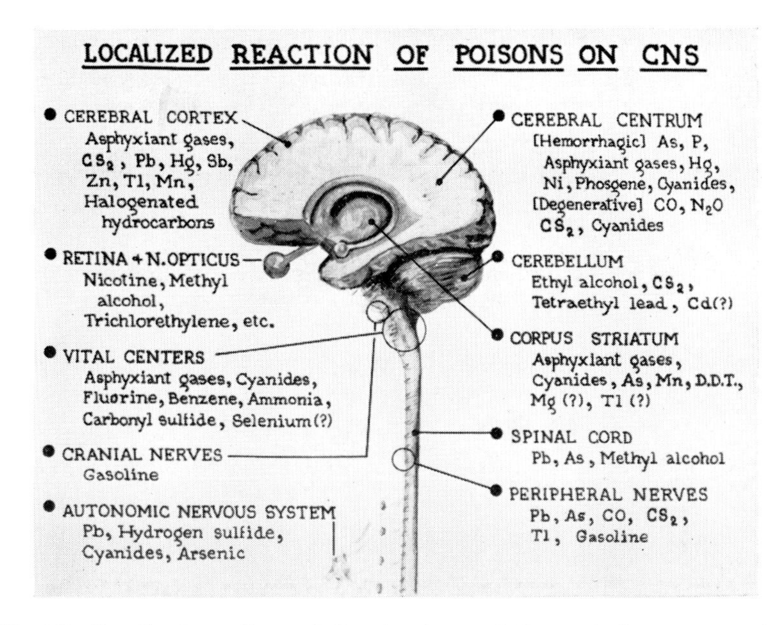

Fig. 52—Localized reactions of the structures of the central nervous system to noxious substances.

and arsenic poisoning produce changes in the anterior horn cells.[2] These changes may be due to a profound "axon reaction" incident to advanced motor neuropathy. Methyl alcohol also seems to produce more severe injury to these cells than to those of the cerebral cortex.

Little attention has been given in the past to the alterations in the cells and fibers of the autonomic nervous system, although in certain toxic states from industrial poisoning symptoms referable to this system do occur (Leschke, 1934) (5). Alterations in this system seem to be evident in cases of acute and chronic poisoning with lead, arsenic, mercury, cyanide, and hydrogen sulfide. Usually the changes seen in the cells of the autonomic ganglia are excessive lipoidal pigmentation and vacuolization, with degenerative changes in the dendrites and axons, such as Cajal and his coworkers have demonstrated.

Localizing cerebral symptoms or signs should suggest to the pathologist where he is most likely to find objective evidence of toxic effects. Specific and detailed attention should be directed to the portion of the cortex or basal ganglia under suspicion. It is often true, of course, that significant changes are not found, either in the suspected area or elsewhere. It is necessary to make a more careful scrutiny when no changes are obvious in cases with long survival (i. e., delayed death after exposure to the asphyxiant gases) or in cases in which death occurs after chronic intoxication (chronic metallic poisonings). This tissue specificity also demands that more attention be given to quantitative microchemical determinations of the specific areas of the cortex or basal ganglia which are under suspicion (Butt, et al., 1954) (6).

Nature of Cerebral Lesions

It would be helpful in the detection of lesions of the brain if the cerebral lesions of each noxious agent or even of each group of agents presented characteristic gross or microscopic changes. Unfortunately, this is not the case. There are often

[2] Any alterations found in the fiber tracts of the spinal cord should be considered as secondary to cerebral, cerebellar, or ganglionic changes. No specific syndrome or lesion complex of the spinal cord has been found, other than in chronic poisoning with ethyl alcohol (Courville and Myers, 1954) (4).

no changes in the nervous tissues which indicate that central damage has been initiated by exposure to a specific lethal agent or poison. It is possible to learn from a critical examination of the tissues of the nervous system what the extent of the insult is, and possibly what parts of the system are specifically affected. With these limitations in mind, the actual lesions consequent to the noxious substances will be surveyed. The alterations will be considered as (1) circulatory, (2) vascular, (3) architectural, (4) cellular, (5) nerve fiber, and (6) interstitial.

Circulatory Alterations—A distinction must be made between *functional* alterations in the circulation of the brain and *structural* changes in the blood vessels themselves. The circulatory changes are congestion, with or without petechial or gross hemorrhages, edema, and ischemia resulting from vasospasm, embolism or thrombosis (Fig. 53). Congestion is very obvious when observed in an unembalmed brain. The small pial vessels and the larger leptomeningeal arteries and veins are engorged and tortuous, so that the vascular pattern of the brain appears to be very complex. Local subarachnoid hemorrhages are often present when the congestion is severe. When the brain is sectioned, the gray matter has a bluish cast. When viewed through a hand lens, the small vessels in the cortex, centrum, and basal ganglia stand out as bluish dots. Microscopically, the venules, arterioles, and capillaries are conspicuous and appear to be increased in number, although they actually are not. Small perivascular hemorrhages (either of the "ball" or "ring" type) may be seen microscopically in the cortical gray matter.

Multiple *focal hemorrhages* may occur as part of the pathological complexes of toxic states and poisonings. These hemorrhages are small, fairly uniform in size, and concentrated throughout the white matter of the brain ("hemorrhagic encephalitis"). They have been described in fatal cases of acute poisoning with heavy metals (mercury, nickel carbonyl, collargol), some metalloids (arsenic, phosphorus, cyanides), some asphyxiant gases (nitrous oxide, carbon monoxide, phosgene), and certain organic solvents (ether, ethyl alcohol, creosote and benzene). Less numerous, larger extravasations are also found in asphyxia due to nitrous oxide and carbon

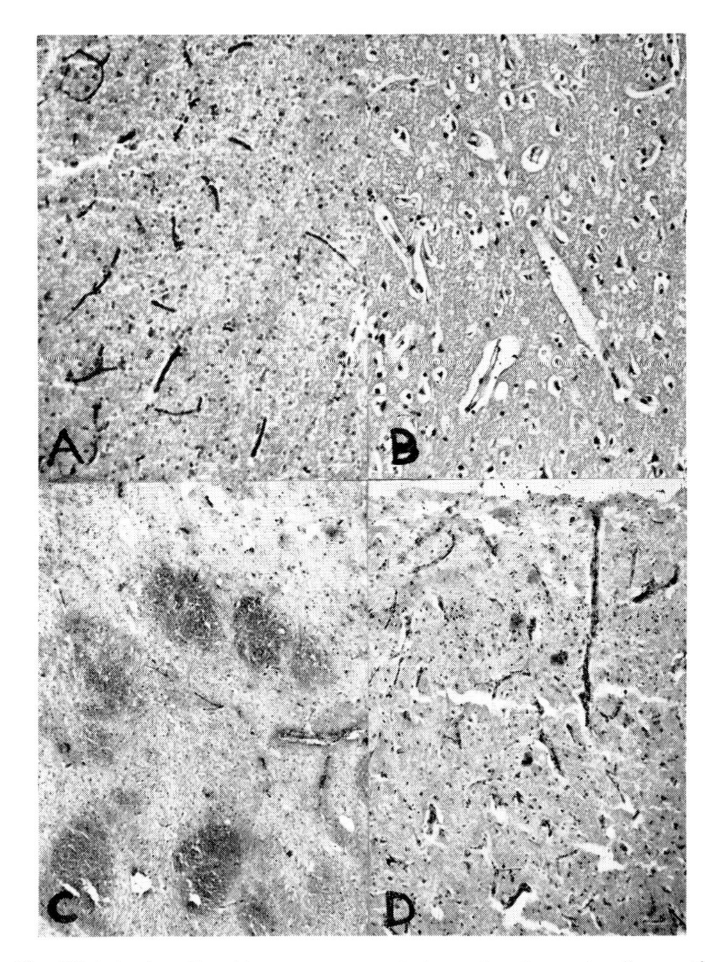

Fig. 53—Histologic alterations consequent to poisoning. A. Congestion in cadmium poisoning. H & E X 75. B. Edema in insecticide poisoning. H & E X 75. C. Petechial hemorrhages in phenol poisoning. H & E X 35. D. Cortical softening in chenopodium poisoning.

monoxide. Gross hemorrhages into the brain have been found in fatal poisoning with lead, nickel carbonyl, collargol, arsenic, phosphorus, and some of the asphyxiant gases (carbon monoxide and phosgene). Subdural hemorrhage rarely occurs in cases of poisoning. In 1948, however, Patty (7) reported the occurrence of subdural hemorrhage in a case of cadmium poisoning. Such hemorrhages must represent rupture and extravasation of blood following degenerative changes in the walls of the blood vessels.

Cerebral edema is an indirect circulatory effect of certain toxic agents. Two types of cerebral edema have been described. A *wet brain* is characterized grossly by excessive amounts of free fluid in the subarachnoid and ventricular spaces, and microscopically by a widening of the perivascular and pericellular spaces and increased vacuolization of the choroid plexus and ependyma. The less common *dry brain* is characterized by dryness of the surface of the hemispheres, flattened convolutions, narrowed sulci, and reduction of the ventricular cavities due to swelling of the tissue. In both wet and dry brain, the oligodendroglia are acutely swollen. Cerebral edema of the wet type has been described as an effect of acute poisoning by alcohol, lead, the arsenicals, fluorine, cyanides, phosgene gas, and ethyl ether (Petri, 1930) (8). Dry brain as an uncomplicated effect of poisoning is rare.

Cerebral ischemia as a direct, isolated consequence of poisoning is rare. Thrombosis of the cerebral vessels with consequent ischemia has been described in cases of acute lead poisoning, and after severe exposure to tetra-ethyl lead, phosgene and carbon monoxide. The focal cortical and subcortical softenings found 6 weeks or more after exposure to carbon monoxide are more likely due to ischemia incident to vasospasm rather than to thrombosis (Courville, 1955) (9).

Patchy loss of nerve cells (Ausfallung) may be seen microscopically in many types of chronic intoxications and poisonings (notably alcohol). This loss may be an effect of transitory ischemias of vasomotor origin. A number of processes (notably asphyxia) are also known to be accompanied by functional aberrations in the small arterioles. Just how poisoning initiates these processes is uncertain. It is likely that the petechial hemorrhages observed in cases of acute poisoning may be explained in some cases by vasomotor dysfunction, initiated by the poison itself, by anoxic processes, or by functional or structural alterations in the blood vessels. Embolisms from the fatty tissues, the lungs, or some post-traumatic infectious focus may also be responsible for these alterations at times.

Vascular Alterations—Physical alterations in the blood vessels of the nervous system as a consequence, direct or indirect, of poisoning have been relatively unexplored. It is known, of course, that in many chronic degenerative processes in the brain, increased amounts of *free fat* are found in compound granular corpuscles in the perivascular spaces (the alcohols) or in the endothelium of the vessels themselves (lead, arsenic, and phosphorus poisoning; asphyxia from carbon monoxide). This indicates the destructive effect of the poison on the tissues, with subsequent breakdown which releases small globules of free fat to be engulfed by macrophages or collected by the endothelial cells of the blood vessels. This seems to be proven by the presence of fatty globules in the nerve cells, the neuroglia, and the interstices, as well as in the endothelium of the blood vessels as characteristic in acute fatal poisoning with phosphorus. It is uncertain whether this breakdown into fat is the direct result of the poison acting on the protoplasm of the cell or whether it represents an interference with the anabolism of the lipoproteins. The presence of abnormal amounts of lipoidal pigment in the nerve cells in poisoning with the asphyxiant gases suggests that impairment of oxygenation plays an important part in the process.

Endothelial proliferation associated with laminar necrosis is a characteristic residual of certain forms of cerebral anoxia. New capillary formation ultimately results in the development of a dense vascular scar in the intermediate layer of the cerebral cortex. Endothelial proliferation occurs typically after exposure to any asphyxiant gas.

Hyalinization of the small arterioles has been described as a consequence of chronic lead poisoning and as a subacute or chronic residual of carbon monoxide poisoning.

Calcification of the muscular coat of the arterioles in the lenticular nucleus or in areas of central necrosis occurs in poisoning with carbon monoxide and other asphyxiants.

Inflammatory changes in the small blood vessels have been described in cases of chronic lead and manganese poisoning. Inflammation is associated with proliferation of the perivascular neuroglia in lead poisoning and with perivascular collections of lymphocytes in poisoning with nitrous oxide and carbon monoxide.

Architectural Alterations—Cortical, ganglionic, or central architectural changes may also be important clues to the cause of cerebral lesions (Fig. 54). This is particularly true after exposure to an asphyxiant gas with survival of three or more days. Focal, laminar, or subtotal necrosis are specific residuals of acute or subacute cerebral anoxia. Irregular cortical atrophy has been described by Meyer (1926) (10) as a late residual (after 16 years) of carbon monoxide asphyxia. Focal scars and cysts have similarly been found in the basal ganglia, particularly in the globus pallidus.

Focal infarctions have been seen in the white matter in cases of carbon monoxide poisoning. These may be consequent to thrombotic interruption of the small central blood vessels. These lesions are associated with small central hemorrhages and are likely the result of impaired circulation. Similar lesions are seen in brain purpura with fat embolism.

Central necrosis of the lenticular nucleus, especially of the globus pallidus, is a characteristic residual of poisoning with the asphyxiant gases (Courville and Myers, 1954) (1), particularly carbon monoxide (Kolisko, 1914) (11). It is most likely the result of ischemia.

Patchy demyelination or *gross softening* of the white matter of the brain may be found in chronic cyanide poisoning (DeChaume and Chambon, 1946) (12) and as a residual of severe asphyxia by carbon monoxide (Grinker, 1925) (13). These seem to result from impairment of the circulation through progressive obliteration of the deep penetrating arteries (Courville, 1953) (14).

Cellular Alterations—Cellular changes incident to noxious substances may be classified as acute-subacute and chronic. The *acute-subacute* changes consist of acute swelling (chromatolysis), pyknosis (shrinkage) of the small pyramidal cell elements and Purkinje cells, ischemia (at borders of focal cortical lesions after a week), pigmentary infiltration (about focal hemorrhages), severe nerve cell loss (about anoxial lesions of the cortex), and lipoidal degeneration (as after acute arsenic or phosphorus poisoning) (Courville, 1955) (15).

The *chronic* changes consist most characteristically of pigmentary atrophy with lipoidal deposits about the nucleus (most extensive after asphyxiation or chronic alcoholic in-

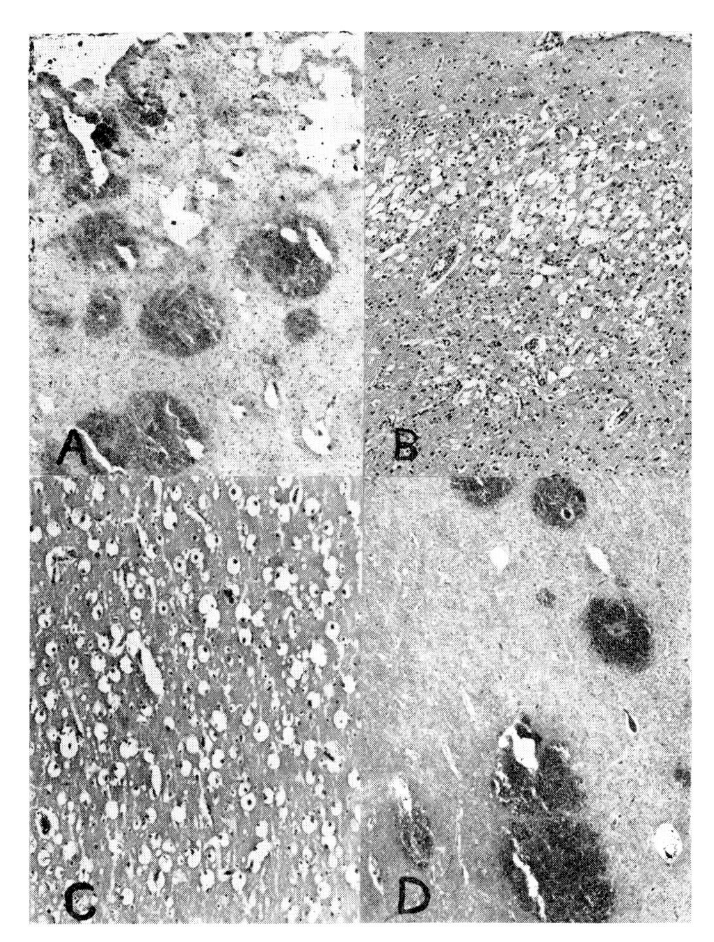

Fig. 54—Architectural changes in the cerebral cortex due to poisoning. A. Hemorrhagic softening in camphor poisoning. B. Status spongiosus in carbon monoxide poisoning. C. Severe edema in salicylate poisoning. D. Severe central hemorrhage in acute morphine poisoning.

toxication) (Fig. 55). Occasionally calcified nerve cells are seen about old anoxial lesions of the cerebral cortex.

Alterations in Nerve Fibers—Alterations in the myelinated fibers of the central white matter and the peripheral neurons may occur after damage to the nervous system. Delayed demyelination and central softening are found in carbon monoxide asphyxiation and chronic cyanide poisoning. The changes seen in peripheral neuropathy are similar to those

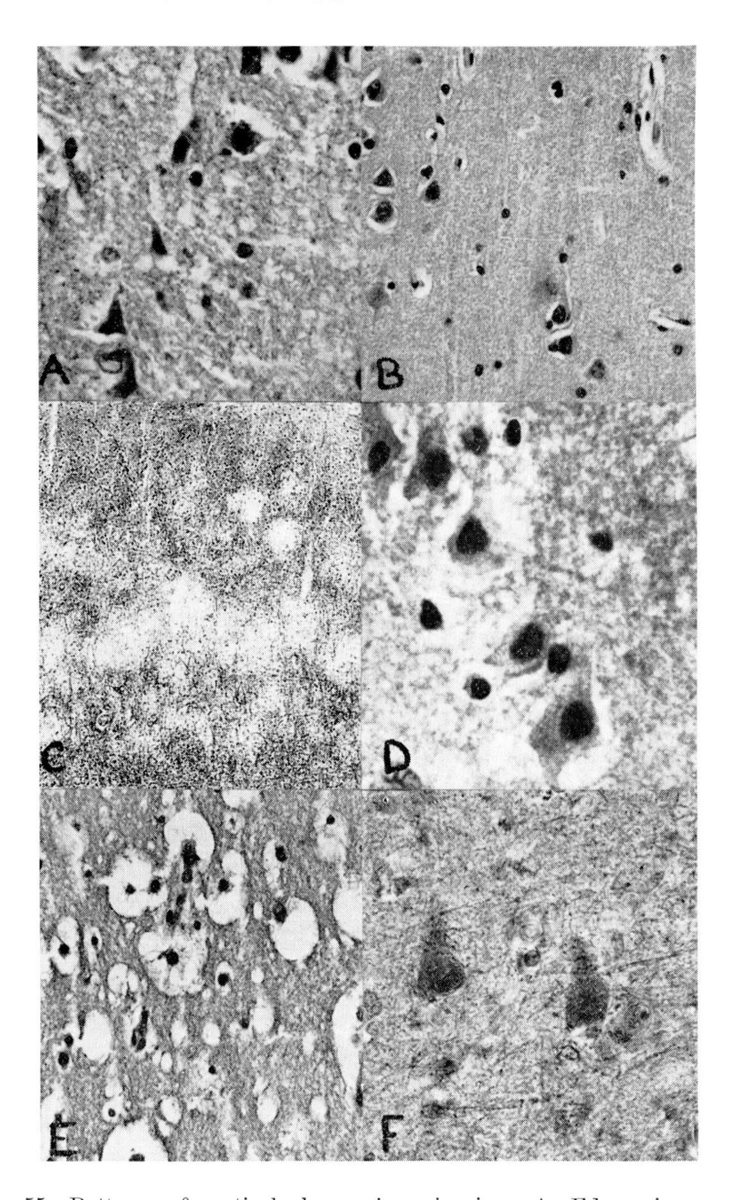

Fig. 55—Patterns of cortical change in poisoning. A. Edema in mercury poisoning. X 500. B. Widespread cell loss in chronic lead poisoning. X 500. C. Focal necrosis in nitrous oxide poisoning. D. Focal cell loss in nitrous oxide, under higher magnification. E. Salicylate poisoning. F. Lipoidal cell change in Korsakoff's psychosis (alcoholic psychosis). X 500.

observed in chronic alcoholism (Courville and Myers, 1954) (4). They consist of fragmentation of the myelin sheaths, with the formation of myelin balls and transformation into free fat. The axis cylinders also become fragmented and granular. It is evident that the peripheral nerves are directly vulnerable to certain noxious agents, notably lead, arsenic, and carbon monoxide.

Interstitial Alterations—The interstitial elements of the central nervous system are generally not affected by noxious substances. Exceptions include acute swelling of the oligodendroglia in any toxic state and perivascular glial proliferation in lead encephalopathy. Fat is deposited in the interstitial elements after acute phosphorus poisoning and iron is deposited in chronic arsenic or phosphorus poisoning.

General Considerations

There are relatively few typical pathological complexes incident to poisoning which are significant. The most outstanding are focal perivascular reaction in chronic lead poisoning with encephalopathy, brain purpura in acute arsenic and phosgene poisoning, necrosis or demyelination of the cerebral white matter resulting from carbon monoxide and cyanide poisoning, neuropathies of arsenic and lead poisoning, and characteristic cortical-ganglionic complexes consequent to asphyxia. Alterations beyond these are ordinarily not specific or remarkable. Acute alterations consist of cerebral congestion or edema and chronic changes consist of patchy loss of nerve cells in the cortex, with or without pigmentary degeneration.

The relatively common occurrence of neurological and psychiatric manifestations in cases of poisoning without any remarkable changes in the nervous tissues, suggests functional rather than structural vulnerability to many of these noxious agents. This accounts for the recovery from such symptoms when an individual is removed from exposure to a noxious substance. The variation of symptoms with the various toxic substances also indicates a specific affinity of these substances for certain structures or regions in the brain. This has not yet been established pathologically.

These effects of poisons should be a challenge to those interested in the pathology of the nervous system. More critical attention must be paid the nervous tissues in fatal acute or chronic intoxication, particularly with respect to the clinical manifestations, whether of general or localizing nature. It is doubtful that even a critical scrutiny will bring out any startling changes, but the tendency to localization of effects of certain poisons may be more precisely evaluated, particularly when histological studies are made in conjunction with quantitative microchemical investigation of the tissues.

Further Note on the Mechanism of Brain Poisons

What little we know about the mechanism of brain poisoning indicates that a number of factors may play a part in the process. In the first place each specific poison results in one or more *types* of change. For example, many poisons result in meningeal congestion, producing in addition to any direct action of the drug or chemical itself, a slowing down of the blood current resulting in a *stagnation anoxia.* On the other hand, poisons that one would expect to produce an anoxia, apparently result in a modified type of an anoxia. As an example, a phosphine gas which one would expect to produce an acutely fatal demise, so rapid in fact that the short survival period does not permit the typical pattern-sequence to develop before death ensues, may show not the usual vesicular-laminar status spongiosis of the cortex but rather a widespread status *microcavernosus* in which most of the nervous tissue is so marked (Hallermann and Pribilla) (1959) (16).

It has already been hinted that when more is learned about the structural effect of poisons on the brain tissue it may be possible to detect the nature of such poisons. A still unexplored field of detections of specific brain poisons will prove to be fruitful when the areas of greatest concentrations of such poisons can be determined. The lesions learned from trace metal concentrations may ultimately help in this regard when it comes to lead, arsenic, etc. whose detection in brain tissue can be determined in very small amounts (see Courville 1964) (17).

As illustrated in the above-cited case, evaluating the mechanism of brain poisons is one of the areas of neuropathology which needs further critical study. In the first place, almost all acute changes in poisonings of such origin are manifested by congestion with hyperemia and variable amounts of subarachnoid hemorrhages. Actual bleeding into the substance of the brain itself also takes place in many poisonings. Whether this congestion is a part of the means by which the organ tries to eliminate the poisonous substance from its tissues is uncertain. Perhaps it is the ultimate residual lesions from which further information is to be gained as to the actual mechanism of tissue change.

Summary

The frequent occurrence of neurological or psychiatric symptoms after poisoning suggests that the nervous system is quite susceptible to noxious agents. Even in fatal cases, however, structural changes in the brain are often minimal and nonspecific. Certain agents do produce structural changes in the brain, sometimes of a necrobiotic effect. When alterations are present it is often difficult to know the exact mechanism by which they were produced. Poisons may directly affect the brain through the circulation or indirectly through the kidneys or liver. The resultant lesions may be classified as those resulting from (1) changes in the circulation or walls of the blood vessels, and (2) specific effects of a noxious agent on the architecture of the brain or the structure of the individual cellular elements. Circulatory effects include congestion and hemorrhage, cerebral edema, focal areas of softening incident to ischemia, and patchy loss of nerve cells probably resulting from vasomotor changes. Alterations in the blood vessels consist of deposits of free fat in the walls, endothelial proliferation, hyalinization, and calcification. Gross architectural alterations occurring as residuals of intoxication include cerebral atrophy, focal cortical-subcortical softening and patchy demyelination or formation of cysts in the cerebral centrum. Cellular changes which occur are not characteristic of toxic states, but the localization of the changes is important because various poisons attack certain portions of the nervous system. Critical microscopic examination indicates that the cerebral cortex (or specific portions of it), the cerebral centrum, the basal ganglia, the cerebellum, the vital centers in the medulla, the cranial or spinal nerves, the spinal cord, and the autonomic nervous system may be selectively injured.

REFERENCES

1. Courville, Cyril B., and Myers, R. O.: Effects of Extraneous Poisons on the Nervous System. III. The Asphyxiant Gases. Bull. Los Angeles Neurol. Soc. 19:197–223 (Dec) 1954.
2. ———: Case Studies in Cerebral Anoxia. I. Cerebral Changes Incident to Hyperinsulinism (Hypoglycemia). Bull. Los Angeles Neurol. Soc. 19:29–35 (Mar) 1954.
3. von Oetingen, W. F.: Toxicity and Potential Dangers of Aliphatic and Aromatic Hydrocarbons. A Critical Review of the Literature. Pub. Health Bull. No. 255:1–135, 1940.
4. Courville, Cyril B., and Myers, R. O.: Effects of Extraneous Poisons on the Nervous System. II. The Alcohols. Bull. Los Angeles Neurol. Soc. 19:66–95 (June) 1954.
5. Leschke, E.: Clinical Toxicology. Trans. from the German by C. P. Stewart and O. Dorrer. Baltimore, William Wood & Co., 1934.
6. Butt, E. M., Nusbaum, R. E., Gilmour, T. C., and Di Dio, S. L.: Use of Emission Spectrograph for Study of Inorganic Elements in Human Tissues. Am. J. Clin. Path. 24:385–394 (Apr) 1954.
7. Patty, F. A.: Industrial Hygiene and Toxicology. New York, Interscience Publ. Inc., 1948. Two volumes.
8. Petri, E.: Pathologische Anatomie und Histologie der Vergiftungen. Berlin, Verlag von Julius Springer, 1930.
9. Courville, Cyril B.: Case Studies in Cerebral Anoxia. IX. The Cerebral Lesion-Complexes Incident to Carbon Monoxide Asphyxia. Bull. Los Angeles Neurol. Soc. 20:139–144 (Sept) 1955.
10. Meyer, A.: Ueber die Wirkung der Kohlenoxydvergiftung auf das Zentralnervensystem. Ztschr. f. d. ges. Neurol. u. Psychiat. 100:201–247, 1926.
11. Kolisko, A.: Die Symmetrische Encephalomalacia in den Linsenkernen nach Kohlenoxydgasvergiftung. Beitr. Gericht. Med. 2:1–16, 1914.
12. DeChaume, J., and Chambon, M.: Leuco-encephalite Toxique par le Cyanure de Potassium. J. de. Med. de. Lyon. 27:753–757 (Nov) 1946.
13. Grinker, R. R.: Ueber einem Fall von Leuchtgasvergiftung mit doppelseitiger Pallidumerweichung und schwerer Degeneration des tieferen Grosshirnmarklagrs. Ztschr. f. d. ges. Neurol. u. Psychiat. 98:433–456, 1925.
14. Courville, Cyril B.: Contributions to the Study of Cerebral Anoxia. Los Angeles, San Lucas Press, 1953.
15. ———: Pathological Changes in the Nervous System from Occupational Causes. With Particular Reference to Industrial Poisons. Bull. Los Angeles Neurol. Soc. 20:41–61 (June) 1955.
16. Hallerman and Pribilla: Personal Communication. 1959.
17. Courville, Cyril B.: Confusion of Presumed Toxic Gas Poisoning for Fatal Granulomatous Meningo Encephalitis, with Severe Progressive Arteritis and Gross Cerebral Hemorrhages. (To be published in the Bull. Los Angeles Neurol. Soc. (June) 1964.)

Chapter IX. Central Effects of Poisoning from Some Common Drugs*

One hazard of drug therapy is that the substance used may produce toxic reactions when administered to sensitive individuals. An overdose or some individual hypersensitivity to a therapeutic dose of a drug may produce severe or fatal results. Individual hypersensitivity has sometimes been described as an "allergic" reaction, even though no purely protein sensitization is involved and no similar manifestations have resulted from previous contact with the substance.

This chapter will be limited to a discussion of the structural changes which take place in the nervous system incident to the administration of excessive amounts of some common drugs, either accidentally or with suicidal intent. An overdose of such a drug may cause disturbances in circulation of the brain (usually an acute effect), alterations in the architecture of the cerebral cortex, or physical changes in the individual parenchymatous and interstitial elements. The earliest effects of drug poisoning, of course, are functional and are usually unaccompanied by any microscopically visible changes. Nevertheless, critical analysis of the tissues of the central nervous system after later changes occur does often give some clues regarding the toxic mechanisms, as well as point out the areas of the brain specifically affected.

Classification of Toxic Drugs

Table II shows the drugs and medicinal agents which caused death in 1,379 cases of poisoning (homicides, suicides, and

---

* In this chapter, at attempt has been made to describe the effects on the nervous system of the drugs capable of producing fatal effects. In many instances the effects on the human nervous system of less serious drugs are not known. Some clues may be found by animal experimentation; references to such articles may be found in the medical indexes.

Table II

Fatal Poisoning with Common Drugs and Medicinal Agents *

	1950–51	1951–52	1952–53	1953–54	1954–55	Total
TOTAL DEATHS INVESTIGATED BY CORONER	7,774	8,134	8,534	8,539	8,634	41,615
Due to Natural Causes	4,972	5,145	5,327	5,521	5,490	26,455
TOTAL POISONINGS (excluding CO and alcohol)	254	241	276	279	328	1,378
Due to Drugs and Medicinal Agents	192	174	220	222	271	1,079
CENTRAL STIMULANTS						
Strychnine	4	1	4	6	4	19
Camphor				1		1
Antihistamines, bronchodilators, etc.	1		2		1	4
CENTRAL DEPRESSANTS						
Sedatives and Hypnotics						
Barbiturates	133	134	160	169	224	820
with alcohol				5	3	8
with other agents or drugs		3	1		1	5
Others						
Amytal	4	1	1			6
Nembutal	5	2	6	9	6	28
Paraldehyde	1		3	2	3	9
Seconal	19	16	13	1	6	55
Tuinal	2	5	3	5	2	17
Various (e. g., Ipral)	2	1	1	1		5
Bromides	4		2	1	2	9
Chloral hydrate	1	1	1	1	2	6
with barbiturates	1					1
Anesthetics (chloroform, etc.)			2	1	1	4
Narcotics						
Codeine				1		1
with barbiturates			1			1
Heroin	1		1	5	1	8
Morphine	2		1	4	2	9
with other agents			3	2		5
Others (e. g., demerol, dilaudid)		1	3		1	5
Analgesics (salicylates and others)	8	3	5	5	8	29
Anticonvulsants (Membaral)		2				2
Sulfa compounds		1				1
Biologicals (insulin)					1	1
OTHER MEDICINAL AGENTS						
Boric acid			1			1
Digitalis		1	3			4
Ferrous sulphate (iron tablets)	1					1
Iodine	1					1
Laxative			1			1
Muriatic acid	2					2
Unknown		2	2	3	3	10
TOTAL DRUG AND MEDICINAL POISONINGS	192	174	220	222	271	1,079

* Of the cases investigated by the Office of the Coroner-Medical Examiner, Los Angeles County, for this five-year period, 63.5 per cent were deaths due to natural causes. Of the total, 3.3 per cent died of poisoning (excluding CO and alcohol). Of the poisonings, 78.3 per cent were due to drugs and medicinal agents. Of these, 76 per cent were due to barbiturates.

accidents), exclusive of carbon monoxide and alcohol, studied by the Coroner-Medical Examiner of Los Angeles County for the five years 1950–51 through 1954–55. Of the 1,379 deaths, 1,079 were due to drugs and medicinal agents. The remainder were due to such agents as chemicals, metals, and gases. These will be considered in another chapter.

It is difficult to classify the action of drugs on the central nervous system because there is overlapping of the effects of unrelated drugs and because all drugs within a therapeutic group do not produce similar structural changes. This is the most satisfactory basis of classification, however, and will be applied here.

A. Central Stimulants

1. Cellular excitants: (a) xanthine group (caffeine), (b) alkaloid group (strychnine, atropine, nicotine, cocaine, ergot, quinine), and (c) camphor.
2. Other analeptics (metrazol).
3. Mild stimulants (amphetamine group).

B. Central Depressants

1. Sedatives and hypnotics: (a) tranquilizers, (b) barbiturates, (c) bromides, (d) chloral hydrate, and (e) marihuana.
2. Narcotics of the alcohol series (see Chapter XII).
3. General anesthetics (see Chapter XI).
4. Local anesthetics.
5. Analgesics: (b) opiates, (b) salicylates.
6. Anticonvulsants (e. g., dilantin, tridione).
7. Anthelmentics (e. g., oil of chenopodium).
8. Bacteriacidals (sulphas and other antibiotic compounds).
9. Antispirochetic drugs (i. e., arsphenamine).
10. Biological products (i. e., insulin).

At least one drug in each of these groups will be considered. Several drugs in some groups, such as the alkaloid group, will be considered because they are more commonly encountered in forensic pathology.

Because of the importance and complexity of the effects of the alcohols on the nervous system, they will be considered separately (Chapter XII). The action of the general anesthetics on the brain will also be discussed in another study, in connection with the asphyxiant gases (Chapter XI). These drugs are included in this outline in order to make the classification complete.

Mode of Action of Drugs on the Nervous System

The action of a particular drug on the nervous system depends upon its physiological properties. The *toxic physiological action* of a drug is the accumulation of the normal responses to therapeutic doses of the drug. The toxic action of a stimulative drug, for example, is the excessive stimulation of sensation (increased frequency and vividness of sensory impressions), motion (hypermotility and increased motor responses to stimuli), reflex action, and psychic functions (increased awareness of surroundings, alertness). The toxic action of a central depressive drug is an excessive slowing down of responsiveness. With both stimulative and depressive drugs, perversions of normal sensory (paresthesias), motor (convulsive activity), or psychic (delusions or illusions) activity may also occur.

Direct Effects.—The effects in the nervous system of exposure to excessive amounts of drugs may be direct or indirect. The nuclear structures are most likely to show the direct effects of drug poisoning in fatal cases. Architectural or cellular changes, however, may be minimal or completely absent in cases in which death occurs within a short time. In order for visible changes to be produced after physical or chemical stress, the survival period must be sufficiently long to permit the development of lesions.

Indirect Effects.—The indirect effects of drug poisoning in the nervous system may be more striking and serious than the direct toxic effects. Circulatory effects are the most conspicuous indirect ones. Congestion and hemorrhage of the meninges and brain occur in many kinds of poisoning (e. g., acute morphine poisoning), and cerebral edema also occurs in some terminal cases (i. e., salicylate poisoning). Profound circulatory collapse or secondary functional changes in the arteries (vasospasm) may result in focal or diffuse softening of the gray matter, with typical loss of nerve cells and proliferation of the vascular endothelium (i. e., oil of chenopodium). It is impossible to evaluate adequately the effects of poisoning without consideration of these intervening circulatory changes.

Toxic Action of Central Nervous System Stimulants

Certain alkaloids other than opium are capable of producing profound toxic nervous reactions, even fatally. Physostigmine, berberine, caffeine, pilocarpine, aconite, strychnine, nicotine, atropine, cocaine and its derivatives, ergot, and quinine may all be fatal. The central effects of some of these drugs will be discussed briefly. Other central stimulants, such as camphor, metrazol, and amphetamine will also be discussed.

Strychnine.—This common, deadly representative of the alkaloid group is derived from the seeds of *Strychnos nux vomica* and the beans of *S. ignatii.* Death may follow ingestion of as small a dose as 0.03 grams. Its action seems to be through sensitization of the synapse, favoring rapid transmission of impulses. In acute strychnine poisoning, the essential gross alterations consist of profound congestion, with extravasations of blood in any part of the nervous system. Microscopic changes consist of loss of Nissl's substance and condensation of nuclear chromatin.

In one case of fatal strychnine poisoning in our series, a 3-year-old child ate two tablets of strychnine. When the brain was examined grossly, congestion was observed. Microscopically, the cortical capillaries were congested and subpial and cortical petechiae were present. The pericellular and perivascular spaces were also widened, indicating an acute cerebral cortical edema. In another case, a child of 5 years died after ingestion of 96 cathartic pills containing strychnine, belladonna and cascara. The child was dead on arrival at the hospital. The cerebral convolutions were flattened and the ventricles narrowed (edema). Microscopically, the perivascular spaces were widened, the cortical nerve cells presented evidence of acute chromatolysis with eccentric and disintegrating nuclei, and the Purkinje cells of the cerebellum showed acute chromatolytic changes.

Nicotine.—This alkaloid, derived from tobacco, has a profound effect on the nervous tissues. Death may follow ingestion within a short time, due to respiratory failure, collapse, and clonic convulsive seizures (Lawes, 1928) (1). In acute poisoning, severe venous congestion of the brain and subpial hemorrhages are noteworthy. In chronic poisoning, only mild congestion occurs. Lewin (see Petri, 1930) (2) found ventricular hemorrhages in the brain of a child who died from nicotine poisoning. Alterations in the nervous structures of the eye are more common and more conspicuous than changes in the brain. Shrinking of the cell bodies, vacuolar transformation of the nuclei, as well as loss of nerve cells and fibers, have been conspicuous in experimental animals. The fibers of the papillomacular bundle seem to be specifically affected. Changes in the walls of terminal arteries have also been described. Other histological changes include alterations in the protoplasm of the anterior horn cells and the nerve cells of the spinal ganglia, such as pyknosis, chromatolysis and vacuole formation.

Cocaine and Its Derivatives.—This alkaloid is derived from the leaves of the coca plant (*Erythroxylon coca*). Poisoning, especially acute fatal, may follow a therapeutic injection or an overdose of a cocaine product (Maier, 1926) (3). In acute poisoning, edema and congestion of the meninges and nervous tissues occur. In experimental animal studies, thrombosis of the small blood vessels of the brain has also been described (Pachonwow) (4). In chronic poisoning, the usual toxic changes are seen, such as fatty changes in the blood vessels, the cortical and ganglionic nerve cells and the microglia. Chromatolysis, vacuole formation and condensation of the nuclear chromatin take place in the nerve cells. The greatest degree of chromatolysis occurs in Ammon's horn.

In one of our cases of acute poisoning with cocaine, death occurred about an hour after an injection of novocain was given to a 17-year-old boy. Early chromatolysis and pyknosis were the only changes noted.

Ergot.—Poisoning with this fungus (*ergota*) originally resulted from contaminated grain. More recently it has been due to ergot products used medicinally. In acute poisoning in animals, epileptic seizures occur, but no changes in the brain have been described in animals or man. In chronic poisoning, degeneration occurs in the dorsal funiculus of the cord. Alterations in the anterior horn cells (vacuole formation), hemorrhage, focal softening, dilatation of the blood vessels, changes in the walls of the blood vessels, and vascular occlusion from hyaline-like masses also occur from ergot poisoning (Barger, 1931) (5). Structural changes in the peripheral nerves were described by Winogradow (6). Because ergot poisoning tends to produce changes in the blood vessels, it seems that alterations in the nervous structures are due to disturbed circulation, rather than to any direct effect of this alkaloid.

Quinine.—This extract of cinchona bark has long been used in the treatment of malaria; its toxic effects were recognized early. Clinical symptoms of severe toxicity are acute delirium, convulsive seizures, and collapse, which suggest some deleterious effects on the cerebral cortex. Ingestion of as little as 2 grams may be fatal.

Grossly, focal hemorrhages are seen in the meninges and brain as a result of quinine poisoning (Stingl, 1952) (7). Edema of the meninges may sometimes be seen. In quinine blindness, toxic alterations in the muscular coat of the arteries have been described. Changes in the nervous elements are probably secondary to ischemia, with resultant swelling and atrophy of the fiber bundles. Edema of the nerve fiber layer and vacuoles in the nerve cells of the outer granular layer of the cortex, as well as alterations in the myelin sheaths, have also been noted.

In one of our cases, an epileptic girl died from an overdose of quinine taken in an effort to produce an abortion. The changes which may have been due to acute quinine poisoning were obscured by the generalized cortical atrophy presumed to be incident to neonatal asphyxia.

Camphor.—This substance is commonly used in the form of camphorated oil, as a counterirritant to the skin. Poisoning usually is incident to accidental ingestion by children who are being treated with a camphor product. Ingestion is followed by convulsive seizures; death results from cardiorespiratory failure. This drug may have a direct effect on the nervous tissues, but death is more likely due to an ischemic-anoxemic mechanism. Severe congestion and hemorrhagic softening of the cortex and basal ganglia are seen in the brain with secondary changes incident to proliferation of the endothelial cells and increased prominence of the small blood vessels. Severe generalized, but nonspecific, change in the nerve cells of the cerebral cortex, basal ganglia, brain stem and cerebellum, with little or no glial reaction, is characteristic (Fig. 56). A faint odor of camphor may be detected in the altered tissue.

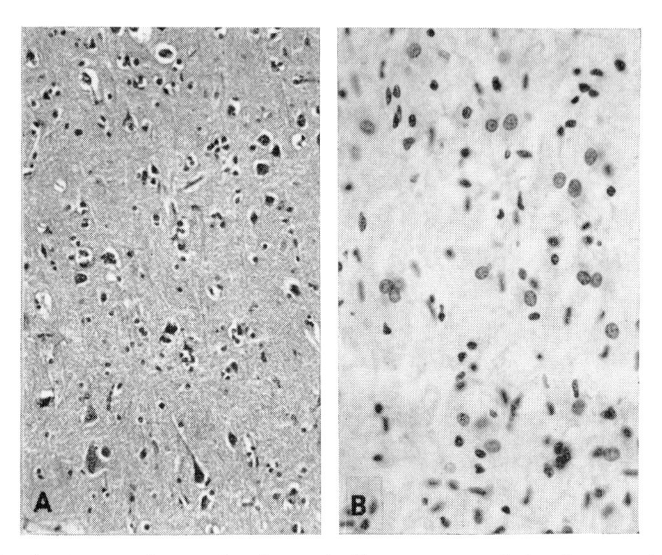

Fig. 56—Acute camphor poisoning. A. Low power photomicrograph showing disappearance of outlines of cortical nerve cells. H & E. B. High power showing same. H & E X 250.

In our series, a boy of 20 months was given, by mistake, a teaspoonful of camphorated oil. The child soon developed generalized convulsive seizures and lapsed into coma. Gastric lavage disclosed oily contents of the stomach. The child remained comatose until death, 24 days later. At autopsy, there was evidence of recent ulceration of the mucosa of the esophagus and stomach. Cloudy swelling of the liver and thrombosis of the veins of the left kidney were disclosed. The meninges seemed to be surcharged with fluid, as the sulci were widened. When sectioned, the cortical gray matter seemed to be softer than normal, while the white matter remained firm. There were no other gross lesions. Microscopically, the cortex was more cellular and more friable than usual. The nerve cells of the cortex and corpus striatum were undergoing severe change, including advanced chromatolysis, lipoidal atrophy, progressive deterioration ("ghost cells"), and structural disorganization. The neurofibrils of the nerve cells had disintegrated. The interstitial cells were increased in number; the microglia showed early swelling of their cell bodies with droplets of fat within their cytoplasm. A profound breakdown of the parenchymatous elements of the cerebral gray matter was the obvious result of poisoning with camphor.

Metrazol.—Most of the remaining central nervous stimulants are grouped as analeptics or drugs that tend to provoke convulsive seizures. Such a drug may be used to stimulate a convulsive seizure so its character may be studied or to aid the cortical activity in older individuals who have deteriorated because of arteriosclerosis. Larger doses have also been used to stimulate convulsive disorder in the treatment of schizophrenia.

In one of our cases, a 41-year-old Caucasian schizophrenic woman had been treated with metrazol. Death occurred during the course of shock therapy even though no excessive amount of metrazol was given. No changes which could be considered as specific for this drug were found in the brain.

Mild Stimulants.—Although the amphetamine and allied drugs act on the central nervous system, fatalities are rare, usually by suicide. The cerebral lesions are usually vascular, such as congestion and subdural and subarachnoid petechiae (Greenwood and Peachey, 1957) (8).

Action of Central Depressants

From the viewpoint of the frequency of poisoning, the drugs which act as depressants of the central nervous system are the most important. They are generally more accessible than the stimulants, and therefore are used more frequently, especially for suicide. In this classification, several groups of drugs are recognized to be toxic: the tranquilizers, the barbiturates, chloral hydrate, the narcotics, and the alcohols (frequently used in connection with the barbiturates).

Tranquilizers.—The tranquilizers are a group of very mild sedatives which are used for the control of agitated or anxious patients. Because of their unusual mildness, they are less likely to be fatal. Any nervous system findings would likely be nonspecific cerebral cortical or corpus striatal changes, secondary to circulatory collapse.

Simple Sedatives (Bromides, Barbiturates).—In spite of their mild sedative effects, such drugs as the barbiturates have become the most common toxic drugs. This is due to their frequent use as soporific agents by high-tension or neurotic individuals. Either because of their tendency to cause patients to forget having taken the usual dose or because they are taken in a deliberate attempt to commit suicide, overdosage frequently results in severe or fatal intoxication.

Three common effects follow overdosage. (1) *Severe, usually fatal intoxication.* In these cases, with short survival periods, the brain shows only acute, nonspecific alterations (chromatolysis) in the cortical nerve cells. (2) *Prolonged survival in a vegetative state.* The cerebral cortex and basal ganglia show all degrees of laminar damage, from cell deterioration to scar formation characteristic of cerebral anoxia (Fig. 57). Depression of the respiratory (and vasomotor) center is so severe that histotoxic anoxia results in the typical changes of cortical-ganglionic softening (Jervis and Joyce, 1948) (10). Death from inanition usually follows weeks or even months of a vegetative state (Courville, 1955) (11). (3) *Chronic barbiturism.* Individuals who have become addicted to one of the barbiturate drugs will ultimately undergo mild intellectual deterioration and a lessening of will power. At autopsy, after death from some intercurrent cause, frontal cortical atrophy of the brain may be seen. This atrophy is a result of progressive deterioration of the cortical nerve cells, with their ultimate disappearance. (Neumann, 1951) (12). There is no responsive gliosis to this loss of cells.

In *chronic bromidism,* the same changes may be seen, though less severe (Fig. 58). The process is slower, the chromatolysis of the cortical nerve cells being slower. Similar changes are to be expected in chloral hydrate (Shoor, 1941) (9) or paraldehyde (McDougall and Wyllie, 1932) (13) addiction.

Marihuana.—Very little is known about the effects of this drug, which is commonly used to the point of addiction in Mexico. The leaves and flowering tops of *Cannabis sativa* are used in cigarettes, so that the smoke is inhaled. One adult

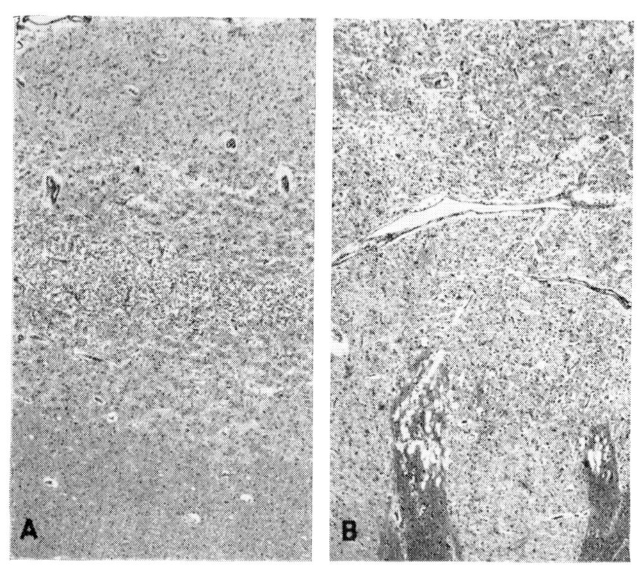

Fig. 57—Barbiturate poisoning. A. Laminar necrosis of cortex, indicative of cerebral anoxia. H & E X 35. B. Central necrosis of lenticular nucleus, also indicating anoxia. H & E X 35.

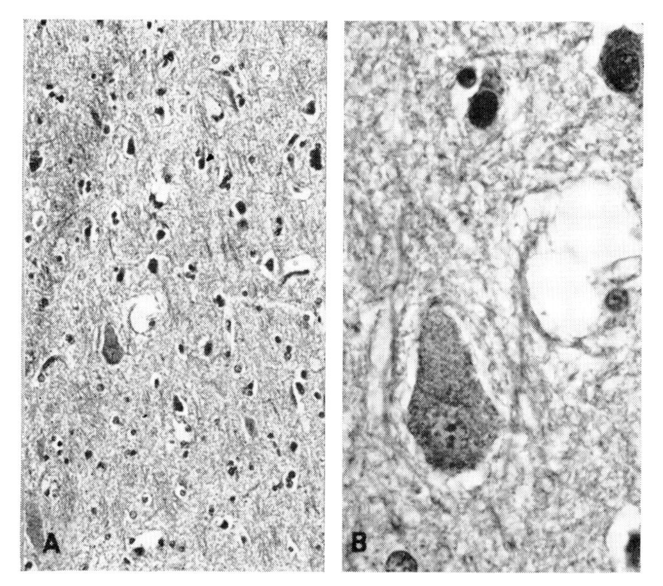

Fig. 58—Chronic bromide intoxication. A. Diffuse loss of cortical nerve cells. H & E X 250. B. Fine granulation of tigroid material in cytoplasm. H & E X 550.

male examined by a coroner's autopsy had experienced mental changes after taking an unknown amount of marihuana ("loco weed"). A few weeks later, he committed suicide by shooting himself through the head. The possibly significant histological changes consisted of neuronophagia and vacuolation of the cytoplasm and nuclei of the cortical nerve cells.

Opium and Its Derivatives.—Opium is obtained from the juice of the poppy *Papaver somniferum,* whose soporific effects have been known in China for centuries. Medicinal poisoning with opium is rare; poisoning is usually due to accidental dosage in children. Chronic opium (e. g., morphine) poisoning is commonly spoken of as "addiction" because of the habit-forming propensities of the drug. It is rarely directly fatal, although it may produce chronic disorders and predispositions.

Acute Morphine Poisoning.—Characteristically, acute morphine poisoning produces severe congestion with diapedesis of the erythrocytes. The blood vessels (particularly the larger veins) are swollen with dark blood. Perivascular hemorrhages may be present, together with excessive free fluid (cerebral edema). In one of our cases, death was due to a large dose of morphine injected intravenously in a successful suicidal try. The white matter of the brain was studded with focal hemorrhages (Fig. 59).

Other cases of chronic opiate addiction studied included addiction to heroin, methadon, and synthetic drugs such as demerol, and demerol with delvinal sodium. Proliferation of either the cap cells or fibrous elements of the leptomeninges, edema of the cortex, and changes in the cortical nerve cells (chromatolysis, lipoidal change, pyknosis, satellitosis and progressive deterioration leading to patchy cell loss) were observed. Mild chromatolysis of the Purkinje cells was also observed in some cases. In individuals who survive large doses of an opiate for a few days, changes occur in the brain similar to those of cerebral anoxia. Weimann (1926) (14) reported an unusual case of acute pantopon poisoning in a child of five years, in which symmetrical softening of the globus pallidus and early softening of the cerebral cortex, including laminar necrosis of Ammon's horn, developed. Whether such changes are the intercurrent effect (depres-

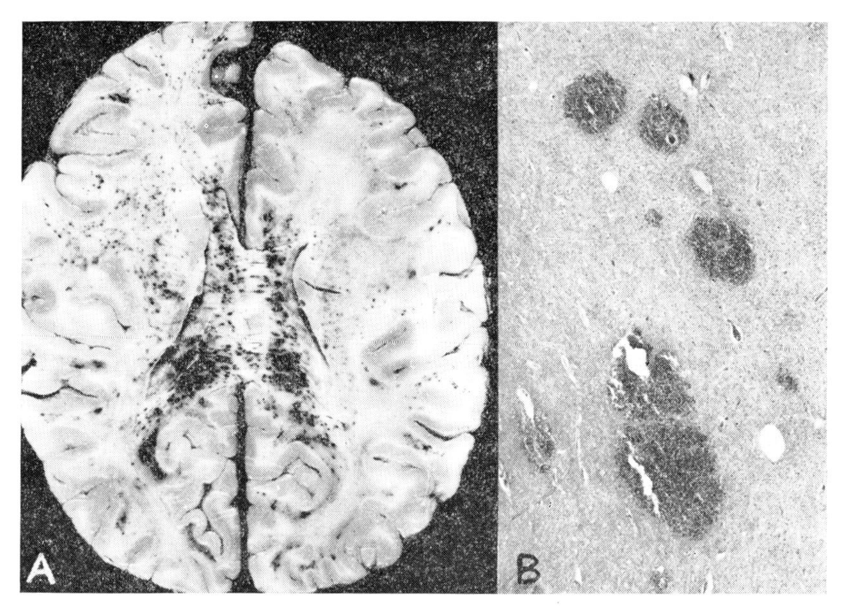

Fig. 59—Acute morphine poisoning. A. Horizontal section of brain, with petechiae. B. Photomicrograph showing multiple hemorrhages. H & E X 15.

sion) on the respiratory and cardiac centers with the resultant anoxic effects, or whether they may be accounted for on the basis of histotoxic anoxia (which may lay a basis for secondary vasomotor effects) is not certain.

Chronic Morphine Poisoning (Addiction).—The chronic effects of opiates on the nervous system are less striking. In addicted individuals of middle age, some atrophy of the frontal cortex is usually seen. Histologically, there is fibrous thickening of the leptomeninges and patchy loss of the nerve cells. The progressive deterioration of the pyramidal cells presumably accounts for the atrophic changes in the convolutions. Lipoidal pigmentation of the ganglion cells, microglia, and endothelial cells of the blood vessels is nonspecific. No remarkable changes occur in the interstitial elements, but widespread fibrous thickening of the walls of the small blood vessels has been described by some observers.

In animal experimentation, various changes have been described, including pyknosis of the small and medium pyramidal cells, loss of tigroid material, swelling, homogenization or vesicle formation in the cytoplasm of the nerve cells, clumping of the nuclear chromatin, bead-like swellings of the dendrites, and focal hemorrhages in various parts of the nervous system (Weimann, 1926) (14).

The nonspecific, chronic alterations which take place in the nerve cells in opiate addiction lead to cerebral cortical atrophy similar to that due to narcotics, barbiturates, and alcohol.

Salicylate Poisoning.—Because salicylates are the most widely used drugs in the world and because all of them are toxic, poisoning with them is not uncommon (Gross and Greenberg, 1948) (15). Many children are poisoned by accidental ingestion or overdosages of salicylates (Troll and Menting, 1945) (16). Poisoning in adults may follow overdosages of a salicylate or excessive intake in a suicidal attempt. Toxic reactions may also result from salicylates applied externally in plasters, lotions, ointments or collodion. Idiosyncracy to the drug is sometimes responsible for untoward symptoms, even after small doses.

The toxic, complex reaction to salicylates is not fully understood. Possibly, stimulation of the respiratory center (hyperpnea and hyperventilation) is first followed by alkalosis and then by acidosis of complex renal and metabolic origin. Interference with cellular carbohydrate metabolism results in histotoxic anoxia of the cerebral nerve cells. The induction of hypoprothrombinemia may be the basic cause of hemorrhagic tendencies manifested in the nervous system by extravasations in the meninges and brain.

The general effects of salicylate poisoning consist of ulceration with hemorrhage of the gastric mucosa, often marked by the characteristic odor of wintergreen, petechiae in the pleura, epicardium, pericardium, peritoneum, and sometimes of the skin, degenerative changes in the renal epithelium, liver cells, myocardium and adrenal cortex, and pulmonary edema.

Cerebral changes consist of congestion, edema, and focal hemorrhages. Edema is characteristically pronounced and generalized in the cortex (Courville and Myers, 1956) (17) (Fig. 60). Focal hemorrhages are found in the meninges, the basal ganglia, the cerebellum, the brain stem, the walls of the third and fourth ventricles, and sometimes in the spinal cord (Dobbs and de Saram, 1938) (18).

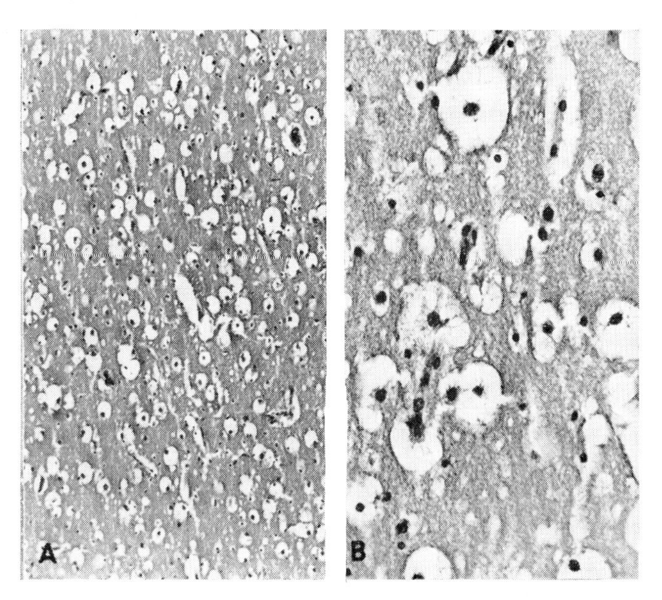

Fig. 60—Acute salicylate poisoning. A. Low power showing characteristic profound cortical edema. H & E X 75. B. High power showing same. H & E X 275.

In the cortex there is a laminar or patchy loss of nerve cells in the intermediate and deep layers. There is similar loss of the cells in the basal ganglia and the Purkinje cells of the cerebellum.

Microscopically, the meninges are distended with fluid, the blood vessels are congested, and focal hemorrhages are often present. In the cortex, small perivascular hemorrhages may be present; congestion of the small vessels is particularly conspicuous. The most characteristic change is profound edema with distention of the perivascular and pericellular spaces, and the formation of interstitial vacuoles. This is associated with severe nerve cell changes, leading to destruction of the parenchymatous elements in the intermediate and deep laminae. The tigroid material is almost universally absent and the neurofibrils undergo hirudiform change or granular degeneration. The cortical nerve fibers are varicose and fragmented, with end-bulb formations.

Similar changes occur in the large nerve cells of the lenticular nucleus and thalamus. Variable changes (e. g., pyknosis, acute swelling) also occur in the Purkinje cells of the cerebellar cortex. In the inferior olivary nucleus, the nerve cells are almost universally pyknotic (Courville and Myers, 1956) (17).

Anticonvulsant Drug Poisoning.—These important drugs come to the attention of the forensic pathologist infrequently. Generally, these drugs are free from "side effects", which are actually toxic symptoms. Fatal poisoning from one of these drugs is, therefore, very rare.

The noxious effects of phenobarbital, the bromides, and allied drugs (i. e., Membaral) have already been described. Some of the other common anticonvulsants will be considered here.

Dilantin sodium (Diphenylhydantoin sodium) is one of the most commonly used anticonvulsants because it is usually well tolerated. Although no clear-cut fatalities are known, side effects are not uncommon and may be severe. Dizziness and ataxia suggest a prominent effect on the cerebellum.

Mesantoin (Thiantoin sodium) exerts its chief noxious effect on the blood cells (pancytopenia), which may be fatal (Weller and Metcalfe, 1949) (19). The bone marrow shows many normoblasts and immature white cells resembling the changes of atypical aleukemic myelogenous leukemia.

Tridione and *Paradione* may produce aplastic anemia and agranulocytosis. Fatal cases of this have been reported (Harrison, et al., 1946; Mackay and Gottstein, 1946) (20, 21). In one 35-year-old man in our series, a bullous lesion developed consequent to his taking tridione for petit mal, two or three capsules a day. At autopsy, cortical congestion and edema of the brain were evident. Petechiae were present in the cortex; there was progressive degeneration of the cortical nerve cells, especially in the superficial layer of the cortex. Whether these changes were due solely to the action of tridione or some other associated condition was problematical.

Mysoline and *Celontin,* two of the newer drugs, are apparently nontoxic; no fatal cases have been reported.

Phenurone (Sedormid) therapy may result in the fatal development of toxic hepatitis.

Zarontin (Ethosuximide), used for petit mal epilepsy, was the apparent cause of fatal poisoning in an 8-year-old girl. Bone marrow aplasia, with petechiae and extravasation over the entire body, developed after therapy with the drug. At autopsy, gross intracranial hemorrhage was found in the right parieto-occipital region (Mann and Habenicht, 1962) (22).

The central nervous changes in toxic (fatal) doses of the anticonvulsant drugs need more critical study than they have had in the past. It is hoped that the chemical and histological changes in any such case coming to autopsy in the future will be completely investigated.

Oil of Chenopodium.—This oil has been used for over a century as a vermifuge, particularly for lumbricales. Its action in this regard is twofold because (1) it is an irritant to the gastrointestinal tract, encouraging evacuation of the bowel, and (2) it is noxious to the worm (Roth, 1918) (23). It has been proven to be fatal in the Orient (Darling, et al., 1918) (24).

The primary action of chenopodium is as an irritation to the gastrointestinal tract. After it is in solution, it is carried to the nervous system, the viscera (liver and kidneys), the lungs, and the heart via the blood stream. It seems to affect the frontal lobes (delirium), the motor system (convulsions, paralysis), the extrapyramidal system (rigidity), the temporal lobe (irrational behavior), the cardiomotor and vasomotor centers (rapid weak pulse, cold clammy extremities, collapse), and the cerebellum (dizziness and incoordination).

In the case reported by Ingham and Courville in 1936 (25), restlessness and sleeplessness were succeeded by delirium and irritable coma, convulsive seizures, and rigidity associated with pathological toe signs. The meningeal and small cortical blood vessels were congested and the cerebral white matter was edematous. There was patchy loss of the cortical nerve cells, with acute and subacute alterations in those that remained. The small pyramidal cells showed pigmentary atrophy and pyknosis and the larger ones chromatolysis and eccentric nuclei. The Purkinje cells were altered by chromatolysis, pyknosis and hyalinization. The blood vessels of the cortex were congested. Early, focal endothelial proliferation of the cerebral cortex was conspicuous (Fig. 61). The microglia in these areas showed early swelling and vacuolization.

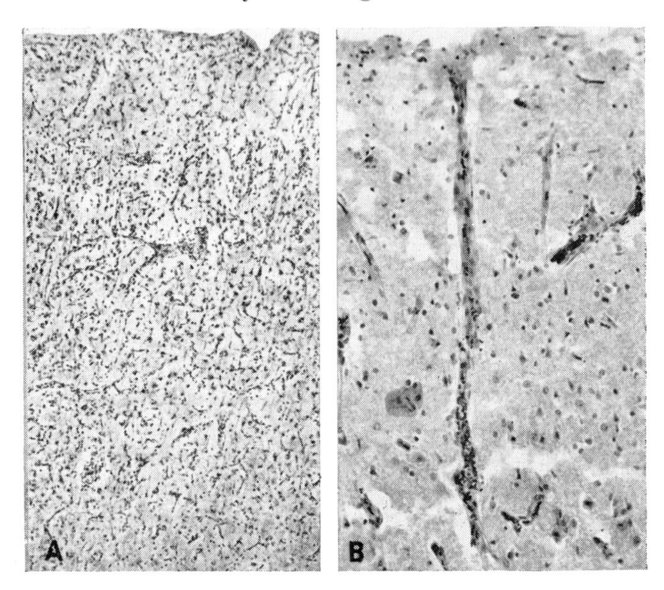

Fig. 61—Oil of chenopodium poisoning. A. Low power view showing acute swelling and proliferation of microglia. Penfield's combined method X 50. B. High power view showing early proliferation of endothelial cells. H & E X 125.

The action of oil of chenopodium on the cerebral and cerebellar cortex suggests an ischemic-anoxic mechanism, probably through the small arterioles. The congestion and cerebral edema may be due to the action of this drug on the respiratory and vasomotor centers.

Sulfa Compounds.—For a brief period prior to the advent of antibiotic substances, the sulfa compounds were used extensively for many of the bacterial diseases. During this time, it was learned that these compounds have a deleterious affinity for the nervous system. Leutscher and Blackman (1943) (26) pointed out that toxic psychosis, convulsive seizures, aphasia, agraphia, stammering, dysmorphopsia, transitory myopia, optic neuritis, and blindness (apparently due to encephalomyelitic, myelitic, and meningeal irritation) sometimes resulted from therapy with the sulfas. These toxic manifestations usually cleared up promptly when use of the drug was discontinued; fatalities seldom occurred. Roseman and Aring (1941) (27) reported one case of poisoning with sulfa methylthiazole. They found multiple petechial hemorrhages throughout the cerebral gray matter, some perivascular lesions, and some changes in the vascular endothelium. There was some doubt about the precise etiology of the lesions, however, because the patient had been an alcoholic and had been exposed to lead. They suggested that these pre-existing intoxications may have predisposed the vascular and perivascular alterations.

In our series, a 38-year-old Caucasian carpenter was given sulfathiazole tablets, 3 grams a day, for a macular rash thought to be due to the use of lead paint. On the third day he complained of generalized aching and developed a fever. On the fourth day the dosage of sulfathiazole was increased to 7 grams. This dosage was continued for at least another day. In five days he received at least 23 grams. The fever, and malaise, persisted. He went into shock on the seventh day and was admitted to the hospital with Cheyne-Stokes respirations and twitching of his extremities. The urine, obtained by catheterization, contained albumin, granular casts, and red blood cells. The cerebrospinal fluid was under a pressure of 250 mm., with 12 cells per cu. mm. Within a few hours after admission, the patient died in an anuric-uremic state. At autopsy, focal necrosis of the liver, kidney, spleen, pancreas and adrenal were found, associated with focal necrosis and hyperemia of the lungs. The kidney contained 11.2 mg. and the liver 5.93 mg. of sulfathiazole per 100 grams of tissue. The brain weighed 1340 grams, and was moderately edematous. Microscopic study of the cortex showed increased friability of the superficial layers, with foci of hemorrhage in the deeper zone (Fig. 62). The nerve cells presented evidence of chromatolysis. The neuroglia were unchanged. The oligodendroglia in the white matter were acutely swollen.

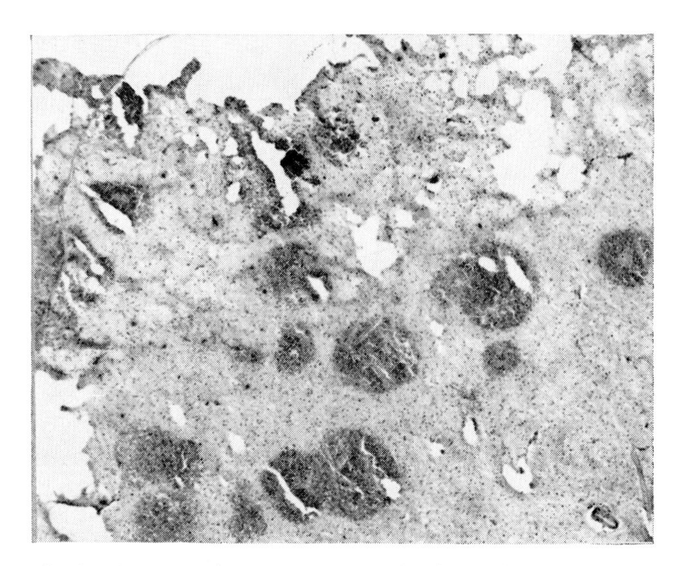

Fig. 62—Sulfathiazole poisoning. Red softening of cerebral cortex with severe damage. H & E X 35.

The mechanism by which structural damage is produced is not clearly established. The serious symptoms of sulfa poisoning seem to stem from condensation of the drug in the kidneys, where an accumulation of crystals appears to cause mechanical occlusion of the uriniferous tubules. Anuria results in a uremic state. The peculiar localization of petechial hemorrhages in the cerebral gray matter, however, is not characteristic of uremia, nor is the tendency to softening of the superficial layers of the cerebral cortex (Fisher and Gilmour, 1939) (28). This change seemed rather to be due to some specific action of the drug on the cerebral gray matter, perhaps through a change in the rich capillary network, as Roseman and Aring (1941) (27) originally suggested.

Antispirochetic Drugs (Arsphenamine).—Occasionally, peculiar encephalic lesions result from intravenous injection of drugs of the arsphenamine group. Such lesions are usually in the form of widely spread petechial hemorrhages (hemorrhagic encephalitis or myelitis, otherwise known as "cerebral purpura", "medullary perivascular necrosis", or "pericapillary encephalorrhagia"), although a variety of hemorrhagic lesions may develop (Courville and Marsh, 1942) (29). These drugs are now used only rarely.

There has been an evolution of opinion as to the mechanism of development of vascular lesions of the brain following injection of arsphenamine. In 1914, Ehrlich (30) postulated that vasodilation is incident to the action of some derivative of arsphenamine (para-aminophenylarsenoxide), accompanied by a deficiency of epinephrine in the circulating blood. The concept of preliminary sensitization, as proposed by Landsteiner and Jacobs in 1936 (31) is supported by the fact that reactions to arsphenamine of this type usually take place after the second or third injection.

Arsphenamine or its by-products affect the endothelium of the capillary blood vessels of the white matter, producing focal hemorrhagic lesions (Globus and Ginsburg, 1933) (32). The influence of personal idiosyncracy is also suggested by the relative rarity of this poisoning. It has been pointed out (Glaser, et al., 1935) (33) that complications develop in one case out of every 28,000 injections, and that one death occurs in 5,390 patients treated.

The general effects on the body of arsphenamine poisoning are manifested by petechiae in the skin and mucous membranes, and associated changes in the lungs, renal cortex and adrenals. Cerebral changes occur in one of four patterns: (1) widespread "hemorrhagic encephalitis", (2) isolated gross hemorrhages, (3) multiple symmetrical foci of hemorrhagic necrosis (Courville and Marsh, 1942) (29) and (4) combinations of these three (Fig. 63). Multiple symmetrical foci of hemorrhagic necrosis seem to have a predilection for the corpus callosum, the internal and external capsules, the hippocampus, the optic radiation, and certain parts of the basal ganglia.

The essential gross lesions are made up of pericapillary ring or ball hemorrhages. Fusion of these small hemorrhages forms the areas of hemorrhagic necrosis. In some cases, only a few lesions occur and survival follows. In such a case, small defects persist in the form of smooth-walled cavities (Ives, 1937) (34).

The reason for the symmetrical location of hemorrhagic foci in the encephalic white matter or basal ganglia has not

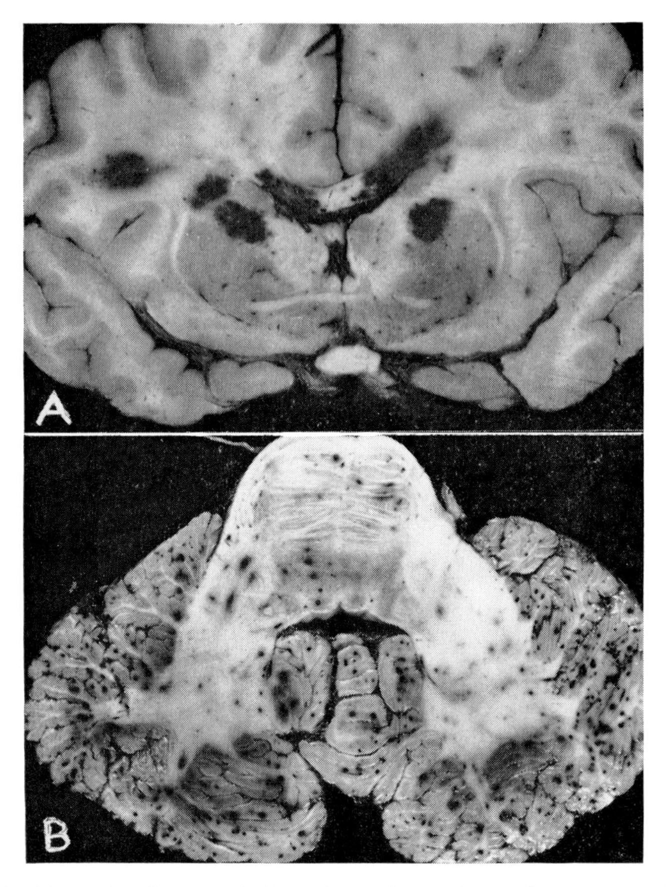

Fig. 63—Hemorrhagic encephalitis of arsphenamine poisoning. A. Section through corpus striatum showing tendency to symmetrical localization of foci of red softening. B. Horizontal section through brain stem and cerebellum.

been adequately explained. Possibly, some more widespread vascular mechanism, under the influence of chemical substances acting on the vasomotor system (absence of epinephrine, as Ehrlich originally postulated, with secondary vasodilating effects of arsphenamine) is responsible. It is uncertain whether this form of hemorrhagic encephalopathy results from the effects of thrombopenia as well as from capillary damage.

Biological Products (Insulin).—The untoward effects of insulin on the nervous system have been observed since it was introduced in the treatment of diabetes mellitus. *Acute effects* have also been observed in cases of insulin shock therapy for certain psychoses (dementia praecox, depressive states) (Scheflen, et al., 1952) (35). *Chronic residuals* occur most often in overdosage in the treatment of diabetes mellitus (Baker and Lufkin, 1937) (36).

The acute effect in the brain of overdosage of insulin is severe congestion, with consequent focal subarachnoid hemorrhages and focal perivascular hemorrhages in the cerebral white matter (Ehrmann and Jacoby, 1924) (37). The chronic residuals are focal softening in the corpus striatum (particularly the putamen) and laminar alterations (from laminar loss of nerve cells to subtotal cortical necrosis). These acute and chronic changes are similar to, if not identical with, those of cerebral anoxia of circulatory or respiratory origin. Olmsted and Taylor (1924) (38) pointed out, however, that there is little or no alteration in the oxygen saturation of the blood. Holmes (1930) (39) demonstrated that large doses of insulin interfere with the utilization of oxygen by the cerebral gray matter and result in decrease in both cerebral glycogen and free glucose.

It is still uncertain why severe congestion occurs in the acute stage of insulin poisoning. It is also uncertain why typical laminar changes suggesting generalized disturbance of vasomotor function are found in residual cortical lesions. It is likely that anoxia incident to hyperinsulinism affects the cells of the vasomotor center, cerebral cortex, and corpus striatum, resulting in dysfunction of the intracranial and somatic circulation. This brings about incomplete but widespread ischemia, which is engrafted upon the primary cellular anoxia. In the acute phase, this vasomotor dysfunction is manifested by severe congestion (probably due to stasis), with diapedesis and focal hemorrhage.

With a survival period of several days, microscopic study reveals that the nerve cells of the cerebral cortex and corpus striatum (especially the putamen) are damaged or lost (Wohlwill, 1928) (40), especially in laminae III and IV of the cerebral cortex (Terplan, 1932; Kobler, 1938) (41, 42). Alterations in the cerebral cortex become more profound with longer survival, when typical focal or laminar loss of nerve cells, status spongiosis, laminar vascular scars, or subtotal necrosis may be found (Ferraro and Jervis, 1939) (43).

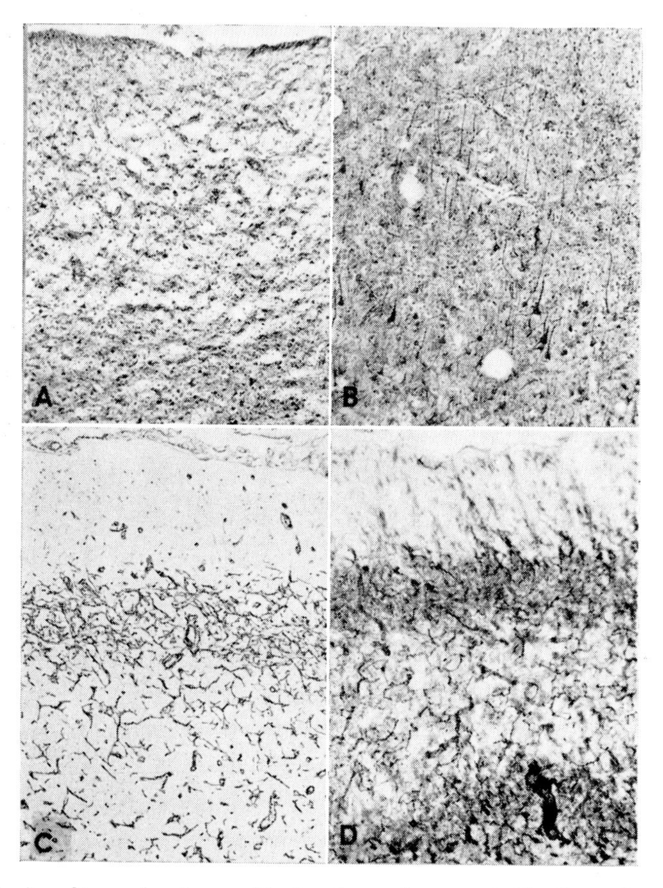

Fig. 64—Insulin poisoning with laminar damage indicative of cerebral anoxia. A. Loss of nerve cells. H & E X 50. B. Loss of nerve cells. Reduced silver preparation X 50. C. Laminar scar. Perdrau stain X 50. D. Laminar deficit. Gold sublimate stain X 50.

In two cases of shock from overdoses of insulin, the patients survived for several months. When the brains were examined at autopsy, the cerebral cortex and corpus striatum (putamen) were profoundly altered (Fig. 64). All degrees of laminar degeneration were found in the cortex, from cell loss to advanced necrosis (Courville, 1954) (44).

A Further Note on Sedative and Hypnotic Drugs

This added thought on this group of drugs seems to be warranted at this particular time because the human race seems to be involved in a conflict between the *stimulants* (or the tonics) on one hand and *sedatives* on the other. From the results of their toxic effects on the nervous system, the *sedatives* seem to be winning out. This obviously is the case if the data found in Table II (page 176) is correct. In the year 1954–1955 death by overdosage of sedatives (notably the barbiturates) in this location reached a total of 224 cases. While it may be possible for tranquilizers to win out, at least in the amounts consumed, over the sedatives, it is likely that atrophic changes in the cerebral cortex will be less severe in the case of tranquilizers. From past experience and deductions therefrom, it is safe to predicate also that a less marked degree of cellular changes will be found in the cerebral cortex, although presumably of similar character.

Summary

The problems presented by the untoward effects of common drugs, even those which predominantly affect the nervous system, are manifold. In this chapter, the effects on the nervous system of the common drugs and medications capable of causing fatal poisoning are discussed. Poisoning with any of these agents might come to the attention of the forensic pathologist. The most common gross and microscopic change encountered in poisoning is congestion, with secondary hemorrhage. Cerebral anoxia is frequently seen, as are more complex methods by which intoxication in its many forms produces havoc in the delicate nervous mechanism. The effects of poisoning on the nervous system should be of special interest to the physician, for sooner or later he will be intimately associated with the unpleasant, if not lethal, effects of a drug which he has hoped will alleviate, if not cure, his patient's ills.

REFERENCES

1. Lawes, F. A. E.: Acute Nicotine Poisoning. Med. J. Australia 1:84, 1928.
2. Petri, Else: Pathologische Anatomie und Histologie der Vergiftungen (Vol. 10). New York: Julius Springer, 1930.
3. Maier, H. W.: Der Kokainismus. Leipzig: George Theime, 1926.
4. Pachonwow: See Petri, Else, 1930.
5. Barger, G.: Ergot and Ergotism. London: Gurney and Jackson, 1931.
6. Winogradow: See Petri, Else, 1930.
7. Stingl, A.: Pyelonephritis e Graviditate unter der Verdachtsdiagnose "Sublimatvergiftung." Zentralbl. Gynök. 74:1000–1003, 1952.
8. Greenwood, R., and Peachey, R. S.: Acute Amphetamine Poisoning; An Account of 3 Cases. Brit. Med. J. 742–744 (Mar. 30) 1957.
9. Shoor, M.: Paraldehyde Poisoning; Report of a Fatality. J. A. M. A. 117:1534–1535 (Nov. 1) 1941.
10. Jervis, G. A., and Joyce, F. T.: Barbiturate-Opiate Intoxication with Necrosis of the Basal Ganglions of the Brain; Report of Case. Arch. Path. 45:319–326 (Mar.) 1948.
11. Courville, Cyril B.: Case Studies in Cerebral Anoxia. VI. Typical Anoxic Alterations in Cerebral Gray Matter After Overdosage of Barbiturates. Bull. Los Angeles Neurol. Soc. 20:16–24 (Mar.) 1955.
12. Neumann, M. A.: Encephalopathy Following Barbiturate Intoxication; Report of Case. J. Neuropath. & Clin. Neurol. 1:145–160 (Apr.) 1951.
13. McDougall, J., and Wyllie, A. M.: Fatal Case of Paraldehyde Poisoning with Post Mortem Findings. J. Ment. Sc. 78:374–376 (Apr.) 1932.
14. Weimann, W.: Gehirnveränderung bei Akuter und Chronischen Morphinvergiftung. Deutsch. z. Gerichl. Med. 8:205, 1926.
15. Gross, M., and Greenberg, L.: The Salicylates, A Cortical Bibliographic Review. New Haven: Hill House Press, 1948.
16. Troll, M. M., and Menting, M. L.: Salicylate Poisoning. Report of Four Cases. Am. J. Dis. Child. 69:37–43 (Jan.) 1945.
17. Courville, Cyril B., and Myers, R. O.: Cerebral Changes in Salicylate Poisoning. Report of Eight Cases. Bull. Los Angeles Neurol. Soc. 21: 124–136 (Dec.) 1956.
18. Dobbs, R. H., and de Saram, G. S. W.: Acute Hemorrhagic Encephalitis Associated with Acute Rheumatism. J. Path. & Bact. 46:437–440 (May) 1938.
19. Weller, R. W., and Metcalfe, J.: Fatal Pancytopenia Following Use of Mesantoin; Report of Case. New England J. Med. 241:17 (July 7) 1949.
20. Harrison, F. F., Johnson, R. D., and Ayer, D.: Fatal Aplastic Anemia Following Use of Tridione and a Hydantoin. J. A. M. A. 132:11–13 (Sept. 7) 1946.
21. Mackay, R. P., and Gottstein, W. K.: Aplastic Anemia and Agranulocytosis Following Tridione; Fatal Case. J. A. M. A. 132:13–16 (Sept. 7) 1946.

22. Mann, L. B., and Habenicht, H. A.: Fatal Bone Marrow Aplasia Associated with Administration of Ethosuximide (Zarontin) for Petit Mal Epilepsy. Bull. Los Angeles Neurol. Soc. 27:173–176 (Dec.) 1962.
23. Roth, D. A.: Some Dangers of the Chenopodium Treatment. South Med. J. 11:733 (Nov.) 1918.
24. Darling, S. T., Barber, M. A., and Hasker, H. P.: The Treatment of Hookworm Disease, J. A. M. A. 70:499 (Feb. 23) 1918.
25. Ingham, S. D., and Courville, C. B.: Diffuse Cerebral Changes in Oil of Chenopodium Poisoning. Bull. Los Angeles Neurol. Soc. 1:152–156 (Dec.) 1936.
26. Leutscher, J. J., and Blackman, S.: Severe Injury to Kidneys and Brain Following Sulfathiazole Administration. Ann. Int. Med. 18:741–756 (May) 1943.
27. Roseman, E., and Aring, C. D.: Encephalopathy Associated with Sulfa Methylthiazole Therapy. New England J. Med. 224:416–420 (Mar. 6) 1941.
28. Fisher, J. H., and Gilmour, J. K.: Encephalitis Following Administration of Sulphanilamide with Note on Histological Findings. Lancet 2:301–305 (Aug. 5) 1939.
29. Courville, Cyril B., and Marsh, C.: Cerebral Lesions Following Administration of Neoarsphenamine. Multiple Symmetrical Foci of Hemorrhagic Necrosis of the Brain. Arch. Dermat. & Syph. 46:512–533 (Oct.) 1942.
30. Ehrlich, P.: Deaths After Salvarsan. Brit. Med. J. 1:1044–1045 (May 9) 1914.
31. Landsteiner, K., and Jacobs, J.: Studies on Sensitization of Animals with Simple Chemical Compounds: Anaphylaxis Induced by Arsphenamine. J. Exp. Med. 64:717–721 (Nov.) 1936.
32. Globus, J. H., and Ginsburg, S. W.: Pericapillary Encephalorrhagia Due to Arsphenamine. The So-Called Arsphenamine Encephalitis. Arch. Neurol. & Psychiat. 30:1226–1247 (Dec.) 1933.
33. Glaser, M. A., Imerman, C. P., and Imerman, S. W.: So-Called Hemorrhagic Encephalitis and Myelitis Secondary to Intravenous Arsphenamine. Am. J. M. Sc. 189:64–79 (Jan.) 1935.
34. Ives, E. R.: Disseminating Areas of Necrosis in the Brain Following Intravenous Injection of Arsphenamine. Bull. Los Angeles Neurol. Soc. 2:140–143 (Dec.) 1937.
35. Scheflen, A. E., Reiner, E. R., and Jetter, W. W.: Fatalities in Insulin Therapy for the Psychoses. Analysis of Eight Cases. Arch. Neurol. & Psychiat. 67:32–43 (Jan.) 1952.
36. Baker, A. B., and Lufkin, N. A.: Cerebral Lesions in Hypoglycemia. Arch. Path. 23:190–201 (Feb.) 1937.
37. Ehrmann, R., and Jacoby, A.: Ueber Blutungen bei im Insulin behandelten Komafällen. Deutsche med. Wchnschr. 50:138, 1924.
38. Olmsted, J. M. D., and Taylor, A. C.: Effect of Insulin on Blood; Changes in Oxygen Saturation, Percentage Hemoglobin and Oxygen Capacity. Am. J. Physiol. 69:142–154 (June) 1924.

39. Holmes, E. G.: Oxidations in Central and Peripheral Nervous Tissue. Biochem. J. 24:914–925, 1930.
40. Wohlwill, I.: Ueber Hirnbefunde bei Insulin—Ueber dosierung. Klin. Wchnschr. 7:344–346 (Feb. 19) 1928.
41. Terplan, K.: Changes in the Brain in a Case of Fatal Insulin Shock. Arch. Path. 14:131–132 (July) 1932.
42. Kobler, F.: Histologischer Gehirnbefund nach Insulinkoma. Arch. f. Psychiat. 107:688–700, 1938.
43. Ferraro, A., and Jervis, G. A.: Brain Pathology in 4 Cases of Schizophrenia Treated with Insulin. Psychiat. Quart. 13:207–228 (Apr.) 1939.
44. Courville, Cyril B.: Case Studies in Cerebral Anoxia. I. Cerebral Changes Incident to Hyperinsulinism (Hypoglycemia). Bull. Los Angeles Neurol. Soc. 19:29–35 (Mar.) 1954.

Chapter X. Common Chemical, Metallic, and Metalloid Poisons*

Poisons which affect the brain can be divided into three major classes on the basis of the sources from which they are obtainable: (1) drug or medicinal poisons, (2) chemical or industrial poisons, and (3) alcohol, the most common and destructive social poison. In Chapter IX the common drug poisons and the brain lesions produced by them were considered. The asphyxiant gases, which may be either chemical or medicinal, will be considered in Chapter XI. Alcohol and its notorious, destructive effects on the brain will be considered in Chapter XII.

This chapter will deal with the more common industrial poisons which affect the nervous system. The industrial poisons most often encountered by the forensic pathologist can be divided into three groups: (1) the organic solvents, (2) the metals and metalloids, and (3) a small but important heterogenous group which may be called miscellaneous. The agents which cause brain symptoms most often will be reviewed and their resultant changes briefly outlined. The organic solvents will be considered first.

Table III shows the distribution of deaths from poisoning by chemical, metallic, and miscellaneous agents during a five year period (1950–1955), as investigated by the Los Angeles County Coroner's Office. (See Table II, Chapter IX, for other data.)

---

* The list of chemical agents capable of producing alterations in the central nervous system is constantly enlarging. This is particularly true of pesticides and chemical products used in the space sciences (missile fuels, etc. See description of central nervous changes in Pentoborane poisoning on pages 220 and 221.)

Table III

Deaths Due to Poisoning with Chemicals, Metals, and Other Agents *

Agent	1950–51	1951–52	1952–53	1953–54	1954–55	Total
Alcohol (isopropal)	1	1		1		3
Ammonia			1	1		2
Arsenic	17	27	20	20	20	104 **
Benedict's solution	1					1
Bichloride of mercury	2	1	2	1	1	7
Carbon tetrachloride	6	2	1	3	4	16
Caustic alkali			1	1		2
Caustic soda					1	1
Chlorodone		1				1
Cleaning fluid					1	1
Cresol			1			1
Cyanide	12	8	10	8	13	51 ***
Dichlorether		1				1
Fluoride	3	4				7
Formaldehyde				1	1	2
Germicide (?)				1		1
Hydrocarbon					1	1
Hydrochloric acid			2			2
Hydrofluoric acid					1	1
Hydrogen sulfide					3	3
Kerosene			2			2
Lead	1	1		1		3
Lye, lysol	4	2	2	6	1	15
Mercury		1		1		2
Methanol		2				2
Methyl bromide		1				1
Nicotine	5	6	8	3	5	27
Nitric acid	1					1
Oil of cedar leaf				1		1
Oxalic acid		1				1
Petroleum (ethyl gas, etc.)	2			1		3
Phenol		1		1		2
Phenol mercuriate			1			1
Phosphorus (1 white P)	1		1	4	1	7
Sodium acid sulfate	1					1
Sodium fluorine, fluoride	1		1			2
Sodium hydroxide	1		1			2
Sodium nitrate					1	1
Sulfide and octophenyl			1			1
Sulfuric acid			1			1
Tetraethyl pyrophosphate		1				1
Triclorethylene					1	1
Unknown chemical		1			1	2
SUBTOTAL						288
BACTERIAL AGENTS						
Botulism	1	5			1	7
Food, unspecified				1		1
Venom, snake	2			1		3
TOTAL	62	67	56	57	57	299

* 21.7 per cent of all deaths due to poisoning, excluding CO and alcohol.
** 36 per cent of poisonings shown here.
*** 17.7 per cent.

Organic Solvents

Of the organic solvents, other than the alcohols, the petroleum derivatives, the coal tar derivatives, the chlorinated hydrocarbons, the esters and the ketones are of greatest interest medicolegally. Their toxicity depends upon a variety of factors, such as their vapor pressure, solubility, volability, concentration, and chemical acuity, which makes it difficult to classify them solely on the basis of their toxicity. Those with low vapor pressure, including the saturated hydrocarbons, ethyl alcohol, benzene, and carbon disulfide, are the most toxic organic solvents.

In this section, brief reference will be made to some related compounds, such as phenol, the aniline compounds (low pressure group), carbon tetrachloride (industrial solvents), and carbon disulfide and methyl bromide (methyl linkages).

Phenol. There were three cases of phenol poisoning in our series. The most interesting one of these was the case of a 24-year-old Japanese man who committed suicide by ingesting cresol because of public exposure as a sexual pervert. At autopsy, he was found to have severe burns of the mucous membranes of the mouth and throat, which were injected and edematous. The stomach was also inflamed, but it had no odor of phenol because of the longer than average survival period. The meninges and cortex of the brain were grossly injected. The white matter of the centrum ovale was marked with a number of miliary hemorrhages (Fig. 65), but only a few such lesions were found in the brainstem and cerebellum.

Aniline. Aniline, or aminobenzene, is not as toxic as other chemical compounds listed here. The various compounds melt at 122 C. to 184 C., are moderately soluble in both water and alcohol, and are chiefly used in the manufacture of dyes for furs, hair, and leather. It is in these industries that intoxication usually occurs. The fate of aniline in the tissues is tied in with its analgesic effect. This is especially true of acetanilid, which is produced by combining glacial acetic acid with aniline (Brodie and Axelrod, 1948) (1). Aniline compounds are also valuable as tissue stains.

Aniline poisoning has become rare. Only one case has been studied in this laboratory. A 66-year-old woman who died of arteriosclerotic heart disease had worked for a fur company

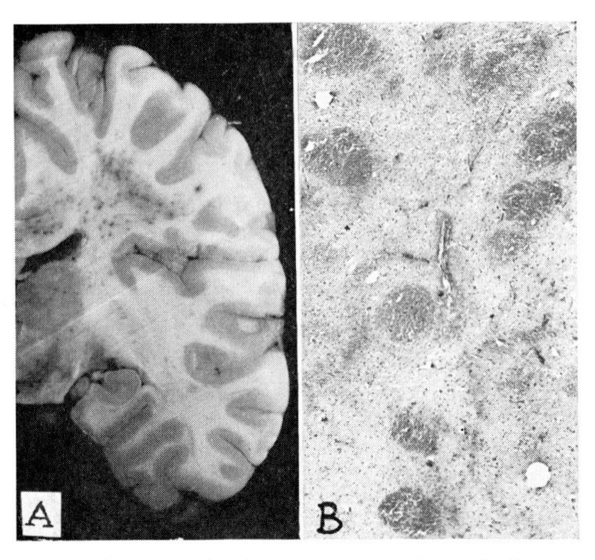

Fig. 65—Phenol poisoning. A. Coronal section through the cerebral hemispheres showing petechiae. B. Microscopic view showing focal hemorrhages. H & E X 35.

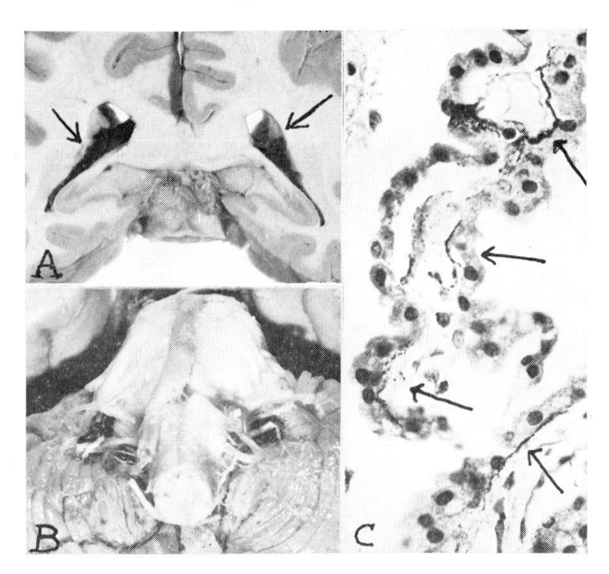

Fig. 66—Aniline poisoning. A and B. Dark pigmentation of choroid plexus in the lateral ventricle (A) and cerebellopontile angle (B). C. Photomicrograph showing aniline pigment in basal membrane of the choroid plexus. H & E X 500.

26 years previously, using one of the aniline dyes in fur preparation. Within a relatively short time, the skin of her face and neck had assumed a dark, bluish color. She spent many years trying to correct the situation without any real success, although the intensity of the color slowly faded. At autopsy, aside from a moderate cerebral atrophy, the only gross evidence of poisoning by the dye was a bluish gray discoloration of the choroid plexuses. Microscopically, the granules of darkly colored pigment were apparent in the basement membrane. To a lesser extent, these granules were present in the subepithelial portions of the stroma and pedicles of the plexuses (Fig. 66).

Carbon Tetrachloride. This substance is a clear, colorless, heavy liquid with a characteristic odor. It boils at 76.8 C. and freezes at 23 C. It is nonflammable, only slightly soluble in water, and freely soluble in other organic solvents. At one time, this compound was most commonly used in dry cleaning, but presently most of the yearly commercial output is used in the manufacture of refrigerants (e. g., "Freon 12") and insecticides (DDT). It is also used in fire extinguishers and in the fumigation of grain.

Prolonged or repeated exposure to air saturated with the fumes of carbon tetrachloride is hazardous. It is readily absorbed by the mucous membranes of the respiratory passages, and to a lesser extent by the skin. Symptoms of acute intoxication are increased salivation, impairment of consciousness, paresthesias, pulmonary edema, and emphysema. The liver is grossly enlarged. In chronic poisoning symptoms include irritation of all mucous membranes, and respiratory and gastrointestinal manifestations (McGill, 1946) (2). In fatal cases, the tissues of the brain are edematous and contain small hemorrhages.

In one case of this series, the patient was a 25-year-old Negro woman who was a chronic alcoholic and had been treated for syphilis and gonorrhea eight years previously. Five days prior to admission to the hospital she cleaned a hat in a closed room, with the contents of a bottle of "Energine" (carbon tetrachloride) in an open pan. Her hands were in contact with the fluid for at least 45 minutes. The following day she complained of severe abdominal pain. Jaundice appeared a few days later.

When admitted to the hospital, she had jaundiced skin and sclerae, and a temperature of 101.6 F. The liver was palpable 12 cm. below the right costal margin and was extremely tender. Her urinary output was inadequate; she was given electrolytes and four units of blood. The clinical impression was hepatic failure due to chronic alcoholism and acute superimposed carbon tetrachloride intoxication. The patient expired after a massive hemorrhage from mouth and nostrils.

The dorsolateral and frontal convolutions of the brain were chronically atrophic. The meninges were thickened and a meningocortical hyperemia was evident. Focal subarachnoid hemorrhages were seen in the dorsolateral areas (Fig. 67, A). The cortical ribbon was narrowed. Microscopically, there was patchy loss of nerve cells in the cortex. There was marked oligodendrogliosis in the cortex and an increased number of interstitial cells in the underlying white matter (Fig. 67, B). The nerve cells in the basal ganglia and hippocampus were

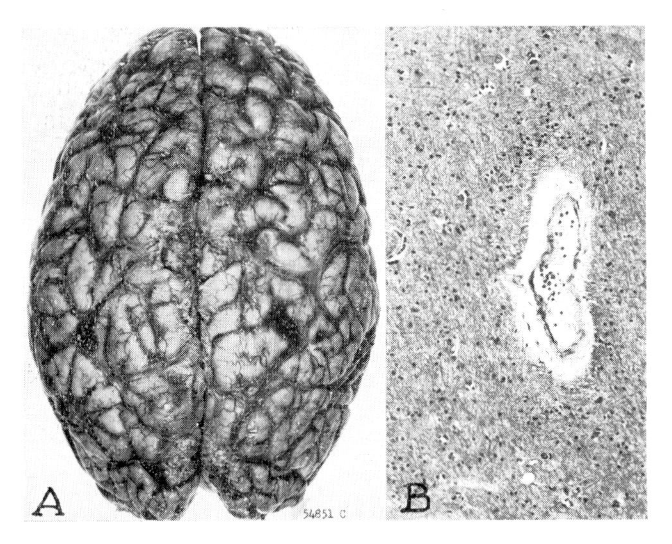

Fig. 67—Effects of carbon tetrachloride poisoning. A. Gross appearance of congestion and focal subarachnoid hemorrhage. B. Photomicrograph showing increased number of acutely swollen oligodendroglia in subcortical white matter. H & E X 125.

reduced in number (probably a result of chronic alcoholism), with change in those remaining.

In this case, the chronic changes in the brain were most likely due to the chronic alcoholism; only the subarachnoid hemorrhage, the tendency to cerebral edema, and the attendant oligodendrogliosis could be attributed to the carbon tetrachloride poisoning.

Dichlorether ("Chlorox"). This allied compound is a colorless liquid with a pungent odor. It is very irritating to the eyes. It is almost insoluble in water, but is soluble in organic solvents. In addition to its uses as an insecticide and soil disinfectant and as an extracting and refining agent, it is valuable in cleaning raw wool and cloth. Its toxic action is largely that of an irritant of the mucous membranes of the eyes and respiratory passages. Its chief toxic effects on the cerebral tissues are those of edema and hemorrhage. Death is usually due to mechanical asphyxiation incident to edema of the lungs.

One fatal case of poisoning with dichlorether was present in our series. In this case, death was primarily due to corrosion of the gastric mucosa. A 39-year-old Caucasian male who had been a heavy drinker ingested an unknown quantity of plant spray containing dichloric ethyl ether. Postmortem examination disclosed injection and corrosion of the gastric mucosa. The brain was grossly normal. Microscopically, there was a moderate degree of oligodendrogliosis, with attendant swelling of the oligodendrocytes in the cerebral centrum. A few phagocytes laden with blood pigment were noted about the blood vessels. There was moderate edema (Fig. 68).

Methyl Bromide. This product is a colorless, nonflammable gas at room temperature and pressure, with little odor. It is soluble in most organic solvents. It is useful as an insecticide and is most often utilized in the fumigation of fruits and vegetables (Mackie, 1938) (3). It is also used as a refrigerant.

Methyl bromide acts on the skin (vesicular dermatitis), the respiratory system (pulmonary edema, bronchitis, bronchopneumonia), the gastrointestinal system, and the liver. Its most serious effects, however, are the results of its noxious action on the central nervous system (Clarke, et al., 1945) (4).

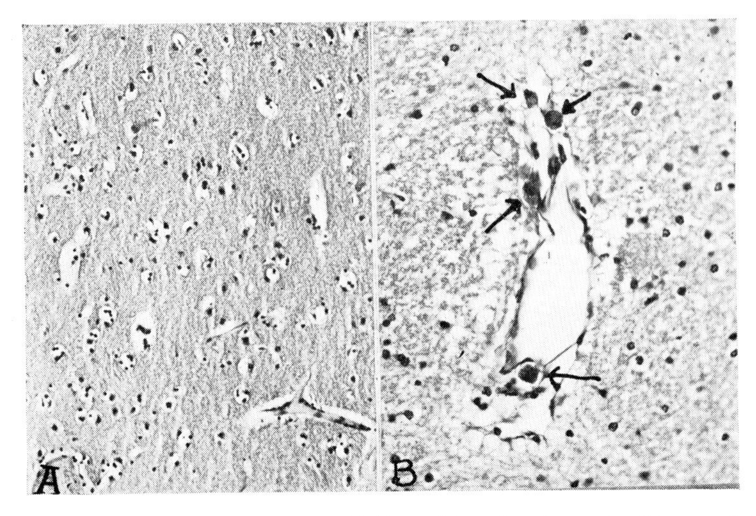

Fig. 68—Effects of dichlorether ("Chlorox") poisoning. A. Edema of lenticular nuclei. H & E X 125. B. Pigment in phagocytes in perivascular spaces. H & E X 250.

Metals and Metalloids

Metals are the most common industrial poisons; many of them can result in toxic symptoms from the time they are taken from the earth until they reach the end stage of manufacture. Even then, improper handling of the manufactured products, such as paint or objects containing lead, may cause poisoning. The metals are, for the most part, toxic in a special way to the tissues of the central nervous system.

As a class, metals are considered as having a potency for diffuse systemic noxious effects on animal protoplasm (Jetter, 1957) (5). Some investigators think that metals may act as enzyme inhibitors, depressing the functions of the pyruvate oxydase system (Peters, 1948; Thompson, 1948) (6, 7). In this sense they may behave similar to a vitamin B_1 deficiency. They exert their severest action at their sites of entry to the tissues and elimination therefrom. The neuropathological changes produced by lead, mercury, arsenic, manganese, and phosphorus are the most important medicolegally, although copper and iron may produce deleterious effects under some circumstances.

Lead. Lead is perhaps the most important metal from the viewpoint of the frequency with which it concerns the central and peripheral nervous system in cases of poisoning. It may be hazardous to those who extract it from the earth, those who manufacture objects or substances from it, or even those who come in contact with the manufactured product. Careless handling of leaden materials by painters or plumbers, or the chewing of lead paint on cribs, toys, or nipple shields by infants may produce lead poisoning. Some individuals are exposed to plumbism by drinking soft water which runs through lead pipes. Bystanders in the vicinity of the burning of discarded batteries may be innocent victims of lead poisoning. Persons who have been shot with leaden missiles may get chronic poisoning from the absorption of lead retained in the tissues.

Lead poisoning can be acute or chronic, giving rise to symptoms of lead encephalopathy. One may find evidences of lead atrophy, hydrocephalus (especially in children), and lead meningitis associated with cirrhosis of the liver. Isolated lead neuropathy may arise in individuals who are unaware of the real source of their poisoning.

Acute lead poisoning in adults is rare. In children, however, it occurs even in sucklings, when it is sometimes mistaken clinically for some sort of a congenital disorder. Structural changes in the nervous tissues are not very marked, but in the spinal fluid the globulin, the cells, and the sugar may be increased.

Chronic lead poisoning (lead encephalopathy) of adults is likewise often associated with cirrhosis of the liver. Grossly, the brain may show minor, nonspecific atrophy of the frontal convolutions with thickening and opacity of the leptomeninges. Microscopically, infiltration of perivascular lymphocytes may be observed. Edema of the cerebral tissues and degeneration leading to patchy loss of the cortical nerve cells is the characteristic change in the nervous tissues. Gliosis and significant alterations in the blood vessels may also be found. Endothelial proliferation in groups of small blood vessels has been reported (Petri, 1930) (8). Pseudocalcification may be found in the lenticular nuclei. Other vascular changes are arteriosclerosis, fatty changes in the capillary endothelium, and hyaline thrombi.

Lead neuropathy is purely motor, but involves the myelin sheaths, the axis cylinders, and the distal portions of the motor fibers and end-plates.

In one typical case of chronic lead poisoning a 63-year-old Caucasian man had been a painter for forty years. An essential part of his work was to squeeze continually a large lump of lead putty in his right hand. He had a rash, believed to be due to a sensitivity to paint thinner, on his hands and face five years before his death. In February of 1953 he began to have episodes of abdominal cramps, with some vomiting, frequent severe headaches, and occasional dizziness (but no ataxia). In May he complained of pain and weakness of his right arm; he was unable to write, paint, or raise his arm. There was also some weakness of the legs. A diagnosis of lead neuropathy and myelopathy was made, and the patient was given a course of treatment to stimulate the excretion of the lead in the urine. He later became quadriplegic and was then readmitted to the hospital. He died at home in March, 1954, due to aspiration of stomach contents in the air passages.

Postmortem examination of the brain disclosed it to be atrophic, with thickened leptomeninges (Fig. 69, A). The blood vessels at the base were not atheromatous; the small vessels were tortuous and lay on the surface of the brain. The brain cut with resistance, suggesting central gliosis. Microscopically, the leptomeninges showed fibrous proliferation, and wandering phagocytes were found in the subarachnoid space. The cortex presented similar changes. The subcortical white matter was mildly edematous. The blood vessels were congested; the normal arrangement had disappeared. Some vessels were hyalinized and showed obstruction, with regional edema. In some areas a vascular proliferation was noted. There was a generalized patchy nerve cell loss (Fig. 69, B), and severe changes (swelling, lipoidal degeneration and atrophy, clumping of tigroid material, atrophy, and chromatolysis) were noted in the cells that remained. Ghost cells were present throughout. The glial cells were increased. Satellitosis was present about the larger nerve cells. The subcortical white matter was also edematous, with an increase in glial

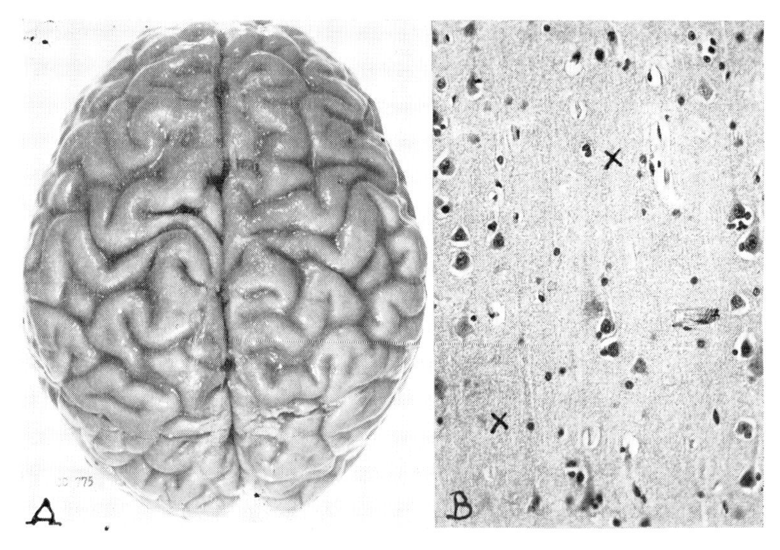

Fig. 69—Effects of chronic lead poisoning. A. Thickening of leptomeninges. B. Patchy loss of cortical nerve cells (x). Several ghost cells can be seen. H & E X 250.

cells. The cerebellum showed congestion and nerve cell changes (swelling, pyknosis) in the smaller parenchymatous elements and chromatolysis of the Purkinje cells. The glial elements of the cervical cord were increased. The myelin sheaths were swollen. The vessels in the cord were distended, surrounded with a perivascular loosening of the ground substance.

Thallium. This metal is usually absorbed through both the skin and the mucous membranes. Poisoning may be acute, subacute, or chronic. In the acute form death occurs in 7 to 15 days. In the subacute form (which occurs particularly in growing children), death occurs in from 6 weeks to 3 months.

Symptoms of thallium poisoning usually appear in the form of a vegetative polyneuritis or a peripheral motor/sensory polyneuropathy manifested by weakness, pain, and trophic disturbances in the hands and feet. One or more of the cranial nerves may be involved—optic, extraocular, facial or auditory-vestibular complex, vagus or bulbar palsies, or retrobulbar neuritis. In some patients, psychotic manifestations described as a thallium psychosis (with hypochondriasis, hysteric behavior or a psychotic overlay of other phenomena), or extrapyramidal or motor signs (including convulsive seizures) may occur. In children, psychotic manifestations seem to be fairly common; neurological symptoms are much the same as in adults.

At autopsy, structural changes in the internal secretions, fatty changes in the myocardium and liver, degeneration of gastric mucosa (with achylia gastrica), and degeneration of the renal epithelium are found. The changes in the brain are presumed to be due to neurotoxicosis or hypo-riboflavinosis.

Grossly, swelling (edema), reddish softening of the cortex, and small perivascular hemorrhages in the white matter are associated with hyperemia and congestion. Alterations seen in children with severe damage include degeneration of the tangential fibers of the cerebral cortex, loss of nerve cells of the frontal cortex (leading to atrophy), gliosis, degeneration of myelin sheaths of the cerebrum, cerebellum, and posterior columns of the spinal cord, and degeneration of nerve cells of the bulbar nuclei and the anterior horn cells of the spinal cord.

No cases of thallium poisoning have been studied in this laboratory.

Mercury. Mercurial poisoning was probably the first industrial disease to be identified. It was apparently quite common in the middle ages, among the gilders of gold, silver, and copper. More recently (the nineteenth century) it has been found among those engaged in the mining of mercury. The characteristic symptoms were seen particularly in those engaged in the manufacture of beaver hats.[1]

Two types of mercury poisoning are presumed to occur: (1) mercury poisoning as such, and (2) mercury *dampf* (Biondi, 1930) (10), which is a form of mercurial encephalitis from inhalation of mercury vapor. Chronic encephalitis affects the respiratory passages. Psychic phenomena are characteristic. Among the symptoms of poisoning are intention tremor (ataxia), choreiform movements, visual disturbances, dysarthria, meningitic manifestations, and neuritis.

---

[1] It was these typical manifestations which led the author of *Alice in Wonderland* to include the "Mad Hatter" in his list of characters (Guillain and Laroche, 1907, 1913) (9).

The acute changes in the brain consist of hyperemia of the meninges and cortex, edema of the brain, petechial hemorrhages, and focal cortical softenings with residual atrophy of the area striata of the occipital lobe and the precentral gyrus. At times, atrophy is also found in the region of the frontal pole. This atrophy seems to affect the cortex in the depths of the sulcus, rather than at the crowns of the convolutions. The cellular changes are nonspecific; perivascular gliosis may be seen. In the cerebellum, there is found at times a symmetrical lobar atrophy. This seems to be due to a selective atrophy of the granular cell layer, at times with preservation of the Purkinje cell layer. The dendrites of the Purkinje cells, however, show stellate bodies when impregnated with silver. A glial proliferation of the molecular layer also takes place. The anterior horn cells show prominent changes in some cases.

Following is a description of a fatal case of acute mercuric poisoning from ingestion of mercuric chloride tablets.

After ingestion of a number of mercuric chloride tablets in a suicidal attempt, a 21-year-old Caucasian woman was admitted to the hospital. A gastric lavage was performed, but she died four days later after clouding of the sensorium and coma. At autopsy, the convolutions of the brain were atrophic, and there was minimal thickening of the meninges. Microscopic examination showed fibrous thickening of the leptomeninges in all areas. Wandering macrophages were present throughout the subarachnoid space. The cortex was mildly congested, with acute nonspecific nerve cell changes. There was some acute swelling, pyknosis, and chromatolysis of the pyramidal nerve cells of the cerebral cortex (Fig. 70, A and B). Some acute vacuolization of the nuclei was noted in the larger cells. The subcortical white matter was intact. In the cerebellum, there were mild changes in the Purkinje cells (acute swelling of the cytoplasm and vacuolization of the nuclei).

Manganese. This poison tends to produce an ultimate clinical picture similar to that of hepatolenticular degeneration. A coarse tremor suggestive of parkinsonism, but of intension type, associated with episodes of uncontrolled laughter has been noted. Casamajor (1913) (11) observed degeneration of some tracts in the brainstem, as well as advanced cirrhosis

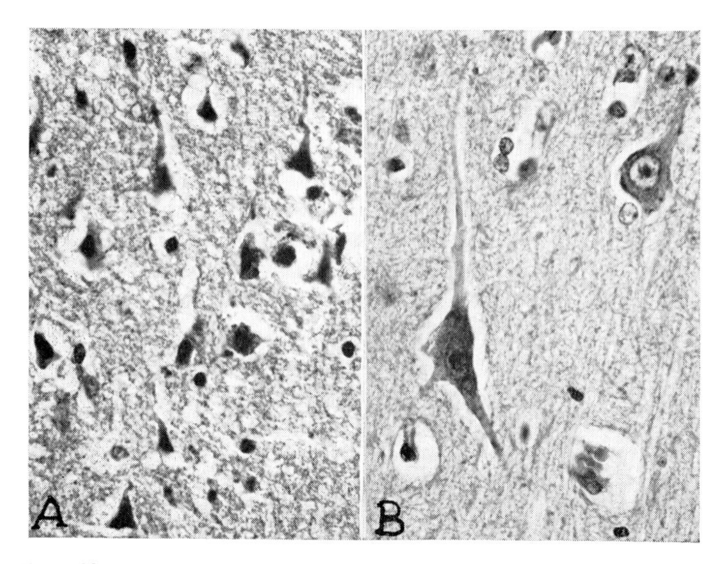

Fig. 70—Effects of mercury poisoning. A. Photomicrograph showing marked pericellular edema associated with pyknosis of the smaller cortical nerve cells. H & E X 250. B. Higher power magnification showing loss of tigroid pigment in larger nerve cells. H & E X 500.

of the liver and chronic interstitial nephritis. Canavan, et al. (1934) (12) observed diffuse degeneration of the nerve cells in the cerebral and cerebellar cortex and, especially, in the basal ganglia, which were considerably shrunken and contained circumscribed glial scars. In Stadler's case (1935) (13), there were focal softenings and scars in the frontal and parietal lobes, as well as a distinct loss of nerve cells in the corpus striatum (especially the globus pallidus). Lobular sclerosis of the cerebellar cortex was also present. The locations of these lesions account for the symptoms referable to the basal ganglia.

Copper. Copper in its metallic state is not considered to be particularly poisonous. Like some other potential poisons, it is essential to metabolism. Pentschew (1958) (14) has pointed out that copper may be a deficient trace metal in the corpus striatum. Courville, et al. (1963) (16), found a decrease of this metal in three cases of Huntington's chorea.

Certain compounds of copper may be toxic. This was shown in a case of poisoning studied in this laboratory in which a

60-year-old Caucasian man ingested three fourths of a bottle of Clinitest tablets (copper sulfate) in a suicidal attempt. He had been a diabetic for 18 years. When he was admitted to the hospital his blood pressure was 240 systolic, 120 diastolic, and his pulse was 100. There was periorbital edema of the right eye, stiffness of the neck, and decreased breath sounds in both lung bases. A left hemiplegia and a Babinski sign on the left were also present. He had an enlarged liver and 3-plus edema of the left leg (the right leg had been previously amputated). He soon developed jacksonian seizures on the right side of his body. On the fourth hospital day he developed hematemesis and melana. He was given transfusions of blood but continued to bleed. He expired on the tenth day after ingestion of the tablets.

The cerebral cortex was atrophic, presumably on an arteriosclerotic basis. The lateral ventricles were enlarged. Microscopically, there was an increase in fibrous elements in the leptomeninges. The blood vessels were moderately thickened. There was patchy loss of nerve cells in the cortex. Some cells displayed central loss of tigroid material. Others were pale, with loss of structural detail. The subcortical white matter showed no change. The intracerebral blood vessels were slightly thickened; some were surrounded by collections of pigmented macrophages. The white matter of the basal ganglia was fragmented and loosened and the nerve cells were pale. One focus of cells showed ischemic change. Patches of golden pigment were present in that area.

The chronic changes in the nervous system in this case were the result of degenerative vascular disease. Whether or not the acute changes in the nerve cells of the cerebral cortex and basal ganglia were the result of the copper compound is unknown.

Arsenic. This poisonous metalloid has been known for its noxious action since about 400 B.C. In the middle ages arsenic, especially white arsenic (arsenic trioxide), was used as a homicidal poison. At the present time, it is theoretically limited as a poison to use on vermin and weeds. Accidental contact, however, does occur, such as in paint or an overdose of a medicinal preparation.[2] The frequency of poisoning may be seen in the statistics from the Los Angeles County Coroner's office for a five year period (1950–1955). During that time there were 104 fatal cases of arsenic poisoning (36 per cent of all chemical or metallic poisonings) among 41,615 cases investigated.

In acute poisoning arsenic seems to have its primary effects as a general protoplasmic poison, acting chemically on the phosphates and structurally on the walls of the blood vessels. Symptoms of arsenical poisoning depend upon the amount ingested. In acute human poisoning abdominal pain is usually experienced within an hour of ingestion of the arsenic. Involvement of the brain is suggested by the onset of headaches, confusion, coma, convulsive seizures, and ultimate signs of increased intracranial pressure. Very little attention, however, has been paid to changes in the central nervous system in fatal cases, except after arsphenamine poisoning. Aside from a hemorrhagic tendency, there is nothing in the microscopic alterations to indicate any specific action of arsenic on the brain.

A 62-year-old man accidentally swallowed one tablespoon of "Antrol" ant poison. He vomited immediately and for approximately the next two hours. Gastric lavage was performed and BAL was given. The left pupil was constricted; the pupils reacted to light. The heart sounds were distant; the abdomen was tender in the epigastrium. The patient expired after three days. Postmortem examination of the brain showed advanced cortical atrophy and meningeal thickening. The third and lateral ventricles were enlarged. These changes were obviously of long standing. Microscopically, there was severe cell loss in the cortex, with pigmentary atrophy and severe cell change seen in many

---

[2] Formerly, a type of arsenical poisoning occurred with the organic compounds (arsphenamine group) used in the treatment of syphilis. These are no longer encountered in this country. In those cases, hemorrhages in the corpus callosum and deep in the white matter near the anterior and posterior horns of the lateral ventricle, in the cerebral peduncles, and in the peripheral parts of the pons and medulla were found. Microscopically, there were foci of demyelination and necrosis in the cerebral cortex and white matter (Courville and Marsh, 1942; Russell, 1937) (16, 17).

remaining cells. The pericellular and perineural spaces were widened, suggestive of edema. The interstitial elements, such as the oligodendroglia, in the subcortical white matter were increased. It is very likely that these changes were due to generalized circulatory changes and not due to any very specific action of arsenic.

Arsenical neuropathy may occur as an independent condition, in which case both the myelin sheaths and axis cylinders are involved (Hassin, 1930) (19).

Miscellaneous

A few common poisons which are not of metallic origin, but which need to be briefly mentioned, will be discussed here.

Phosphorus. Although phosphorus poisoning is not considered a common form of intoxication, several fatal cases have been investigated by the Los Angeles County Coroner's office in the recent past. The usual sources of this element are rat poison (suicidal attempts), phosphorescent paints, and the fumes of phosphoric oxide (industrial intoxication).

This toxic agent quickly results in fatty degeneration of the tissues in all the viscera, including the brain. This change in the nerve cells of the brain is not profound, however (Ferraro, et al., 1938) (20). Typical of most forms of cortical degeneration leading to atrophy, is patchy cell loss, often in the vicinity of blood vessels, and swelling and early proliferation of the vascular endothelium, often associated with hemorrhage. The oligodendroglia and microglia show acute swelling (Pentschew, 1958) (14) (Peters, 1952) (15).

Cyanide. The cyanides constitute one of the larger groups of fatal poisons. Over a recent five year period there were 51 fatal cases investigated by the Los Angeles County Coroner's office. Most of these were suicides. Industrial poisoning occurs from contact with sodium or potassium cyanide in metallurgy. Cyanogen chloride is used as an insecticide.

The earliest symptoms of cyanide poisoning are due to its local action (pain and tingling of the mucous membranes of the mouth), rather than to some influence on the brain (convulsions and impairment of consciousness). Its action on the nervous tissues produces histotoxic anoxia (internal asphyxia), rendering the nerve cells unable to utilize the available oxygen in the circulating blood. Structural changes in the cerebral cortex are rarely marked because of the usually short survival period. When present, they appear chiefly as areas of focal necrosis of the cortex, with more or less total absence of tigroid material in the cytoplasm of the nerve cells.

One 22-year-old man was found unconscious in a fumigation tent spread over an orange tree which had just been sprayed with a cyanide solution. He had been seen alive and rational only a few moments before, and it was presumed that he had carelessly stepped into the tent. Postmortem examination of the brain revealed it to be grossly normal. Microscopically, all the cortical nerve cells showed either mild swelling or pyknosis, total loss of tigroid material, and shrinkage of the nuclei. Occasional neuronophagia was also seen. Sections from the hippocampus, in particular, showed areas of focal necrosis, characteristic of cerebral anoxia. Sections from the cerebellar cortex showed early softening of the molecular layer with loss of structural detail and loss of tigroid staining of the Purkinje cells.

Because of its peculiar action as an agent productive of histotoxic anoxia, this poison will also be discussed as an asphyxial agent in Chapter XI.

Pentoborane. One case of poisoning occurred by exposure to this extremely toxic boron compound, found only in combinations of borax and boric acid. It is used now as a solid propellant in jet propulsion. A 63-year-old Caucasian man was accidentally exposed to its fumes. Following momentary inhalation, he had a tonic and clonic convulsion and was unconscious for 15 to 30 minutes. He was pale, cyanotic, and sweating diffusely. When he regained consciousness, he complained only of dizziness, weakness and feeling "flushed". Approximately 12 hours later, he had another convulsive seizure. He became disoriented, wandering away from the hospital after breaking loose from restraints. When he was returned to the hospital, he appeared calm, but was confused. He had intermittent periods of unconsciousness and hyperirritability. He deteriorated to complete toxic psychosis, with ultimate respiratory depression and hyperthermia, and died 59 hours after the exposure. When the brain was examined, the vessels over the dorsolateral surface were congested

(Fig. 71, A). The frontal cortex was slightly thinned. The white matter was dusky; the veins were evident as dark spots in some areas. The cerebellum and brainstem also showed evidence of congestion. Microscopically, the cortical vessels were congested. The pericellular and perivascular spaces were widened. The neurons were lost in some areas; the others showed vacuolization of cytoplasm, swelling, lipochrome pigmentation, and chromatolysis (Fig. 71, B). There was a slight loss of Purkinje cells in the cerebellum.

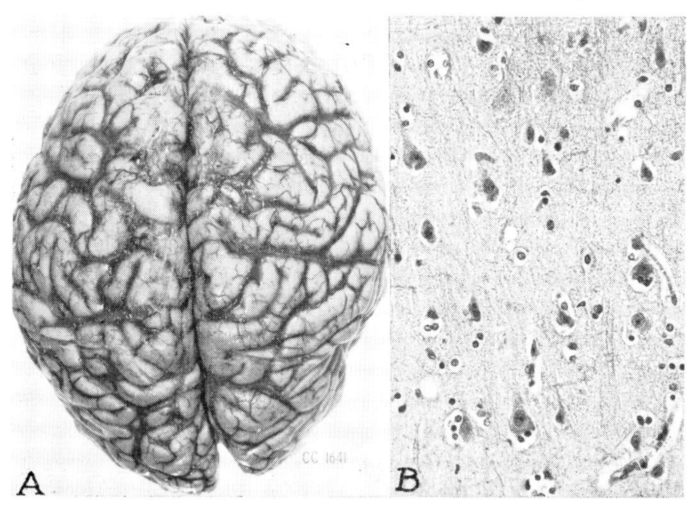

Fig. 71—Central effects of pentoborane poisoning. A. Gross leptomeningeal-cortical congestion. B. Acute nonspecific changes in cortical nerve cells. H & E X 250.

Nicotine. Poisoning with nicotine sometimes occurs incident to the processing of tobacco or the handling or application of insecticides containing nicotine. Over a period of five years, the Los Angeles County Coroner's office investigated 27 fatal cases of nicotine poisoning. Nicotine is available as a free base or as a sulfate. The fatal dose of nicotine is about one drop, the quantity contained in two cigarettes. This substance first stimulates and then depresses the nerve cells of the autonomic ganglia and the nuclei of the brainstem and spinal cord. Poisoning by ingestion of this virulent substance leaves no characteristic signs of its noxious action on the brain.

The effects of this substance on the nervous system are essentially physiological. Therefore, nonspecific architectural or cellular changes are to be expected in any part of the nervous system, although focal meningeal and ventricular hemorrhages and nonspecific cell changes may be found. Following is a description of a case of nicotine poisoning.

A 36-year-old Caucasian man was found dead in a hotel room. He had recently been discharged from the Marine Corps for medical reasons. Witnesses stated that he had been drinking and acting strangely. He was thought to have ingested "Black Leaf 40", as two one-ounce containers for this substance were found in his room. Nicotine tartrate, 0.79 gm. per liter of blood, and ethanol, 0.211 mg. per cent, were found. There was no external lesion of the brain, but the cortex was atrophic and the arachnoid was thick and opaque, both evidently long-standing changes. The lateral ventricles were slightly enlarged. The cortical atrophy was presumably postalcoholic and due to areas of nerve cell loss in the cerebral cortex. Some nerve cells showed pyknotic changes. Satellitosis was present. The oligodendroglia in the white matter were increased, as were the fibrous astrocytes.

Summary

Organic solvents and metals are common poisons which affect the nervous system. The degree of toxicity of the solvents is variable. The least toxic are the phenolic and aniline compounds and the most toxic are alcohol, benzene and carbon disulfide. The heavy metals as a class are presumed to have a potency for diffuse noxious effects on protoplasm. Some investigators believe that they also depress the functions of the pyruvate oxydase system. Of the metals, lead causes poisoning most often. Its action on the human nervous system is multiple. Thallium, manganese, and mercury seem to produce the most characteristic structural alterations. Arsenic apparently does not have a specific action on the brain, but does produce an unusually persistent structural change in the peripheral nerves.

Phosphorus poisoning may be fatal, but no profound changes are produced in the brain. Cyanide is a common industrial poison, but because of the usually short survival period few changes are found in the brain. Pentoborane, a newer toxic substance derived from borax for use as a solid jet propulsive agent, produces congestion and other cerebral changes. Nicotine is a potent poison but it leaves no characteristic signs.

REFERENCES

1. Brodie, B. B., and Axelrod, J.: The Fate of Acetanilide in Man. J. Pharmacol. & Exper. Therap. 94:29–38 (Sept.) 1948.
2. McGill, C. M.: Death and Illness from Use of Carbon Tetrachloride. Northwest Med. 45:169–172 (Mar.) 1946.
3. Mackie: Methyl Bromide—Its Expectancy as a Fumigant. J. Econ. Entomal. 31:70, 1938.
4. Clarke, C. A., Roworth, C. G., and Holling, H. E.: Methyl Bromide Poisoning; Account of Four Recent Cases Met with in One of H. M. Ships. Brit. J. Indust. Med. 2:17–23 (Jan.) 1945.
5. Jetter, W. W.: Chemical Injury, in Pathology, 3rd ed., edited by W. A. D. Anderson, St. Louis, C. V. Mosby Co., 1957, pp. 145–152.
6. Peters, R. A.: Development and Theoretical Significance of British Anti-Lewisite (BAL). Brit. M. Bull. 5:313–319, 1948.
7. Thompson, R. H. S.: Therapeutic Applications of British Anti-Lewisite. Brit. M. Bull. 5:319–324, 1948.
8. Petri, Else: Pathologische Anatomie und Histologie der Vergiftungen. Berlin, Verlag von Julius Springer, 1930.
9. Guillain, G., and Laroche, G.: Sur la Pathogénie du Tremblement Mercuriel. Revue Neur. 15:137, 1907. Sur la Nuture du Tremblement Mercuriel. Bull. Soc. Méd. Hôp. Paris 947, 1913.
10. Biondi, C.: Úber die Vergiftungen durch Quecksilberdampf und Quecksilberverbindungen und die symptomatologischen und physiopathologischen Differenzen. Arch. Gewerbepath. 1:745, 1930.
11. Casamajor, L.: An Unusual Form of Mineral Poisoning Affecting the Nervous System: Manganese? J. A. M. A. 60:646, 1913.
12. Canavan, M. M., Cobb, S., and Drinker, C. K.: Chronic Manganese Poisoning. Report of Case, with Autopsy. Arch. Neurol. & Psychiat. 32:501–512 (Sept.) 1934.
13. Stadler, H.: Histopathologische Untersuchungen zur Frage der Beziehungen zwischen Leber und Gehirn Krankheiten. Ztschr. f. d. ges Neurol. u. Psychiat. 154:626–657, 1935.
14. Pentschew, A.: Intoxikationen (Vol. 13, Part II, Section B: Nervensystem. Zweiter Teil—Erkrenkungen des Zentralen Nervensystem. Hundbuch der Speziellen Pathologischen Anatomie und Histologie). Berlin, Springer-Verlag, 1958.
15. Peters, G.: Über Spätverenderüngen im Zentralnervensystem nach Intoxication mit Arsen und Phosphor. Ztschr. f. nerventr. 168:281–304, 1952.

16. Courville, Cyril B., Nusbaum, R. E., and Butt, E. M.: Changes in Trace Metals in the Brain in Huntington's Chorea. Arch. Neurol. 8:481–489 May 1963.
17. ———, and Marsh, C.: Cerebral Lesions Following Administration of Neoarsphenamine. Multiple Symmetric Foci of Hemorrhagic Necrosis of the Brain. Arch. Derm. & Syphil. 46:512–533 (Oct.) 1942.
18. Russell, D. S.: Changes in the Central Nervous System Following Arsphenamine Medication. J. Path. & Bact. 45:357–366 (Sept.) 1937.
19. Hassin, G. B.: Symptomatology of Arsenical Polyneuritis. J. Nerv. & Ment. Dis. 72:628–636 (Dec.) 1930.
20. Ferraro, A., Jervis, G. A., and English, W. H.: Pathological Changes in the Brain in Cases of Experimental Phosphorus Intoxication. Psychiatric Quart. 12:294–305 (Apr.) 1938.

Chapter XI. The Asphyxiant Gases*

Although the effects of the various asphyxiant agents are largely concentrated in one system of the body, their ultimate effects vary considerably. It is possible to trace out certain structural tendencies in the residuals of anoxia after exposure to noxious agents—each one is marked by its own peculiar stamp which distinguishes it from other agents. These differences are accounted for on the basis of the inherent stresses of each agent on the vasomotor system.

Classification of Noxious Gases

There is no completely satisfactory classification of the noxious gases. Henderson and Haggard (1943) (1) divided all such gases and vapors into four groups: Group I, the irritants; Group II, the asphyxiants; Group III, the volatile drugs and drug-like substances; and Group IV, the inorganic and organometallic gases. They subdivided the *irritant gases* into primary and secondary irritants, depending on whether or not the systemic toxic effects were in concentrations sufficient to cause death. They subdivided the *asphyxiants* into the simple asphyxiants (inert gases) and the chemical asphyxiants, which result in asphyxia because of their chemical affinities. They classified the hydrocarbons and general anesthetic agents as *volatile drugs and drug-like substances* and pointed out that the *inorganic and organometallic gases* are absorbed through inhalation, but are neither directly nor indirectly asphyxiant in their action. Preti (1925) (2) reported that many industrial poisonings result from inhalation of gases in this group.

---

* Received for publication April 17, 1963. This chapter is a simplification and reduction of a paper by Dr. Richard O. Myers and the author published in the Bulletin of the Los Angeles Neurological Society, Vol. 19, No. 4, Dec., 1954, pp. 197–223.

In this study the various noxious gases, fumes or vapors capable of producing cerebral anoxia will be divided into the direct and the indirect asphyxiants. The *direct asphyxiants* will be subdivided into (1) the simple asphyxiants (smoke, fumes and inert gases), (2) the chemical asphyxiants (e. g., carbon monoxide, cyanide), and (3) the central depressants (chiefly the general anesthetics). The *indirect asphyxiants* are chiefly irritant gases whose action is largely due to changes in the air passages and lungs which interfere with the interchange of oxygen and carbon dioxide. These indirect asphyxiants may be subdivided into (1) the industrial gases and (2) the war gases. Some of these agents exert their asphyxiant effects through two or even three mechanisms, but their classification in this chapter is based upon their chief effects.

The Mechanism of Cerebral Anoxia

Divided on the basis of their physiology, there are four types of anoxia: (1) the anemic form, (2) the stagnant form, (3) the anoxic form, and (4) the histotoxic form. The disturbing symptoms of *anemic anoxia* arise because there are not enough erythrocytes to transport an adequate amount of oxygen. This type of anoxia rarely results in permanent brain damage, except when severe hemorrhage occurs (Courville, 1953) (3). In *stagnant anoxia,* the slowed blood current likewise fails to carry a sufficient amount of oxygen to satisfy the normal metabolic needs. The most common, *anoxic anoxia,* is of particular interest because is occurs in asphyxiation by the various noxious gases. Although this type of anoxia may result from obstruction of the air passages (i. e., mechanical block), or from an interference with the interchange of oxygen and carbon dioxide (i. e., pneumonia, pulmonary edema), the asphyxiant gases act by excluding adequate amounts of oxygen from the blood stream (nitrous oxide), by preventing the passage of oxygen through the alveolar walls (phosgene), or by interfering with its transportation in the blood stream (carbon monoxide). The fourth type of anoxia, *histotoxic anoxia,* is most commonly produced by another toxic vapor (hydrogen cyanide), although many nongaseous agents also cause this type of anoxia. Histotoxins interfere with the utilization of oxygen by the nerve cells, even though an abundant supply is available in the blood stream. The mechanisms by which anoxia may occur are briefly discussed at the end of this chapter.

The Direct Asphyxiants

The direct asphyxiants include those agents whose predominant, primary and direct effect on the organism is asphyxiation. In this group are involved (1) the simple asphyxiants, which act by simple replacement of oxygen in the inspired air (smoke, fumes, vapors and inert gases), (2) the chemical asphyxiants, whose action interferes with transportation or utilization of oxygen (carbon monoxide, cyanide), and (3) the central depressants, which produce asphyxia by their narcotic action on the cerebral cortex or basal ganglia (general anesthetic agents). The direct asphyxiants will be considered in this order.

Simple Asphyxiants. According to the definition used here, the simple asphyxiants are gases acting by replacement of oxygen in the inspired air. The most common of these is smoke. "Smoke" is an inexact term used to describe gaseous products of combustion rendered visible by particles of carbon. The name is also used to designate mixtures of various materials resulting from incomplete combustion or to designate a cloud resembling such products of combustion (Patty, 1949) (4).[1]

The noxious effects of smoke are incident to the exclusion of oxygen from the inspired air, as well as to the presence of certain irritant chemical substances in the smoke. Naturally, the danger is greatest when combustion occurs in an enclosed space. If combustion is complete, the components of smoke include carbon dioxide, nitrous acid, ammonia and

[1] The following definitions were offered by Patty in 1949: A *gas* is any material in the gaseous state at 25 C. and 760 mm. Hg. pressure. A *vapor* is the gas of a substance ordinarily liquid or solid at 25 C. and 760 mm. Hg. pressure. A *dust* is composed of solid particles dispersed by disintegration. A *mist* is made up of liquid particles that have condensed in the atmosphere (condensates). *Fog* is made up of liquid particles of condensates. An *aerosole* is a dispersion or suspension of fine solid or liquid particles in the air or some gaseous medium.

sulfur dioxide. Incomplete combustion produces carbon monoxide, various hydrocarbons, formaldehyde, formic acid, phenolic compounds, methyl alcohol, acetone, acetic acid, and hydrogen sulfide (Chajes, 1930) (5). Carbon monoxide is undoubtedly the most dangerous and important component. Naturally, the type of material consumed will determine the nature of the toxic products evolved. Burning celluloid may produce hydrogen cyanide in dangerous amounts. Hamilton and Hardy (6) estimated that the fumes from a burning comb would be sufficient to poison a human being. Acrolein [2] is produced by the thermal decomposition of neutral fats. This was produced by the burning of the leatherette chairs in the Cocoanut Grove fire and was probably responsible for the pulmonary damage sustained in that disaster (Dutra, 1949) (7).

Carbon dioxide poisoning is occasionally reported. The gas is heavier than air and collects in the lower levels of unused wells and brewing vats, cellars, manholes, caves, silos, and the holds of ships. Gonzales, et al. (1937) (8), reported fatal asphyxiation in the hold of a ship in which "dry ice" was used as a refrigerant. Several fatalities have occurred when brewery or winery workers entered brewing vats (Hamilton and Hardy) (6). Toxic effects of air in closed or poorly ventilated rooms are due to oxygen depletion, moisture, and heat, more than to the increased amounts of carbon dioxide (Gonzales, et al.) (8).

Carbon dioxide is usually described as a simple asphyxiant. This is an oversimplification, however, since in concentrations of 5 to 10 per cent or more it has a definite narcotic action. Susceptible individuals may become unconscious after breathing 7 to 10 per cent carbon dioxide for a few minutes, or a concentration above 10 per cent for less than a minute (9).

Nitrogen is rarely a threat to human well-being. In the physiological-pathological situation encountered in compressed-air illness, the central effects are produced by bubbles of nitrogen in the cerebral arteries. The gas has been used

---

[2] Acrolein (Propenal, Acrylaldehyde, Acrylic aldehyde) is a colorless, inflammable liquid with a pungent odor. It is used in the manufacture of synthetic perfumes, in the manufacture of allyl alcohol, the synthesis of plastics, and to accelerate vulcanization.

experimentally to produce asphyxia in animals (Thorner and Lewy, 1940; Lucas and Strangeways, 1952) (10, 11).

The danger of simple oxygen lack must not be overlooked in several occupational situations. If a manhole, for example, is situated in silty loam soil where the oxygen demand of the soil is very high, a dangerous reduction of oxygen may occur. Workmen descending into such a manhole may die of simple oxygen deprivation. The oxygen concentrations in such manholes has been recorded as low as 3.2 per cent to nothing, with a carbon dioxide content somewhat higher than normal (12). The contents of silos may demand a high oxygen level and dangerously deplete the oxygen content of the silo. One such situation occurred in an elevator in which flaxseed was stored (Hamilton and Hardy, 1949) (6).

Several other asphyxiant gases masquerading under popular names merit brief mention. "Choke damp" found in coal mines, is largely carbon dioxide. "Black damp", also encountered in coal mines, consists of about 87 per cent nitrogen and 13 per cent carbon dioxide. "Fire damp", another gas occurring in mining operations, is an explosive mixture of methane and oxygen. Methane is the principal component of "marsh gas" found in the miasmata arising from marshes and swamps.

The Chemical Asphyxiants. In this second group of direct asphyxiants, the chemical action of the particular gas interferes with some specific phase of respiratory activity.

Carbon monoxide forms a firm union with the hemoglobin in the erythrocytes, which precludes the transportation of oxygen to the brain. Thus, even the small amount of oxygen which may be inspired with the gas cannot reach the brain cells (anoxic anoxia). The cyanide gases interrupt the normal respiratory process in another stage, preventing the utilization of oxygen by the cortical and ganglionic nerve cells (histotoxic anoxia). In both cases there is probably a superimposed vasomotor factor which accentuates and prolongs the anoxic state (Courville, 1953) (3).

Carbon monoxide poisoning is the most common poisoning due to the asphyxiant gases. It has been known from antiquity (Lewin, 1909) (13).

During a recent five year period (1950–1955) there were 875 deaths due to carbon monoxide poisoning among 41,615 cases investigated by the Los Angeles County Coroner's office. More than two thirds of the 875 deaths were suicides. Carbon monoxide deaths accounted for 2.1 per cent of all cases investigated. (See Table II, Chapter IX and Table III, Chapter X, for other data.)

Carbon monoxide is produced whenever carbonaceous materials are incompletely burned. It is, therefore, a source of danger in nearly every situation where combustion occurs. The incomplete combustion of fuel gas, particularly if the flame plays against a cold surface, produces dangerous amounts of this odorless, colorless gas. Unvented gas heaters burning in closed rooms are especially hazardous in this connection. Illuminating gas usually contains 6 to 30 per cent carbon monoxide and can be lethal if from leakage or is burned improperly. Natural gas usually does not contain free carbon monoxide. As occurred in the Los Angeles area during the war, however, carbon monoxide-containing materials may be added to it to raise its thermal value.

Exhaust from piston-type gasoline engines or diesel engines frequently causes carbon monoxide poisoning. Incapacity and death have resulted from the exhalation of gases from blast furnaces and kilns, from locomotive smoke, and following the detonation of explosives. Even the atmosphere of machine gun pits can become lethal.

Most persons who die in a conflagration are killed by carbon monoxide before burning occurs (Dutra, 1949; Fisher, 1952) (7, 14). The presence of carbon monoxide in the blood establishes that a burned body was alive when the fire started.

The poisonous effects of carbon monoxide are derived from its double action in the production of asphyxia. An excessive amount of it in inspired air excludes oxygen and then forms a stable compound with the hemoglobin. Furthermore, carboxyhemoglobin interferes with the dissociation of any oxyhemoglobin which still remains in the erythrocytes. The removal of carbon dioxide is also hindered because the insufficient oxyhemoglobin cannot act as a catalyst in the liberation of carbon dioxide. Damage done by carbon monoxide to the tissues is indirect because it results from histotoxic anoxia secondary to anoxemia. There is no evidence that carbon monoxide damages the tissues, particularly the nervous tissues (Dutra, 1952) (15).

The effects of carbon monoxide seen postmortem vary with the length of survival. These effects may be considered as acute, subacute, and chronic. The progressive changes, seen grossly and microscopically during the three stages, will be considered.

The *acute effects* of asphyxia incident to carbon monoxide depend upon the length of survival. In patients who die from acute, severe asphyxia, the brain appears congested and has a livid color due to the presence of carboxyhemoglobin in the red cells. The pattern of the small superficial vessels is readily seen. Patchy subarachnoid or subpial hemorrhages may also be evident. Congestion is manifest on cross section by the reddish blue discoloration of the white matter, the overfull vessels and, at times, by petechiae scattered through the cerebral centrum.

When death occurs within a few days, physical changes take place in the basal ganglia. Most commonly this change involves the globus pallidus, sometimes the head of the caudate nucleus and putamen (corpus striatum), and rarely the optic thalamus. This alteration is first manifest as either a granular appearance of the nuclear mass or red softening. Later, the central part of the nucleus undergoes necrosis, the involved tissues appearing granular and friable in a pocket of yellowish tissue fluid (Fig. 72).

Microscopically, the globus pallidus (or any other involved nuclear mass) first appears to be friable. It also lacks its normal staining qualities. Within the first week, hemorrhage into these tissues may be seen, and compound granular cells may be seen in the softened region, sometimes associated with early endothelial proliferation, which makes the vessels seem more prominent. By the end of the second week, either actual softening, with large numbers of phagocytic cells, or a network of newly formed capillaries will be found. These changes have been described in detail by Hiller (1924) (16), who attributes them to alterations in the local blood supply. Whether this vascular change is functional and incident to

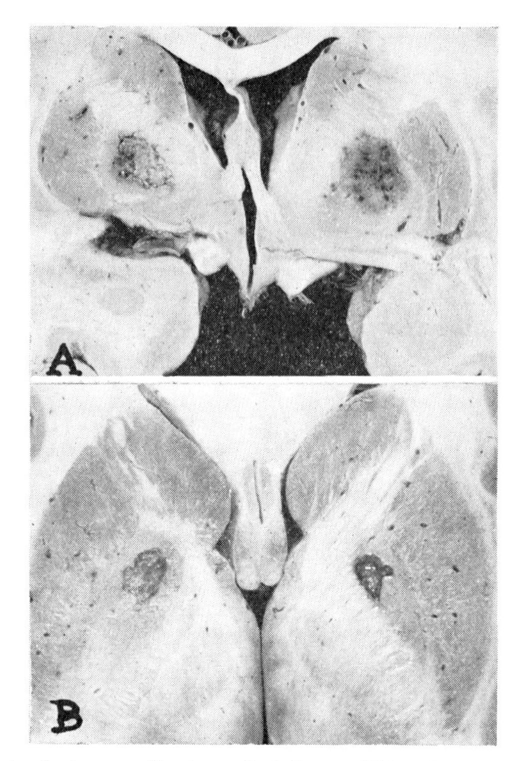

Fig. 72—Kolisko lesion—softening of globus pallidus from carbon monoxide intoxication. A. Survival period of 5 days. B. Survival period of 33 days.

an atonic dilatation of the arterial walls, or structural and the result of changes in the intima or the tunica media, with fatty degeneration or hyaline change (Herzog, 1920) (17), is not yet clearly established. These changes continue into the subacute stage.

During the first two weeks no cortical change is evident grossly. Microscopically, however, areas of focal cell loss begin to appear, with progressive deterioration of the pyramidal nerve cells within these areas. Special staining shows that these acellular areas are also avascular.

Three types of lesions may be found grossly in the brain during the *subacute stage*, from two to six weeks. The first of these is rare; localized, circumscribed areas of cortical-subcortical softening (Fig. 73) are found, most often on the dorsolateral surface of the central or parieto-occipital regions. The affected cortex first becomes slightly swollen and granular, and appears yellow-orange. This is followed by necrosis of the cortex and the underlying white matter. After a longer survival period, the cortex and subcortex appear grayish yellow and are necrotic. Microscopically, the areas of softening are characterized by progressive breakdown of the gray and white matter, with infiltration of compound granular corpuscles. At the margin of the softening the cortex may show laminar necrosis with the early formation of a vascular scar. The usual reactive proliferation of astrocytes and the transformation of microglia into phagocytes are also seen.

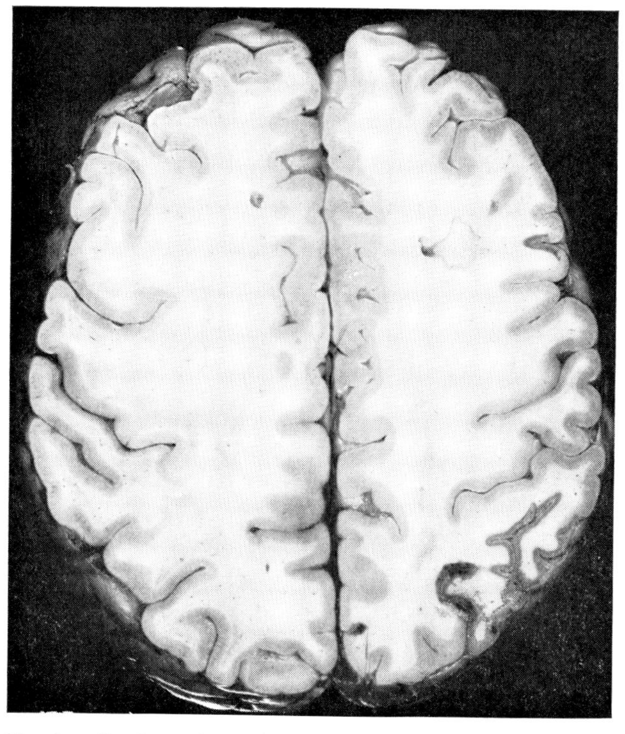

Fig. 73—Focal softening of cerebral white matter and softening of right parietal cortex after carbon monoxide intoxication.

The second, more common, lesion, results from the continuation of the necrotic process in the basal ganglia, which begins in the acute phase. After two weeks, granular change (with the formation of new blood vessels) or central necrosis leading to cyst formation is well defined, constituting one of the hallmarks of this disorder (Kolisko, 1914) (18). This change is characterized histologically by the destruction of all interstitial and parenchymal elements within the limits of the necrotic center, which has a bordering glial scar. There may be an increase in the number of newly formed capillaries. Local perivascular collections of lymphocytes are occasionally seen. Rings of iron and calcium are typically seen in the muscular layer of the arterioles.

The third lesion, gross areas of softening in the cerebral centrum, is also rare. Only two examples have come to our attention and it has rarely been reported by other investigators. At autopsy, coronal sections of the brain show large, irregular, and discontinuous foci of softening in the deep centrum of the cerebral hemispheres. These foci are often symmetrical in the two hemispheres. The characteristic lesion in the globus pallidus is also usually present. Microscopically, progressive degeneration of the white matter surrounds the central defect. Necrosis seems to be a matter of coalescence of numerous foci of degeneration and cyst formation. The absence of blood vessels in these degenerative foci suggests that loss of blood supply is a prerequisite to their formation. Demyelination is also characteristic of this process, although the areas about the preserved blood vessels and the subcortical zones are spared. Subacute central necrosis seems to occur between four and eight weeks after asphyxiation with carbon monoxide. Even when the cortex is grossly unaltered, patchy areas of loss of pyramidal cells are evident microscopically in the middle cortical layers. True focal laminar necrosis, however, is evidently rare. The mechanism of this process has been discussed elsewhere (Courville, 1953) (3).

It is not common for patients to survive into the chronic stage, in which *residuals* of carbon monoxide poisoning are seen. Individuals may survive for several months and then succumb after a progressive downhill course (progressive demyelination), they may live for months or even years with a characteristic striatal syndrome (central necrosis of the globus pallidus), or they may survive with only occasional epileptiform seizures or an organic pyschosis (widespread nodular cortical atrophy).

Progressive demyelination which leads to death in from three months to a year has long been recognized. Typical cases have been described by Grinker (1925) (19), Meyer (1928) (20), and Hsü and Ch'Eng (1938) (21). This change does not occur until seven weeks or more of survival. Courville (1953) (3) has pointed out that demyelinization is only a slowly developing form of cystic central degeneration already described (Fig. 74). Basically, the pathogenesis of the two lesions is the same, degeneration being the direct result of a progressive ischemia of the deeper portions of the cerebral white matter, and demyelination being a delayed result of the process.

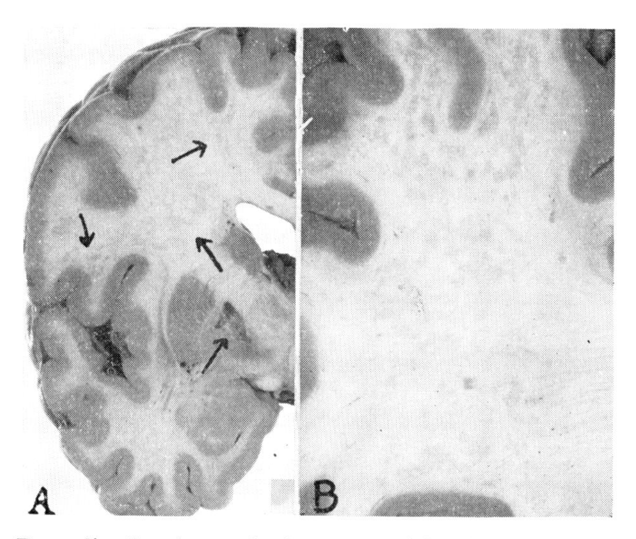

Fig. 74—Demyelination in cerebral centrum following severe asphyxiation with carbon monoxide. Survival of 77 days. A. Irregular cyst in globus pallidus. B. Enlarged view showing spotty demyelination.

Histologically, the white matter shows a progressive degeneration of myelin, greatest in the central areas. The subcortical zone, which is better supplied with blood vessels, is spared. Associated with the loss of myelin, occurring as a parallel if not a predisposing change, is narrowing, subsequent collapse, and complete disappearance of the deep penetrating arteries. Zones of preserved myelin are found about the blood vessels which remain. This observation suggests a possible connection between asphyxia and the demyelinating disorders of infancy and childhood (diffuse sclerosis, encephalitis periaxialis diffusa).

In patients who survive for months or years with a Parkinson's syndrome, there is usually found a small, irregular, fluid-filled, smooth-walled cyst in the globus pallidus. Microscopically, a narrow glial scar borders this cyst. Iron-calcium rings are commonly observed in the tunica media of the regional blood vessels.

In one interesting case a man of 69 years had been asphyxiated by carbon monoxide at the age of 19 (Courville, 1953) (3). He developed convulsive seizures some years after the episode. An old precentral cortical cyst and multiple old cystic cavities of the globus pallidus seen at autopsy were presumed residuals of focal softening which had occurred following the asphyxial insult (Fig. 75).

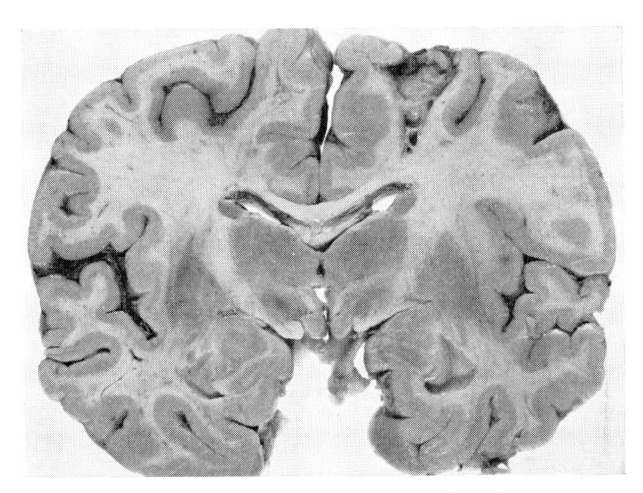

Fig. 75—Focal cortical-subcortical cyst—residual of carbon monoxide asphyxiation. Survival period of 50 years.

Carbon monoxide might be a *precipitating cause of other diseases,* accentuating clinical manifestations of other organic diseases. This is particularly true in elderly individuals already subject to atherosclerotic degeneration of the cerebral blood vessels. General paresis seems to have been accentuated in this way (Skolnick, 1936) (22). Myocarditis (Ehrich, et al., 1944) (23), diabetes (Rogers, 1931) (24), and anemia (Killick, 1940) (25) have been reported as residuals of asphyxia incident to carbon monoxide.

It is evident that the length of the survival period generally predicates what cerebral lesions will develop after carbon monoxide poisoning. It is also evident that a considerable variety of lesions result from a mechanism that seems to be basically simple.

Natural gas as an asphyxiant is occasionally used successfully in suicide. Acute accidental asphyxiation, usually involving workmen in subterranean areas, has also occurred. Natural gas is composed of the following: methane, 80 to 86 per cent; ethane, 10 to 16 per cent; nitrogen, 4 per cent; propane, less than 1 per cent; butane, less than 1 per cent; and oxygen, 0.1 per cent.

Methane, ethane, propane and butane are gaseous saturated hydrocarbons of the paraffin series and are inactive chemically. Methane is inactive biologically also and causes death only by the displacement of oxygen. Ethane in concentrations of 4.7 to 5.5 per cent by volume may cause drowziness and irregular respiration in guinea pigs. Propane has some anesthetic action but has unpredictable effects in lowering blood pressure and causing respiratory arrest. Butane may result in stupor, irregular respiration and some depression when administered to experimental animals in concentrations of 5.0 to 5.6 per cent for 30 minutes (von Oettingen, 1940) (26). No known studies of the specific neuropathological changes following asphyxiation by these gases have been made. For practical purposes, natural gas may be considered a simple asphyxiant, killing or damaging the nerve cells through exclusion of oxygen.

The possibility that natural gas may be incompletely oxidized, producing carbon monoxide, has already been emphasized. It is sometimes questioned whether or not natural gas burning in a closed room can dangerously vitiate the atmosphere in the absence of carbon monoxide. This seems to be very unlikely. Experiments indicate that a gas burner using 8 cubic feet of natural gas per hour would require one and one-half hours to reduce the oxygen content of the air in a 1000 cubic foot, tightly closed room to 18 per cent. The flame of natural gas would not burn in a concentration below 15.5 per cent oxygen, while a resting individual can tolerate much lower concentrations of oxygen without dangerous results. In addition, the additional carbon dioxide produced would probably act to stimulate respiration (1926) (27).

Hydrogen cyanide gas is sometimes used in the fumigation of fruit trees. Exposure to it may result in fatal asphyxiation. Its anoxic effects are not due to lack of oxygen, but rather to the direct action of cyanide on the nerve cells. It interferes with the utilization of oxygen (histotoxic anoxia), specifically by inhibiting the enzyme of cytochrome oxidation. This enzyme is essential for tissue respiration and acts in the oxidation of cytochrome by the oxygen of the blood. Tissue anoxia occurs as soon as cyanide interferes with this enzyme. This explains the usually rapid course of cyanide poisoning—sometimes a matter of seconds—but does not explain the acute vasomotor changes or the chronic alterations in the blood vessels. Cyanide does not combine with hemoglobin (although it does combine readily with methemoglobin) and the blood remains fully oxygenated. This explains the frequently described bright red color of the blood and tissues in cyanide poisoning (Walker, 1950) (28).

Hydrogen cyanide is also employed to fumigate ships and buildings, and to kill parasites in seeds and nuts before packaging for distribution. The gas is a toxic by-product of many industrial operations in which organic nitrogen containing materials are incompletely burned. The alkaline cyanide salts are widely employed in metallurgy, electroplating, steel processing, photography and silver polishing. These salts may produce hydrogen cyanide in the presence of acids or they may be ingested. In the stomach they are hydrolyzed, becoming hydrocyanic acid, whose toxic action is like hydrogen cyanide, although slower.

Toxic amounts of cyanide can be absorbed through the intact skin; therefore, a gas mask is not adequate protection in a contaminated atmosphere. Fatalities have resulted even from wearing inadequately aired clothing after cyanide fumigation (Hamilton and Hardy, 1949) (6).

In one case of cyanide poisoning, a young man at work with a spraying crew was found unconscious in a tree-tent filled with cyanide gas. He died three days later. When examined postmortem, the brain was grossly normal, though microscopic areas of loss of nerve cells were noted in the cerebral cortex (Fig. 76).

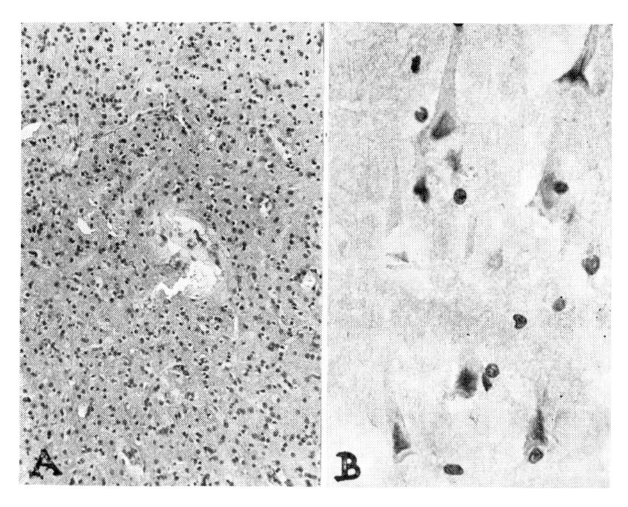

Fig. 76—Acute asphyxiation from cyanide gas. Focal cortical necrosis (A) and focal degeneration of pyramidal cells in hippocampal gyrus (B).

Cyanide poisoning produces not only acute and subacute changes in the cerebral cortex characteristic of anoxia, but also, after prolonged survival, cyst formation and demyelination in the cerebral centrum (Jedlowski, 1938) (29).

Central Depressants (General Anesthetics). The third group of direct asphyxiant gases are those whose chief primary action on the brain is that of narcosis. They produce anoxia either directly by their depressant action (which is reinforced by attendant vasomotor aberrations) on the nerve cells of the cerebral cortex and basal ganglia or indirectly by depression of the respiratory, cardiac, and vasomotor centers. Because nitrous oxide is the most culpable anesthetic agent and its noxious effects are best known, predominant attention will be given to it.

Nitrous oxide has been recognized for over a century to produce cerebral symptoms. The untoward effects of nitrous oxide anesthesia on the nervous system were reported by Löwenberg, et al., and Courville in 1936 (30, 31), and several times later (Courville, 1938, 1939, 1947–48, 1950) (32–35).

The action of nitrous oxide has been considered elsewhere (Courville, 1936, 1939) (31, 33). Studies on the physiological action of this gas suggest that its narcotic action is minimal and that its behavior as a central depressant is chiefly due to its asphyxiant qualities. When it replaces oxygen sufficiently, the functions of the cerebral cortex and corpus striatum are depressed. It also depresses the cardiac and respiratory centers, superimposing one form of anoxia on another with disastrous results. The affected patient either remains in coma with signs of cerebral irritation (convulsions) associated with decorticate rigidity after withdrawal of the mask, or lapses into a maniacal state. The patient may either die after a variable interval, survive with crippling residuals for many years (Courville, et al., 1953) (36), or recover with or without minimal psychic phenomena (Fletcher, 1945) (37).

The acute effects of nitrous oxide occur within the first two weeks, the subacute effects within six weeks, and the chronic residuals during the later months and years of survival.

The *acute effects* of severe asphyxia under nitrous oxide anesthesia resemble those of acute asphyxia from most other causes. Grossly the brain appears congested, with focal subpial extravasations. The cerebrospinal fluid is not increased in amount.

When sectioned, the cerebral tissues appear to be intensely congested, the cortex and basal ganglia often appearing bluish. During the first week or ten days numerous petechiae are at times seen in the white matter, particularly in the subcortical regions (Fig. 77).

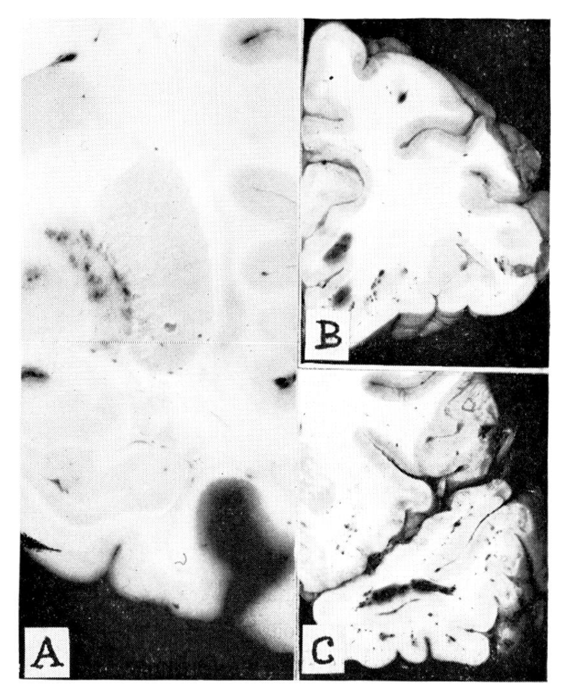

Fig. 77—Focal hemorrhages in lenticular nucleus and white matter after nitrous oxide anesthesia. Survival period of 6 days, 13 hours.

Gross alterations may be visible in the basal ganglia after a few days. The globus pallidus, which is affected more often than the caudate nucleus and the putamen (corpus striatum), first assumes a ground glass appearance, then becomes granular and, finally, grossly softened. These changes become more evident during the subacute stage.

During the acute phase the microscopic architectural and cytological alterations are particularly significant. The architectural alterations involve progressive destruction of foci of nerve cells in the intermediate laminae (III to VI), with ultimate laminar necrosis.

The circumscribed foci in the cortex become apparent as early as 36 hours after asphyxiation. The pericellular spaces become enlarged, the enclosed cells seem shrunken and darkened and the interstitial tissues appear fenestrated (Fig. 78).

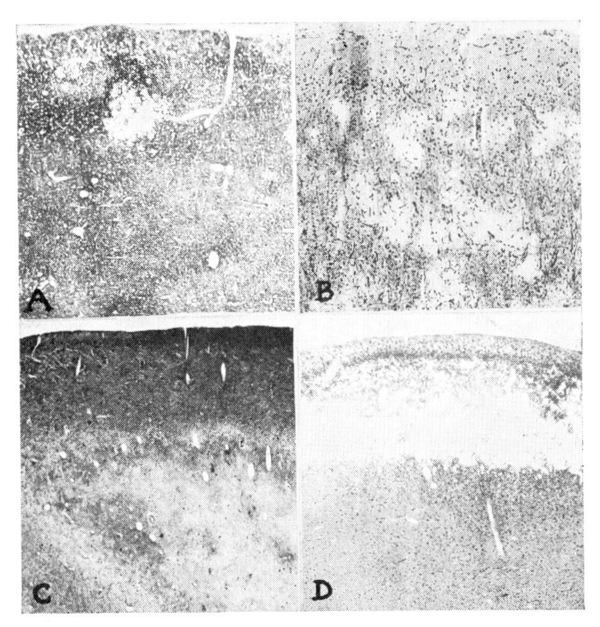

Fig. 78—Cortical changes after nitrous oxide anesthesia. A. Area of focal necrosis. B. Fusion of areas of focal necrosis. C. Laminar necrosis. D. Subtotal cortical necrosis.

Coalescence of these foci forms sharply outlined areas in which the pyramidal nerve cells are severely damaged or absent. These areas of necrosis are irregularly distributed in one or more of the cortical laminae. They are particularly striking in the reduced silver preparations in sections from patients who have survived from three to five days.

Fusion of several larger foci leads to laminar necrosis. Bands of degeneration appear within the central zone of the cortex, which is the zone of greatest vasculature. Early endothelial proliferation leading to the formation of new capillaries is usually seen in the brains of patients who survive. Subtotal cortical degeneration may also be seen after long survival.

The essential cytological changes in the acute stage are progressive disintegration of the nerve cells and interstitial elements within the areas of focal (or laminar) necrosis and early transformation and proliferation of the regional astrocytes and microglia. The nerve cells (in the foci of necrosis) soon show evidence of severe cell change; those between the foci show acute swelling, with loss of tigroid substance. The interstitial elements of all types within these degenerative foci promptly break up and disappear. The astrocytes, especially in the subpial glial layer, show signs of proliferation. Astrocytes in the deep cortical layer show evidence of proliferation and fibrous transformation. The microglia become progressively swollen, lose some of their processes, and presumably form the compound granular corpuscles seen in individuals who survive longer. The oligodendroglia become acutely swollen.

Few individuals survive from two to six weeks, but several features mark the characteristic *subacute effects*. The early laminar necrosis may involve the occipital lobe (Fig. 79) (Courville, 1939, Case 19) (33) or be very widespread (Courville, 1953, Case 5) (3). Granular change is grossly visible in the gray matter, appearing as a yellowish zone or an actual horizontal cleft in the cortex. A characteristic intermediate vascular scar or subtotal cortical necrosis is seen. The globus pallidus usually shows a central cystic defect or a yellow vascular scar.

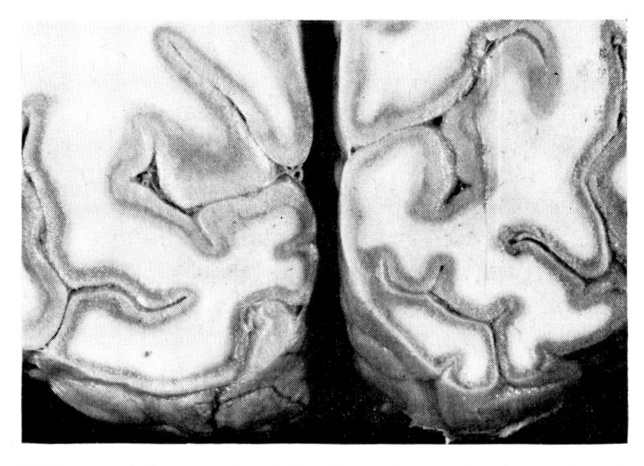

Fig. 79—Diffuse laminar necrosis incident to cerebral anoxia after nitrous oxide anesthesia. Survival period of 26 days.

Histologically, the layer of cortical necrosis is characteristic. A diffuse vascular scar of variable width is made up of a meshwork of new capillaries. In this zone, even though the gross conformation of the cortex has been preserved, the nerve cells have largely disappeared. In less damaged areas, some of the nervous elements may be seen in the superficial and deep zones, particularly in reduced silver preparations. Proliferation of astrocytes continues in the subpial glial and deep layers of the cortex, as well as in the underlying white matter.

Central demyelinization has been observed early in this stage in one or two cases.

Chronic residuals of asphyxia incident to nitrous oxide anesthesia are not well known, because seriously asphyxiated patients do not survive very long. One case verified at autopsy was that of Steegmann (1939) (38), who studied the brain of an asphyxiated patient who survived for 16 months. Vascular scars in the cortical laminae and globus pallidus and extensive demyelination of the cerebral centrum (chiefly the posterior portion) were noted. Observation of the pneumoencephalograms of another patient who survived for over 20 years revealed irregular cortical atrophy, specifically in the parieto-occipital region (Courville, et al., 1953) (36).

Cyclopropane is a gaseous general anesthetic agent which rarely provokes cerebral anoxia. One case was reported by Gebauer and Coleman in 1938 (39). Cerebral damage due to cyclopropane is probably best accounted for by circulatory failure, rather than any asphyxial qualities of the gas. The effects on the cerebral cortex and basal ganglia appear to be identical to those of nitrous oxide.

Acetylene, once used for illumination and anesthesia, is now employed chiefly in welding and in many organic syntheses. It acts as a simple asphyxiant unless mixed with oxygen, when some degree of narcosis seems evident. Excitement followed by coma, cyanosis, weak and irregular pulse, and memory failure have been described in man following inhalation of the gas (Fairhall, 1949) (40). The toxic action of this gas was first recognized in industry rather than in anesthesia. Holtzmann (1928) (41) described the case of a welder using hydrogen-acetylene who became acutely ill and died after four days. At necropsy, there was early pneumonia and symmetrical softening and hemorrhage in the brain, which confirm its asphyxial action.

Commercial acetylene may contain arsine, hydrogen sulfide, and phosphine. The presence of these impurities may explain some cases of poisoning (Fairhall, 1949) (40). Other types of poisoning may also occur in welders if the material worked upon is vaporized by the welding flame (Hamilton and Hardy, 1949) (6).

The Indirect Asphyxiants

The chief anoxic action of the indirect asphyxiant gases is their irritation of the membranes lining the air passages and pulmonary alveoli. The asphyxiant action of these gases is threefold: (1) they replace oxygen in inspired air (usually of secondary importance), (2) they produce swelling of the membranes lining the air passages and edema of the lungs and, at times, (3) they produce respiratory standstill through their irritant action on the trachea and bronchi. The second of these is of greatest importance in the production of asphyxia. Swelling of the membranes with secondary inflammation results in mechanical occlusion of the air passages, and edema of the lungs prevents an adequate interchange of oxygen and carbon dioxide through the alveolar walls. There is danger of the patient drowning in his own secretions.

For practical purposes, this group of noxious gases may be divided into (1) the industrial gases and (2) the war gases. The industrial gases are hydrogen sulfide, sulfur dioxide and ammonia. The more common gases used in World War I were dichlorethyl sulfide ("mustard gas"), chlorine gas, and phosgene. These will not be discussed in this chapter, because they are not likely to be encountered in a forensic situation.

The Industrial Asphyxiants. Hydrogen sulfide, the familiar "rotten egg" gas of chemical laboratories, is almost as toxic as hydrogen cyanide (Haggard, 1925; Yant, 1930) (42, 43). This gas, produced by sulfur-containing organic materials, is best known in connection with the putrefaction of dead animals. It is also formed in coal mines when iron pyrites decompose or following blasting operations, in sulfur mines, and in oil fields and refineries where sulfur petroleum is processed. Workmen in sewers and sewerage plants have been killed by hydrogen sulfide (Fairhall, 1949; Hamilton and Hardy, 1949) (40, 6), sometimes when acid was added to sewer lines (Freireich, 1946; Hurwitz and Taylor, 1954) (44, 45). Other trades dangerous in this regard are tanning, glue-making, fur-dressing, felt-making, meat packing, beet sugar manufacturing and, particularly, manufacturing of artificial silk by the viscose process.

Acute poisoning with hydrogen sulfide is characterized by direct and rapid paralysis of the respiratory centers (Haggard, 1925) (42). In low concentrations, it depresses the nervous system. In higher concentrations, stimulation supervenes with resultant hyperpnea. As inhalation continues, hyperpnea increases and terminates in respiratory failure (carbon dioxide content of blood is lowered, with resultant apnea vera). It has not been possible to find a report on the neuropathological changes observed in fatal hydrogen sulfide poisoning.

Subacute poisoning is characterized by irritation of the conjunctiva and respiratory passages due to the formation of sodium in these membranes. Part of such alkaline sulfide formed enters the blood stream and is hydrolized to liberate hydrogen sulfide again. In the blood this is rapidly oxidized to sodium sulfate. Systemic poisoning will not occur if the capacity to detoxify is not exceeded.

Union with hemoglobin does not occur. Spectroscopic examination of the blood is unreliable in suspected acute poisoning by this agent. Combination with methemoglobin occurs readily and accounts for the bluish green color seen in cadavers. There is no significant absorption of hydrogen sulfide through the skin.

Sulfur dioxide is an intensely irritative asphyxiant gas. It is produced when sulfur is burned. In the liquid state, it is used as a refrigerant, fungicide and fumigant, to bleach wool, straw and wood pulp, and in petroleum refining. It is a by-product of the smelting of lead, iron, zinc, and copper ores containing sulfur (Fairhall, 1949; Hamilton and Hardy, 1949) (40, 6). Fatalities are rare.

Sulfur dioxide is probably an important and sometimes dangerous irritant in fog and smog. It is injurious to vegetation. Bronchitis, bronchopneumonia and edema of the respiratory tract and lungs have been reported after exposure, which has sometimes caused death. Concentrations of 400 to 500 parts per million of air are dangerous even with short exposure (Henderson and Haggard, 1943) (1). The effects of sulfur dioxide in the nervous system have not been described in the medical literature, but there is no reason to suppose that the changes following acute exposure would be different from those of asphyxia due to other causes.

Ammonia is another irritant gas which does not act directly on the nervous system. In high concentrations, its reflex action on the upper respiratory tract produces cessation of respiration (Henderson and Haggard, 1943) (1). Most of the reported deaths from ammonia gassing resulted from pulmonary edema and bronchopneumonia. In 13 deaths following leakage of ammonia into an air raid shelter in London during World War II, toxic and degenerative changes in the liver and kidneys were described. Unfortunately, the nervous system was not studied (Caplin, 1941) (46).

Other Asphyxiant Agents

Cerebral anoxia is produced by many mechanisms in addition to the asphyxiant gases, although the changes in the brain follow a characteristic gross and microscopic pattern. The other mechanisms by which anoxia is produced are outlined in Table IV.

The important aspect in the comprehension of these mechanisms is the recognition of the disastrous results of inadequate oxygenation of the brain. The essential differences in the end-results of anoxia are dependent upon (1) the speed with which anoxemia develops, (2) the extent to which it develops, (3) its constancy, (4) the multiplicity of anoxic factors working at one time, and (5) the degree and persistence of concomitant vasomotor dysfunction. The total picture of cerebral anoxia has never been fully understood because of the complexity of these five factors.

Table IV

Mechanisms by which Anoxia Occurs

A. Birth Process (paranatal anoxia)
B. Mechanical Asphyxiation
    1. Throttling (hanging)
    2. Drowning
    3. Plugging of upper air passages with bolus of food
    4. Pulmonary diseases (pneumonia, asthma)
    5. Congenital cardiac disease
C. Failure of Circulation, Respiration
    1. Prolonged shock
    2. Cardiorespiratory failure or standstill (especially under anesthesia, anterior poliomyelitis)
    3. Exsanguination
D. Histotoxic Anoxia
    1. Narcotic poisoning (sedatives and opiates)
    2. Cyanide poisoning
    3. Hyperinsulinism (insulin shock) or hypoglycemia (oxyachristia)

Summary

Noxious gases or vapors which produce untoward manifestations in man may be divided into the direct asphyxiants, whose toxic effects are due mainly to replacement of oxygen, and the indirect asphyxiants, whose toxic effects result from absorption of poison through the air passages. There are three types of direct asphyxiants: simple asphyxiants (smoke, fumes, and inert gases), chemical asphyxiants (carbon monoxide and cyanide gas), and central depressants (the anesthetic gases).

The primary effect of the simple asphyxiants is the exclusion of oxygen from the lungs. The chemical asphyxiants produce anoxia either by preventing the transportation of oxygen in the blood stream or by interfering with its utilization by the nerve cells of the brain. The central depressants produce anoxia by direct narcotic action on the cortex and basal ganglia, or by the precipitation of cerebral or respiratory failure and superimposition of other types of anoxia.

The indirect asphyxiants are divided into the industrial gases and the war gases. The most common industrial gases are hydrogen sulfide, sulfur dioxide, and ammonia.

In acute asphyxiation (survival up to two weeks), the brain is severely congested, with focal hemorrhages in the leptomeninges and white matter. Distention of the small blood vessels, perivascular hemorrhages and acute changes in the nerve cells occur. The parenchymatous elements and the Purkinje cells may also show acute change. Focal or laminar necrosis of the cortex and central necrosis of the basal ganglia are often associated with proliferation of the endothelium of the small blood vessels.

In the subacute stage (two to six weeks), a variety of cerebral lesions develop. Congestion may be present and focal cortical and subcortical softening may be seen. The cerebral cortex may have a diffuse granular appearance or may show a thin yellow zone of necrosis. Usually, softening of some portion of the basal ganglia will be found. Patchy, focal, laminar or subtotal necrosis occur in the cerebral cortex, with changes in the astrocytes and microglia, and proliferation of the vascular endothelium. The arterioles of the lenticular nucleus may contain rings of calcium or iron. The unmyelinated cortical nerve fibers, the myelinated sheaths of the corticofugal nerve fibers, and the white matter may show degenerative changes. The Purkinje cells may be changed and reduced in number. Deterioration of the granule cell layer may also occur.

The residuals of severe anoxia may be only minor, diffuse leptomeningeal thickening and cortical nerve cell loss, or they may be irregular cortical atrophy, cyst formation due to focal softenings, and central softening and demyelination. Microscopically, the cytological alterations observed in the subacute stage are present, as are iron deposits in the nerve cells.

REFERENCES

1. Henderson, Y., and Haggard, H. W.: Noxious Gases and the Principles of Respiration Influencing Their Actions. American Chemical Society Monograph Series, No. 35, 2nd ed. New York, Reinhold Publ. Corp., 1943.
2. Preti, L.: Industrial Poisoning by Inhalation. J. Indust. Hyg. 7:124–143 (Mar.) 1925.
3. Courville, Cyril B.: Contributions to the Study of Cerebral Anoxia. Some Observations on Its History, Its Mechanics and Nature, the Im-

portance of Its Circulatory Component and Its Significance in the Evaluation of Certain Chronic Diseases of the Brain of Infancy and Early Childhood. Los Angeles, San Lucas Press, 1953.
4. Patty, F. A.: Industrial Hygiene and Toxicology. New York, Interscience Publ., Inc., Vol. I, 1948, Vol. II, 1949.
5. Chajes, B.: Firemen in Occupation and Health. Am. Encyclopedia of Hyg., Path. & Soc. Welfare, Geneva, International Labor Office, 1930, pp. 755–759.
6. Hamilton, A., and Hardy, H. L.: Industrial Toxicology. New York, Paul B. Hoeber, Inc., 1949.
7. Dutra, F. R.: Medicolegal Examination of Bodies Recovered from Burned Buildings. Am. J. Clin. Path. 19:599–607 (July) 1949.
8. Gonzales, T. A., Vance, M., and Helpern, M.: Legal Medicine and Toxicology. New York, Appleton-Century Co., 1937.
9. Committee on Aviation Toxicology. Aero-Medical Association: Aviation Toxicology. New York, The Blakiston Co., 1953.
10. Thorner, M. W., and Lewy, F. H.: Effects of Repeated Anoxia on Brain; Histopathologic Study. JAMA 115:1595–1600 (Nov. 9) 1940.
11. Lucas, B. G. B., and Strangeways, D. H.: The Effect of Intermittent Anoxia on the Brain. J. Path. & Bact. 64:265–271 (Apr.) 1952.
12. Manholes as Mantraps. Annotation. Lancet 1:1120–1121 (May 29) 1954.
13. Lewin, L.: Die Geschichte der Kohlenoxydvergiftung. Arch. f. Gesch. d. Med. 3:1–35, 1909.
14. Fisher, R. S.: How the Pathologist Can Aid the Arson Investigator. J. Crim. Law & Criminol. 43:237–245, 1952.
15. Dutra, F. R.: Cerebral Residua of Acute Carbon Monoxide Poisoning. Am. J. Clin. Path. 22:925–935 (Oct.) 1952.
16. Hiller, F.: Ueber die krankhaften Veränderungen in Zentralnervensystem nach Kohlenoxydvergiftung. Ztschr. f. d. ges. Neurol. u. Psychiat. 93:594–646, 1924.
17. Herzog, F.: Cited by Hiller.
18. Kolisko, A.: Die symmetrische Encephalomalacia in den Linsenkernen nach Kohlenoxydgasvergiftung. Beitr. gericht. Med. 2:1–6, 1914.
19. Grinker, R. R.: Über einen Fall von Leuchtgasvergiftung mit doppelseitiger Pallidumerweichung und schwerer Degeneration des tieferen Grosshirnmarklagers. Ztschr. f. d. ges. Neurol. u. Psychiat. 98:433–456, 1925.
20. Meyer, A.: Experimentelle Erfahrungen über die Kohlenoxydvergiftung des Zentralnervensystems. Ztschr. f. d. ges. Neurol. u. Psychiat. 112:187–212, 1928.
21. Hsu, Y. K., and Ch'Eng, Y. L.: Cerebral Subcortical Myelinopathy in Carbon Monoxide Poisoning. Brain 61:384–392 (Dec.) 1938.
22. Skolnick, M. H.: Asphyxia as a Factor in Paresis; Medicolegal Significance. J. Michigan M. Soc. 35:455–457 (July) 1936.
23. Ehrich, W. E., Bellet, S., and Lewey, F. H.: Cardiac Changes from CO Poisoning. Am. J. M. Sc. 208:511–523 (Oct.) 1944.
24. Rogers, H.: Carbon Monoxide Diabetes; Report of a Case. Calif. & West. Med. 34:411–412 (June) 1931.

25. Killick, E. M.: Carbon Monoxide Anoxemia. Physiol. Rev. 20:313–344 (July) 1940.
26. Von Oettingen, W. F.: Toxicity and Potential Dangers of Aliphatic and Aromatic Hydrocarbons. A Critical Review of the Literature. Pub. Health Bull. No. 255:1–135, 1940.
27. The Investigation of Gas Poisoning and Asphyxiations Resulting from the Use of Gas Heating Appliances in Los Angeles and Vicinity. (Report of Technical Subcommittee of the Mayor's Committee, Los Angeles, possibly printed in 1926.)
28. Walker, J. T.: Medical Progress. Toxicology. New England J. Med. 242:22–25, 56–61 (Jan.) 1950.
29. Jedlowski, P.: Sull' encefalomielopatia sperimentale da cianuro di potassio. Riv. pat. nerv. e. ment. 51:231–275 (Mar.–Apr.) 1938.
30. Löwenberg, K., Waggoner, R., and Zbinden, T.: Destruction of the Cerebral Cortex Following Nitrous Oxide-Oxygen Anesthesia. Ann. Surg. 104:801–810 (Nov.) 1936.
31. Courville, Cyril B.: Asphyxia as a Consequence of Nitrous Oxide Anesthesia. Medicine 15:129–245 (May) 1936.
32. ———: The Pathogenesis of Necrosis of the Cerebral Gray Matter Following Nitrous Oxide Anesthesia. Ann. Surg. 107:371–379 (Mar.) 1938.
33. ———: Untoward Effects of Nitrous Oxide Anesthesia, With Particular Reference to Residual Neurologic and Psychiatric Manifestations. Mountain View, Calif., Pacific Press. Publ. Assn., 1939.
34. ———: Cerebral Anoxia and Its Residuals. M. Arts & Sc. 1:16, 35, 68 (Apr., July, Oct.) 1947; 2: 67–79 (Apr.) 1948.
35. ———: Contributions to the Study of Cerebral Anoxia. I. Asphyxia in Legend, Folklore and History. II. The Mechanism and Nature of Consequent Structural Alterations. III. Neonatal Asphyxia and Its Relation to Certain Degenerative Diseases of the Brain in Infancy and Childhood. Bull. Los Angeles Neurol. Soc. 15:99–195 (Sept.) 1950.
36. ———, Sanchez-Perez, J. M., and Amyes, E. W.: Prolonged Survival After Cerebral Anoxia Incident to Nitrous Oxide Anesthesia. Report of Clinical Follow-up After an Interval of Twenty-two Years. Bull. Los Angeles Neurol. Soc. 18:136–140 (Sept.) 1953.
37. Fletcher, D. E.: Personality Disintegration Incident to Anoxia; Observations with Nitrous Oxide Anesthesia. J. Nerv. & Ment. Dis. 102:392–403 (Oct.) 1945.
38. Steegmann, A. T.: Encephalopathy Following Anesthesia; Histologic Study of Four Cases. Arch. Neurol. & Psychiat. 41:955–977 (May) 1939.
39. Gebauer, P. W., and Coleman, F. P.: Postanesthetic Encephalopathy Following Cyclopropane. Ann. Surg. 107:481–485 (Apr.) 1938.
40. Fairhall, L. T.: Industrial Toxicology. Baltimore, The Williams & Wilkins Co., 1949.
41. Holtzmann, F.: Gefahr bein Schwiesse mit Acetylensauerstoff. Zentralbl. f. Gewerbehyg. 5:233 (Aug.) 1928.

42. Haggard, H. W.: The Toxicology of Hydrogen Sulphide. J. Indust. Hyg. 7:113–121 (Mar.) 1925.
43. Yant, W. P.: Hydrogen Sulphide in Industry; Occurrence, Effects, and Treatment. Am. J. Pub. Health 20:598–608 (June) 1930.
44. Freireich, A. W.: Hydrogen Sulfide Poisoning; Report of Two Cases, One with Fatal Outcome, from Associated Mechanical Asphyxia. Am. J. Path. 22:147–155 (Jan.) 1946.
45. Hurwitz, L. J., and Taylor, G. I.: Poisoning by Sewer Gas with Unusual Sequelae. Lancet 1:1110–1112 (May 29) 1954.
46. Caplin, M.: Ammonia-Gas Poisoning; 47 Cases in a London Shelter. Lancet 2:95–96 (July 26) 1941.

Chapter XII. The Alcohols*

Alcoholism in its various forms is the most common poisoning known. The number of cases of alcohol poisoning exceed those of all other types of intoxications. Because of its effects on the human organism, alcoholic intoxication is one of the greatest of all hazards to life and health. This is true not only because of the direct effect of alcohol on the tissues and organs of the body, and the number of diseased states to which it predisposes, but also because of certain indirect effects incident to physical violence. It has been pointed out (Umiker, 1949) (1) that fatalities from acute alcoholism may either result directly from alcoholic intoxication or indirectly from some complication incident to aspiration of a foreign body, from accidental injury, from homicide or suicide, from an accentuation of the effects of some other poison, from certain infections (notably pneumonia), or from the exaggeration of existing disease. In chronic alcoholism death may be indirectly due to the effects of trauma to the head (e. g., chronic subdural hematoma), cirrhosis of the liver, or malnutrition, or directly due to changes in the central nervous system.

Major attention will be directed in this chapter to the effects of intoxication with ethyl alcohol ingested in the form of beverages. Poisoning incident to methyl alcohol and to higher alcohols, which are of interest only as occasional accidental or industrial intoxications, will be discussed only briefly.

Methyl and the Higher Alcohols

Poisoning with Methyl Alcohol—The effects of methyl alcohol on the nervous system are much the same as those of

* This chapter is a revision of a paper by Dr. Richard O. Myers and the author published in the Bulletin of the Los Angeles Neurological Society, Vol. 19, No. 2, June, 1954, pp. 66–95.

ethyl alcohol, except for the greater toxicity and the specific action of methyl alcohol on the ganglion cells of the eye (Pick and Bielschowsky, 1912) (2). This toxicity is not due to impurities in the alcohol, as was once suspected, but to its inherent nature. A distinguishing feature is its slow elimination (incident to slow oxidation) from the nervous tissues. In fatal cases of acute poisoning, variable degrees of tenseness of the dura mater are noted on removal of the calvarium. The brain usually shows an increase in weight (cerebral edema). There is either an excess of fluid in the subarachnoid space ("wet brain") or a flattening of the convolutions ("dry brain"), with some degree of herniation of the cerebellar tonsils into the foramen magnum. The small pial vessels are markedly engorged.

Microscopically, there is a variable degree of edema and hyperemia of the cerebral tissues (Menne, 1938) (3). The small blood vessels in the cortex are engorged. The perivascular spaces, and at times the pericellular spaces, are widened. The nerve cells show central chromatolysis, the remaining tigroid granules being ragged and frayed. Even in young individuals who survive, lipochrome pigment is deposited in the cells. The margins of the cells are often irregular, the nuclei at times being eccentric in position. Perinuclear vacuoles appear and rupture of the nuclear membranes also occurs. With survival for some days, the pericellular and perivascular oligodendrocytes are increased. In all cases these elements are acutely swollen. The neuroglia remain essentially unchanged. The brain stem and cerebellum are edematous, with variable degrees of chromatolysis of the Purkinje cells. Early degeneration of the granule cells of the cerebellar cortex may also occur.

In more severe poisoning, extensive degeneration of the pyramidal nerve cells and vascular endothelium has been observed, as well as petechial hemorrhages in the midbrain, pons, and medulla (Weil, 1933) (4).

Alterations in the retina and the optic nerves and chiasm are particularly noteworthy. Punctate hemorrhages may also be seen in the optic chiasm. Microscopically, extravasations of erythrocytes are found about the blood vessels. The optic nerves are hyperemic and edematous. The nerve cells in the ganglion cell layer of the retina are irregularly stained, the cellular outlines are frayed, and there is central chromatolysis, at times associated with vacuolization. These alterations occur particularly in the vicinity of the optic disc (Menne, 1938) (3).

Propyl, Caprylic, Allyl, and Iso-amyl Alcohol—Intoxication with these higher alcohols usually occurs as an industrial hazard but cases of fatal intoxication are rare. It has been observed that the degree of toxicity of these alcohols increases with the size of the molecule (Richardson's law). In fatal cases the brain is congested (Patty, et al., 1936) (5). The alterations in the nerve cells are probably the same as in methyl alcohol poisoning.

General Pathology of Alcoholism

In cases of death from acute alcoholism, the changes in the viscera are chiefly due to congestion and edema. The stomach may be hemorrhagic, as well as hyperemic, and in extreme cases, ulceration of the mucosa may occur. The liver and kidneys may be congested; the renal epithelium may show cloudy swelling. The lungs are congested and focal hemorrhages are frequently present; pink colored (blood stained) edema may be found in the alveola and smaller air passages (Wright, 1941) (6).

The postmortem findings in chronic alcoholism are more varied. Glossitis, stomatitis, chronic gastritis and, at times, peptic ulcer may be found. Fatty changes in the liver, heart muscle, and renal capsule, cirrhosis of the liver, and complications of these disorders constitute another group of post-alcoholic lesions (Edmondson, et al., 1956) (7). Chronic pancreatitis with calculi, chronic malnutrition, and possibly the so-called "fatty heart" and arteriosclerosis are at times residuals of chronic alcoholism.

Renal disease with uremia may be an indirect effect of cirrhosis. Less important are changes in the skin (e. g., xerosis conjunctivae, "red nose", cyanotic rhinophyma, acute edema, erythromelalgia), muscles (polymyositis alcoholica), joints (swelling), and bones (yellow eccentric bone atrophy) (Petri, 1930) (8).

Actions of Alcohol on the Nervous System

The actions of alcohol differ greatly in intensity, in sequence, and in the nature of the physical responses evoked in the various tissues. These actions are immediate and direct or delayed and indirect.

The direct action of alcohol on the nervous tissues is first of all *narcotic,* inhibiting the functions of individual cells. Alcohol increases the permeability of the cell membranes, which retards the conduction of electrical charges on the surface of the cells. *Metabolically,* it acts by modifying the viscosity of cytoplasm, to which the cellular activity is directly related. The inhibitory mechanism seems to be due to an interference with oxidation—a type of histotoxic anoxia. Since the metabolism is dependent upon the supply of glucose and vitamin B as well as of oxygen, the excessive use of alcohol interferes with cellular metabolism in any of these three ways. The resultant changes may be irreversible.

Circulatory changes in the form of congestion and hemorrhage produce stagnant anoxia, which is aggravated by edema and accentuated by any alteration in the blood vessels themselves (endothelial proliferation).

Indirectly, the action of alcohol on the nervous tissues is the result of *vitamin deficiency.* Thiamin deficiency results in peripheral neuropathy similar to beriberi. A lack of niacin favors the development of a pellagra-like state. Wernicke's hemorrhagic encephalopathy, which has been produced experimentally in pigeons (Alexander, 1940) (9), has also been considered to be due to a vitamin B deficiency.

Anemia is another less common indirect effect of alcohol. Changes in the spinal cord, which appear to be identical with those resulting from pernicious anemia, occur apparently from secondary atrophic gastritis with resultant deficiency of hydrochloric acid.

Association with other poisons, either introduced through methods of preparation of the beverage or accidentally ingested (carbon tetrachloride, nitroglycerine, phosphorous, nitrobenzene, aniline, mercury, lead, carbon disulfide, and phenol), reinforces the action of alcohol. Courville (1936, 1939) (10, 11) described the disturbing association of alcohol and general anesthetic agents such as ether or nitrous oxide. Jetter and McLean (1943) (12) described "knock-out drops", commonly formed by adding phenobarbital to alcohol.

Cerebral Changes in Acute Alcoholism

The effects of acute alcoholism are usually transitory, although a number of fatal poisonings by ethyl alcohol have occurred, especially in children. The acute effects may be serious because of indirect or associated results, and because of the cumulative effects of repeated insults to the kidneys, the liver, and the brain.

The gross alterations in the brain in acute alcoholism are neither remarkable nor characteristic. Marked congestion, excessive subarachnoid fluid, and a characteristic odor are apparent (Lesser, in Petri, 1930) (8). Some investigators believe the type of beverage consumed can be determined by the odor present.

Congestion of both the arterial and venous pial vessels is usually marked in the unfixed brain. The small pial network stands out and is often associated with focal subpial hemorrhages. When sectioned, the cortex and basal ganglia have a dark purplish hue from an increase in blood cells. The larger superficial veins and those in the cerebral white matter stand out. Petechial hemorrhages are often prominent in the cerebral white matter, but this is uncommon unless craniocerebral trauma or pneumonia has occurred as a complicating factor. The choroid plexus is also turgid and its vessels are prominent.

Hemorrhage into the meninges and brain in fatal cases of acute alcoholism is not unusual. In most instances focal subarachnoid bleeding may be regarded as an accentuation of severe congestion. On the other hand, subdural hemorrhage or hematoma, widespread subarachnoid hemorrhage, or gross bleeding into the brain is usually dependent upon an intercurrent injury to the head. When craniocerebral trauma occurs in individuals under the influence of alcohol, bleeding is always excessive and beyond what would ordinarily result. This excessive bleeding may determine the fatal outcome of the case. Encapsulated subdural hemorrhage, with repeated bleeding (pachymeningitis hemorrhagica interna) is a result of trauma when associated with chronic alcoholism. In rare instances some other predisposing factor, such as a lack of vitamin C or K or associated liver damage may be responsible for initiating the bleeding.

Edema of the brain is manifested by excessive free fluid in the subarachnoid space. "Weeping" through the arachnoid into the subdural space sometimes occurs, especially if trauma is a factor. The brain drips fluid in excess as it is removed from the cranial cavity ("wet brain"). The convolutions may show some degree of flattening and the cortex may feel boggy. The ventricles may be dilated due to excess fluid.

Microscopic alterations in the brain in acute alcoholism are not characteristic. They are usually minor and confined to the nerve cells, the oligodendroglia, the ependyma and choroid plexus, and the blood vessels (Fig. 80). The alterations in the nerve cells are acute swelling with tigrolysis of the central portions of the cells, early stages of pyknosis with condensation of the cytoplasm and shrinkage of the cell body, or mild edema with the formation of vacuoles in the nucleus. The pericellular spaces may be enlarged. The oligodendroglia are acutely swollen, and appear in routine sections as rounded nuclei with clear "halos" through the cortex. All these changes are indicative of acute circulatory changes in the cerebral tissues.

The *vascular changes* consist of dilatation and engorgement of the capillaries and veins of the leptomeninges and choroid plexus. Diapedesis of erythrocytes may be evident, especially in the vicinity of the pial vessels. Tiny vacuoles may be seen in the endothelial cells under higher magnification, but these are not conspicuous.

Alterations in the ependyma and choroid plexus are noteworthy. The epithelial cells are increased in size (especially in their vertical diameter) and an increased number of them

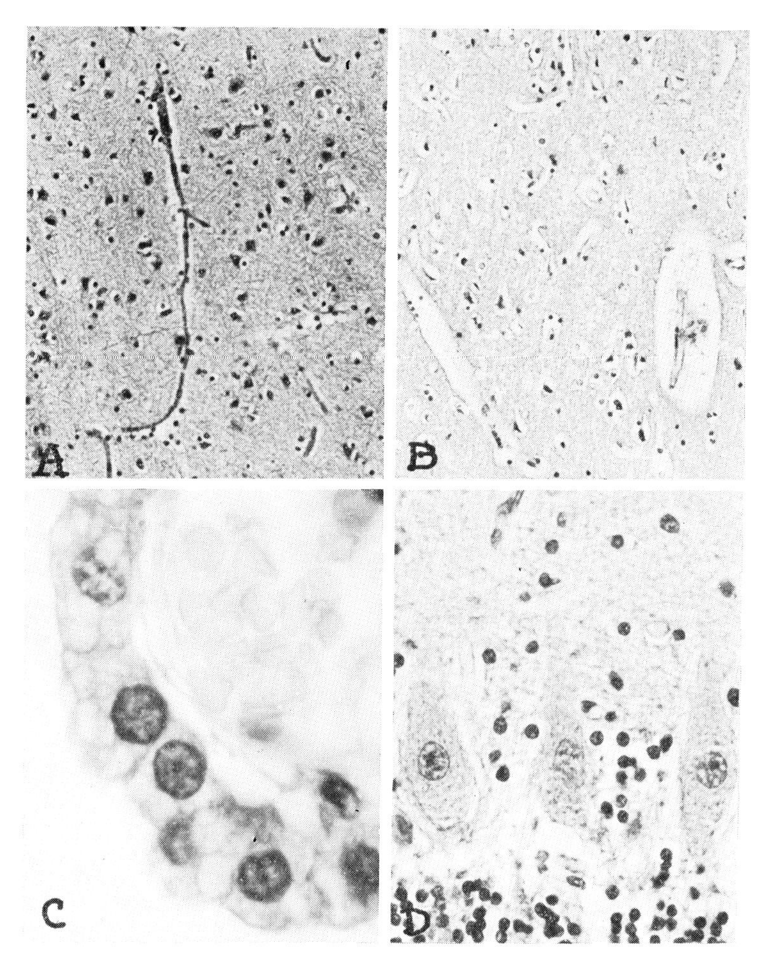

Fig. 80—Histological changes in the brain in acute alcoholism. A. Congestion of small cortical vessels. H & E × 100. B. Edema of cerebral cortex. H & E × 100. C. Increased vacuolization of cells of choroid plexus. H & E ×1100. D. Acute swelling of the Purkinje cells of the cerebellar cortex. H & E × 285.

contain vacuoles or meshworks of small droplets in their cytoplasm. The nuclei may also contain vacuoles. Irregular spaces beneath the basement membrane and the individual cells, or in the stroma itself suggest collections of fluid in the pedicle of this structure. The blood vessels are filled with closely packed red cells. Diapedesis into the regional perivascular spaces is sometimes observed.

Alterations in the Brain in Delirium Tremens

The condition commonly known as "delirium tremens" may be defined as an acute psychotic episode, characterized by delirium and hallucinations, occurring in the course of an alcoholic bout in a chronic alcoholic. This acute episode is superimposed on a chronic substrate.[1] Acute and reversible alterations in the nerve cells, associated with chronic alterations in the nervous system, are generally found at autopsy in these cases.

Alterations in the cortical nerve cells in delirium tremens are of three types: (1) pyknotic change in the small pyramidal cells of the superficial cellular layers, (2) acute swelling of the large pyramidal cells of the deeper layers, and (3) progressive deterioration of the intermediate pyramidal cells leading to patchy cell loss. Pyknosis of the small pyramidal cells of the superficial layers is characterized by shrinkage of the cells in their long axis, pinkish purple cytoplasm which sometimes obscures the deep purple contracted nuclei, and twisted apical dendrites (Fig. 81). The perivascular spaces seem to be enlarged.

The larger nerve cells of the deeper layers of the motor cortex show swelling and chromatolysis. The tigroid granules appear as faint blotches in the cytoplasm, which has a boiled or coagulated appearance. There are small vacuoles in the cytoplasm and larger ones in the nuclei.

Patchy, progressive deterioration of the intermediate pyramidal cells results in the formation of "ghost cells" and the ultimate disappearance of the cells.

Increased perineuronal glial elements (satellitosis), increased perivascular oligodendrocytes, early proliferative

---

[1] Edmondson, et al. (1956) (7), pointed out the invariable association, at least in fatal cases, of fatty disease of the liver with alcoholism in cases of delirium tremens. They suggest that this clinical syndrome may be the combination of the effects of an acute alcoholic episode and some disturbance of liver function, possibly an inability to use glycogen.

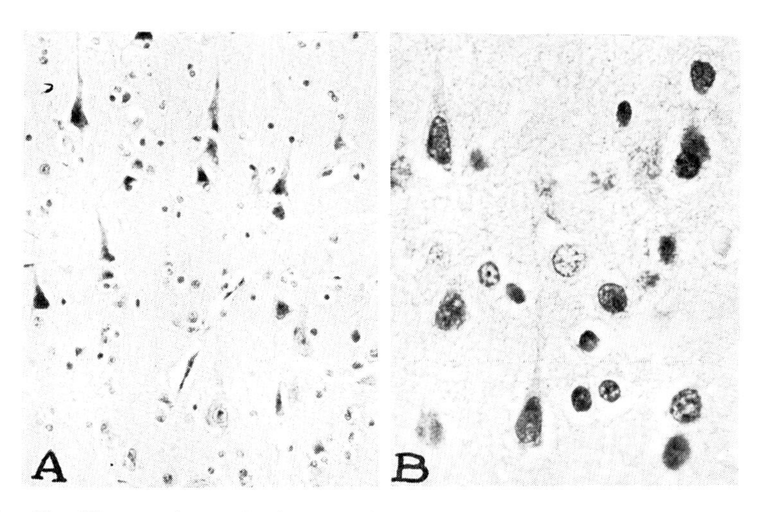

Fig. 81—Changes in cerebral cortex in a patient who died in the course of delirium tremens. A. Low power view showing pyknotic change in small superficial pyramidal cells. H & E × 125. B. High power view showing details of this change. H & E × 500.

changes in the endothelium of the small blood vessels, fatty changes in the larger vessels (Petri, 1930) (8), and congestion and pericapillary hemorrhages may indicate the association of these alterations with those of Wernicke's encephalopathy. The Purkinje cells show loss of tigroid substance, shrinkage and darkening of their cytoplasm and nuclei, or progressive deterioration leading to loss of these cells. Degenerative changes in the nerve fibers of the cerebellar cortex, particularly the vermis, have also been observed.

Peripheral Neuropathy

The most common subacute or chronic change in the nervous system due to alcoholism is peripheral neuropathy. In most cases the structural changes are indistinguishable from those of beriberi (Shattuck, 1928) (13). It is generally assumed that they are actually induced by avitaminosis, but they may develop in spite of an adequate diet when certain wines (notably muscatel) are consumed (Courville, 1950) (14).

In advanced cases, changes in an affected nerve are grossly visible. The nerve appears smaller than normal, with an irregular contour. It is grayish yellow in color. On cross section under a hand lens it appears mottled, with intermingled foci of translucent (degenerated nerve fibers) and grayish matter (proliferated connective tissue).

Special stains reveal the medullary sheaths to be varicose or broken down into segments or balls of myelin, with interposed globules of free fat. In more advanced cases myelophages are loaded with the broken down myelin or fat. The axis cylinders persist longer but also become varicose, segmented, and ultimately broken down into lines of argentophilic granules. The sheath cells proliferate to form band fibers and, at times, there is irregular proliferation of the connective tissue stroma with or without regional collections of lymphocytes (Fig. 82).

Fig. 82—A. Changes in peripheral nerves in alcoholic neuropathology. H & E × 135. B. The same. Myelin sheath preparation × 135.

Alcoholic Atrophy of the Cerebral Cortex

One characteristic result of chronic alcoholism is atrophy of the convolutions of the upper dorsolateral surface of the frontal lobes and central area. Chronic alcoholism seems to be the most common cause of cortical atrophy in the fourth and fifth decades of life. It may appear early in the third decade in some individuals, particularly if psychotic manifestations have occurred. It is not so apt to occur in individuals with cirrhosis of the liver (question of more efficient detoxification).

The atrophy is uniform in the convolutions of the upper dorsolateral surface of the frontal lobes, but is not necessarily equal in both hemispheres. It later extends to the middle and lower frontal convolutions, then to the precentral and postcentral gyri, and finally into the superior parietal lobule (Fig. 83). Thickening and opacity of the overlying leptomeninges are usually associated changes, but are not as extensive as in senile atrophy or general paresis. Alcoholic pseudoparesis similar to general paresis sometimes occurs. It is

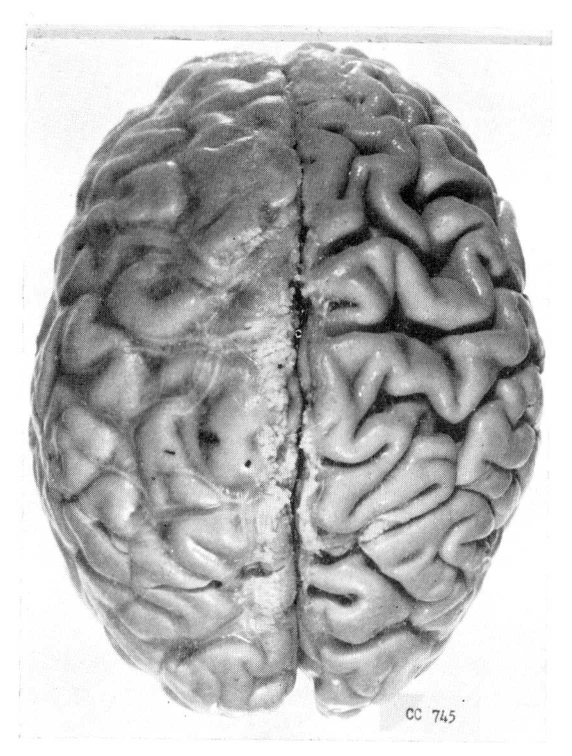

Fig. 83—Atrophy of cerebral cortex as a consequence of chronic alcoholism.

usually associated with the more profound atrophy seen in older individuals.

Microscopically, the architectural and cellular changes in the atrophic cortex are characteristic. There is a moderate proliferation of the cap cells and the fibrous elements of the leptomeninges. Acute swelling, chronic lipoidal change, and irregular loss of the smaller pyramidal cells of the superficial and intermediate laminae are typical (Fig. 84, A). These deficits are similar to those found in the brains of mentally defective, epileptic, and palsied children injured by asphyxia at birth. The nerve cells in or bordering these foci undergo progressive deterioration, becoming "ghost cells" before disappearing entirely (Fig. 84, B).

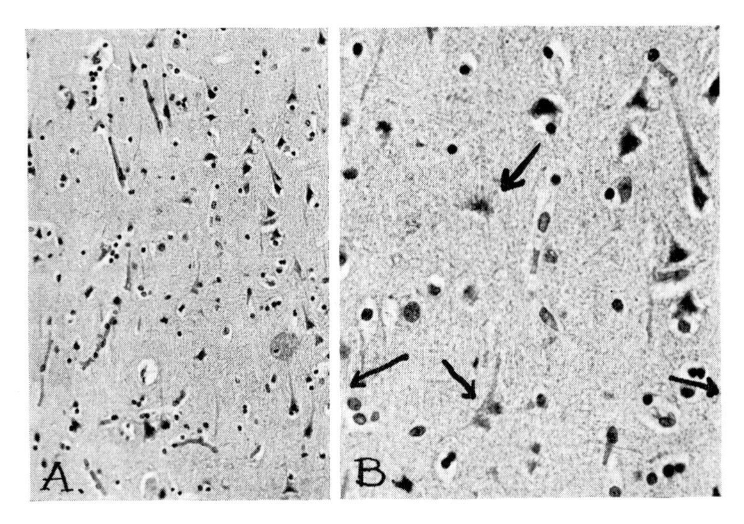

Fig. 84—Histopathology of alcoholic cerebral cortical atrophy. A. Patchy loss of nerve cells. H & E × 120. B. Progressive deterioration leading to formation of "ghost cells". H & E × 265.

There is an almost invariable satellitosis (microglia and oligodendroglia) about the larger nerve cells of the deeper cortical layers and the blood vessels of the white matter. An increase in astrocytes may occur, particularly in the cerebral centrum, but not to the degree encountered in general paresis.

Alterations in the small cortical blood vessels may be present if chronic alcoholism is complicated by hemorrhagic encephalopathy. Congestion, and even microscopic perivascular diapedesis, may be present if there was an acute ante mortem episode of alcoholism.

Korsakoff's Syndrome

This peculiar psychiatric syndrome is characterized by memory deficits and a tendency to confabulation. It is found most often in chronic alcoholics, and is presumed to be the direct result of alcoholism, particularly if associated with a consequent deficiency state. No gross changes occur in the brain, aside from cortical atrophy. Microscopically, excessive deposits of lipochrome are seen in the cortical nerve cells, the neuroglia and microglia, and in and about the blood vessels of the prefrontal and motor cortex (Carmichael and Stern, 1931) (15) (Fig. 85). There is loss of tigroid substance

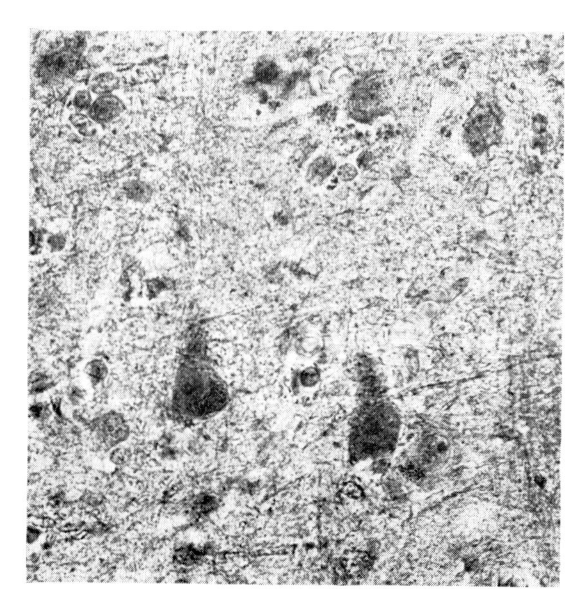

Fig. 85—Cerebral cortical changes in Korsakoff's psychosis. Deposits of lipid material in cortical nerve cells. Scarlet red preparation × 550.

in the Betz cells of the motor cortex. These alterations are sometimes associated with hemorrhagic encephalopathy (Gamper, 1928) (16). They are similar to those of alcoholic pellagra and are presumed to be due to some closely related, if not the same, process.

Alcoholic Pellagra

Leudet (1869) (17) suspected that alcohol often played an important part in the production of pellagra. Kraepelin (1887) (18) pointed out that the characteristic physical and psychic manifestations could not be attributed to alcohol alone. A distinction was made, therefore, between the genuine form and that consequent to chronic alcoholism (pseudopellagra). Tuczek (1882) (19) and Babes and Sion (1901) (20) were among the first to state that poor nutrition was an important predisposing factor. It has been shown that this disorder can be relieved by a diet rich in vitamins, particularly vitamin B.

The histological changes in the nervous system in fatal cases of pellagra have been studied by several investigators (Singer and Pollock, 1913; Ostertag, 1925; Winkelman, 1926; Pentschew, 1928) (21–24). Zimmerman, et al. (1934) (25), found consistent but nonspecific changes in the brain in three cases of the postalcoholic variety. No architectural alterations were found; the essential changes were cellular. Swelling of the cortical nerve cells, loss of tigroid substance, hyaline appearance of the cytoplasm, and eccentration of the nuclei were present in the larger nerve cells (particularly in the Betz cells of the motor cortex), the cells of the dentate nucleus, the nuclei of the fasciculi gracillus and cuneatus, the pontile nuclei, and the anterior horn of the spinal cord. Pyknotic and ischemic changes were found in the cerebral cortex (especially in the cells of Ammon's horn) and in the Purkinje cells of the cerebellum.

Most characteristic in this condition was the abundance of lipochrome pigment in the nerve cells. Large, well delineated, conglomerate masses of lipoidal globules were present in the perineuronal cytoplasm, obviously in excess of the pigment normally found in middle or late adult life.

This lipoidal pigment is similar to the substance found in increasing amounts in later adult life and senescence. This pigment is also found in excessive amounts in young individuals who survive for several days or more a severe asphyxial episode (Courville, 1936, 1939) (10, 11). This suggests that this lipoidal material results from an interference with the normal oxidative processes of the nerve cells. Whether due to a lack of oxygen (cerebral anoxia), a deficiency of vitamin B or some of its constituents, or a decreased supply of dextrose (hypoglycemia), the end result seems to be much the same.

Astroglial change, proliferation of endothelial elements, and hyalinization of the smaller blood vessels have been described. Peripheral neuropathy and subacute combined degeneration of the spinal cord, similar to that in primary anemia have been complicating factors (Pentschew, 1928) (24).

The cellular changes in the brain in postalcoholic pellagra can probably be attributed to a decrease in consumption of vitamin B or impairment of its assimilation consequent to chronic alcoholic gastritis (Zimmerman, et al., 1934) (25).

Hemorrhagic Encephalopathy

When Wernicke (1882) (26) described this syndrome he reported three cases of it. Two cases were postalcoholic and one followed pyloric stenosis caused by sulfuric acid poisoning. He found petechial hemorrhages of symmetrical distribution in the gray matter about the cerebral aqueduct and the floor of the fourth ventricle. The association of these changes with other complications of chronic alcoholism (peripheral neuropathy and changes in the spinal cord) was reported by Jacobäus in 1894 (27). Bonhoeffer (1889) (28) pointed out that these lesions were not inflammatory and that the syndrome was sometimes associated with delirium tremens or Korsakoff's psychosis. The limitation of the hemorrhages to the gray matter adjacent to the ventricular passages in a series of 22 cases was pointed out by Hunt (1906) (29). Creutzfeldt (1928) (30) noted that hemorrhagic foci in these locations were also associated at times with cellular changes in the cortex of the frontal lobes. The detailed descriptions of Gamper (1928) (16) and Neubürger (1931) (31) of the pathological picture of the disease are now generally considered as standard. Bender and Schilder (1933) (32) suggested that because the lesions were adjacent to the ventricles and cerebral aqueduct they were the result of some noxious agent in the cerebrospinal fluid. They concluded that the various clinical syndromes (extraocular palsy, cerebellar disturbances, acute catatonic states, delirium tremens, polioencephalitis with polyneuritis) were the result of lesions in specific locations. Bender (1934) (33) also reported that similar hemorrhagic lesions were sometimes found in the gray matter of the spinal cord. The frequency of the lesions in the various locations was reported by Campbell and Biggart in 1939 (34). The histological details were reported from the Cajal Laboratory by Bailey in 1946 (35).

The frequent association of hemorrhagic encephalopathy with chronic alcoholism has led to the presumption by some that this disorder is a specific postalcoholic syndrome. One of Wernicke's first cases, however, was due to malnutrition. Neubürger (1936, 1937) (36, 37) emphasized its occurrence in cases of gastric carcinoma and chronic gastritis. In their series of 12 cases, Campbell and Biggart (1939) (34) noted the typical findings in gastric carcinoma (three cases), severe anemia (two cases), hyperemesis (two cases), bronchiectasis and chronic myocardial failure, chronic pyosalpinx, chronic dyspepsia, and whooping cough. In only one of their cases was the patient a chronic alcoholic. The occurrence of hemorrhagic encephalopathy in the so-called human milk intoxication (Tanaka, 1934) (38) in Japan, where beriberi was common, and in other chronic diseases, such as Hodgkin's disease (Környey, 1932) (39) and pulmonary abscess and malaria (Neubürger, 1936) (36) suggests a deficiency syndrome.

The experimental production of these lesions in rats (Davison and Stone, 1937) (40) and pigeons (Alexander, 1940) (9) confirmed the work of Bender and Schilder (1933) (32) and Jolliffe, et al. (1941) (41), who believed them to be the result of a vitamin B deficiency. A lack of nicotinic acid (niacin) seems to be the most significant factor (41), although a lack of thiamin (ophthalmoplegia) and riboflavin, as well as a deficiency of carbohydrate, may all be significant.

The locations of the lesions as described by Campbell and Biggart (1939) (34) are generally accepted as correct. They found that the lesions are always present in the corpora mammillaria (100 per cent of cases), and in decreasing frequency in other hypothalamic nuclei, especially the nucleus parafasicularis (75 per cent), posterior colliculi (75 per cent), peri-aqueductal gray matter (particularly the oculomotor nuclei) (67 per cent), juxta-ventricular zone of the thalamus (especially of the medial nucleus) (58 per cent), floor of the fourth ventricle (particularly the vagus nuclei and anterior part of the corpus striatum) (25 per cent), anterior colliculi, habenular nuclei and cerebellar cortex (17 per cent), and substantia nigra (8.5 per cent). These lesions are usually bilateral and symmetrical.

The common pattern of hemorrhages of this condition is shown in the accompanying figure (Fig. 86).

The histological alterations are constant in type, but may vary in severity, distribution within an area, and stage of development. They consist of primary vascular changes, secondary reaction of the parenchymatous elements and, at times, a reaction of the interstitial cells. The vascular changes consist of congestion and hemorrhage, and proliferation of the endothelial cells of the small blood vessels, leading to irregularity in the lumina and partial occlusion. Bead-like swellings follow, on rare occasions, actual budding of newly formed capillaries. Some vessels may be dilated. Less often, proliferation of adventitia occurs, associated with increased reticulin in the arteriolar walls. Recanalization of blood vessels is sometimes observed in prolonged cases.

Focal hemorrhages in hemorrhagic encephalopathy are perivascular, ball or ring in type. They may be due to diapedesis or actual rupture of dilated, thin-walled capillaries. Thrombosis followed by focal glial reactions occurs rarely. (Neubürger, 1931 (31) described "pigmentary softening of the substantia nigra".) Occasionally, perivascular round cell infiltration is observed. These circulatory changes may lead to focal loosening of the interstitial tissues or even to their

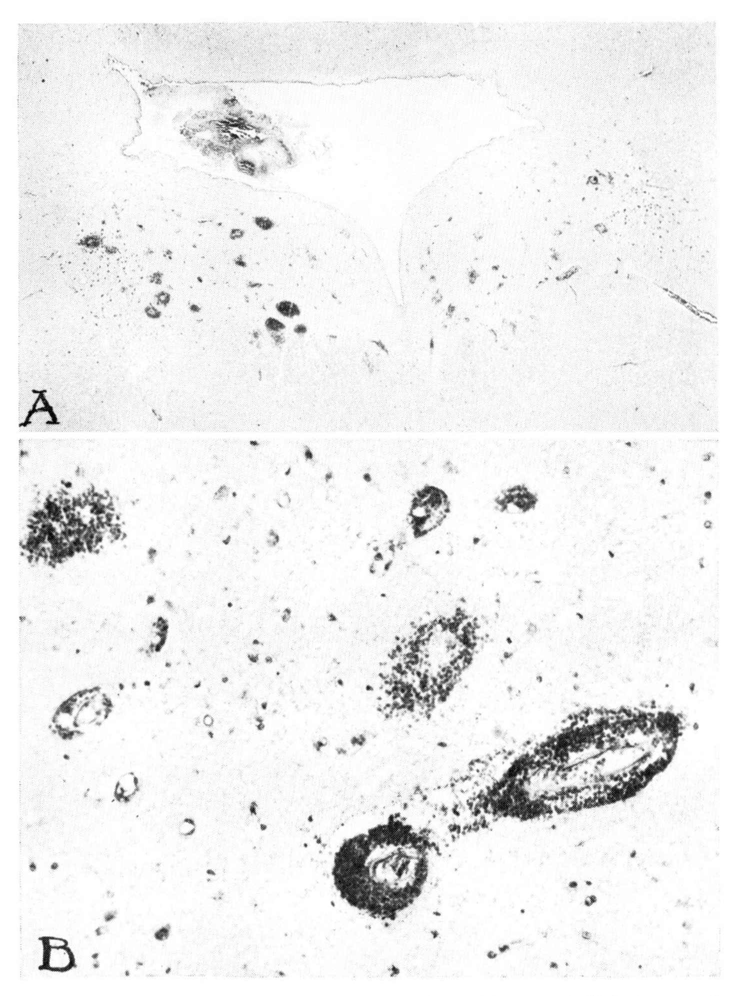

Fig. 86—Focal hemorrhages in brain stem in polioencephalitis hemorrhagica superior (Wernicke's disease). A. In gray matter below cerebral aqueduct. H & E × 7. B. Enlarged view of hemorrhages showing perivascular location of red cells. H & E × 250.

disorganization (pseudomalacia of Neubürger). Rarely, collections of compound granular corpuscles are seen.

The interstitial cells also show varying degrees of degenerative change. The reaction of the astrocytes is characteristically transformative, proliferative and then degenerative, depending on their relation to regional lesions. The microglia show early swelling of their cytoplasm, and in the presence of degenerative lesions and hemorrhage are transformed into compound granular corpuscles. At times, early changes in cells cause them to resemble rod cells. Glial nodules are occasionally seen.

Peripheral neuropathy and changes in the spinal cord (Bender, 1934) (33), as well as pyknosis and lipochrome alteration in the cortical nerve cells (Neubürger, 1931) (31), may occur in some cases of hemorrhagic encephalopathy.

Marchiafava-Bignami Disease

A peculiar form of central necrosis of the corpus callosum, other commissural bundles, and the cerebral white matter was first reported by two Italian pathologists in 1897. A written report by Marchiafava and Bignami, however, did not appear until 1903 (42). The disease occurs in chronic alcoholics, especially in those with inadequate diets. It was once presumed to have a specific national predisposition. It is progressive and characterized by mental and moral deterioration leading to dementia in from several months to a number of years. Bohrod (1942) (43) reported a case in a Swiss-American and found records of 42 cases in the Italian literature. Nielsen and Courville (1943) (44) described a classic case in an American man addicted to Italian red wine, which seemed to disprove the theory of national limitation, and suggested that some toxic substance in the crude wine and malnutrition were the associated causes of its occurrence. They suggested the intervention of some vascular disorder. Similar lesions have been produced in dogs given deficient diets (Testa, 1929) (45).

The gross lesions in this disease are sharply outlined grayish zones of necrosis in the central portion of the corpus callosum, the anterior commissure, and occasionally the optic chiasm, the subcortical white matter (King and Meehan, 1936) (46), and the middle cerebellar peduncles (Lolli, 1941) (47). Lesions never occur in the internal capsule, corona radiata, or subcortical association fibers. The middle fibers of the rostrum and genu of the corpus callosum are primarily affected, leaving an intact marginal zone (Fig. 87). In the splenium of this structure, either multiple discrete areas in the midline or two separate zones in symmetrical positions just lateral to the midline may be found instead of a central lesion. Midline foci of degeneration may also occur in the anterior commissure and optic chiasm.

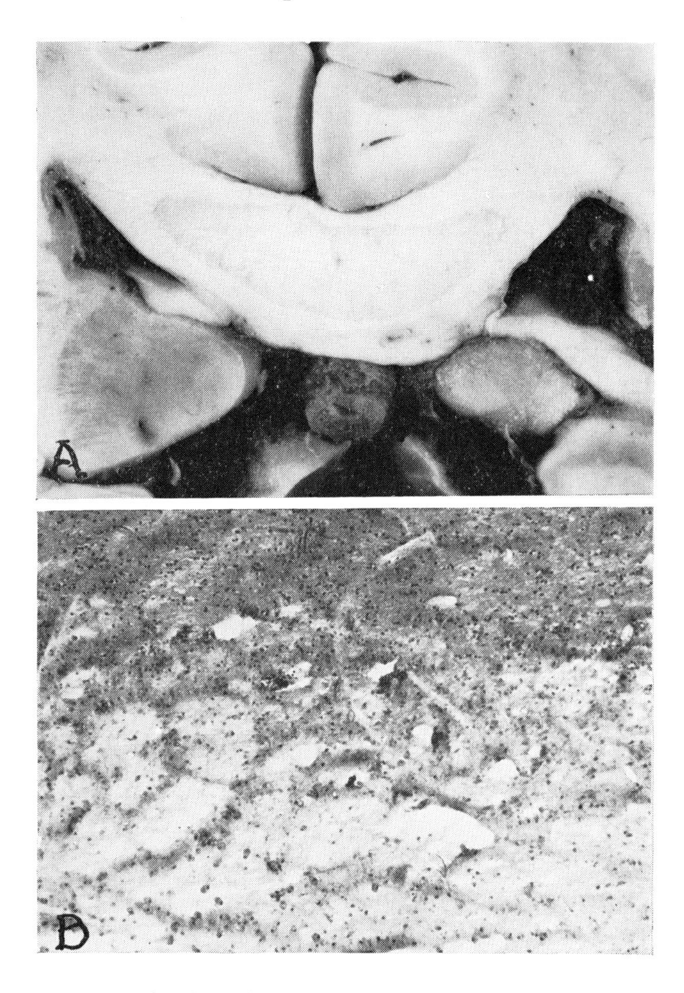

Fig. 87—Central softening of the corpus callosum (A) in chronic alcoholic state from Italian red wine (Marchiafava-Bignami disease). Case of Nielsen and Courville, Bull. Los Angeles Neurol. Soc. 8:81–88 (Sept.) 1943. B. Microscopic appearance of margin of degeneration. H & E × 65.

Symmetrical foci and necrosis sometimes appear in the cerebral white matter just beneath the zone of subcortical association fibers, most commonly in the centrum beneath the second and third frontal convolutions and beneath the middle third of the precentral and postcentral gyri. These areas may be large. They tend to form irregular cystic cavities (King and Meehan, 1936; Merritt and Weisman, 1945) (46, 48). This necrosis has also been designated as "alcoholic phthisis of the brain" (Lolli, 1941) (47).

Microscopically, the lesions are fairly sharply outlined zones of degeneration, characterized by a looseness of the white substance, in which the myelin has largely disappeared. Occasionally fibers with preserved or slightly altered sheaths are found in these areas, particularly at the periphery. The axis cylinders may persist for some time in the degenerative areas, although they usually become varicose. Later, segmentation and granular degeneration occur. The astrocytes may be slightly swollen, with early proliferation and varicose fibrils. There is a well defined reaction of myelophages with phagocytosis of free fat.

The blood vessels within the foci of necrosis are thickened and hyalinized, with a consequent reduction or occlusion of their lumina. Neither the endothelium nor the adventitia show signs of proliferation. These vascular changes may be primary, the necrosis resulting from the progressive local ischemia of the white matter.

Alcoholic Cerebellar Degeneration

Selective atrophy of the cerebellar cortex is a relatively rare residual of chronic alcoholism. Although a reduction in size of the cerebellum and the pons may occur with cerebral cortical atrophy in cases of chronic alcoholism, isolated cortical atrophy of the cerebellum occurs rarely. Attention was first called to this condition by Thomas (1905) (49), who noted progressive degeneration of the Purkinje cells. The association of alcoholism and this degeneration was stressed by Stender and Lüthy (1931) (50). Lhermitte, et al. (1938) (51), produced the degeneration in animals and Lhermitte (1935) (52) pointed out that in some cases of chronic alcoholism the cerebellum was greatly reduced in size, with the most marked changes in the superior vermis and adjacent portions of the hemispheres. Microscopically, the Purkinje cells were absent or had undergone pyknotic change, with nuclear shrinkage and loss of processes. This change in the Purkinje cells is selective, however; with silver impregnation the fibers of the "baskets" about them appear to be normal or even slightly hypertrophic. The ramifications of the Purkinje cells show peculiar tortuosities (snake-like cells). The axis cylinders are distorted and swollen. The nerve cells of the molecular layer and granular cell layer are altered very little. The neuroglial fibers in the white matter are moderately increased in number.

In some cases, physical alteration of the cells of the inferior olivary nucleus is found together with shrinkage of these cells and atrophy of the olivocerebellar fibers. The absence of individual Purkinje cells is, therefore, almost the rule in chronic alcoholics.

The Purkinje cells are known to be particularly sensitive to almost any noxious process. Why they are so selectively and profoundly damaged as to result in gross atrophy of the cerebellar cortex in cases of alcoholism is unknown. It is suspected that a nutritional disorder may be more important in the development of the atrophy than the direct effects of alcohol (Romano, et al., 1940) (53).

Atrophy of the layer of granular cells is also found in approximately a fourth of cases of chronic alcoholism (Courville, 1963) (54). One unsolved question is why the Purkinje cells show greater damage in some cases and the granule cells in others (Fig. 88).

Summary

The effects of alcohol on the nervous system may be either acute or chronic. The acute effects occur in the form of congestion (at times with petechial hemorrhages) and edema and are usually reversible with restoration of the normal processes. When reinforced by malnutrition and vitamin deficiency, these changes are translated into cellular and architectural changes which are accompanied by more or less characteristic syndromes. Delirium tremens is associated

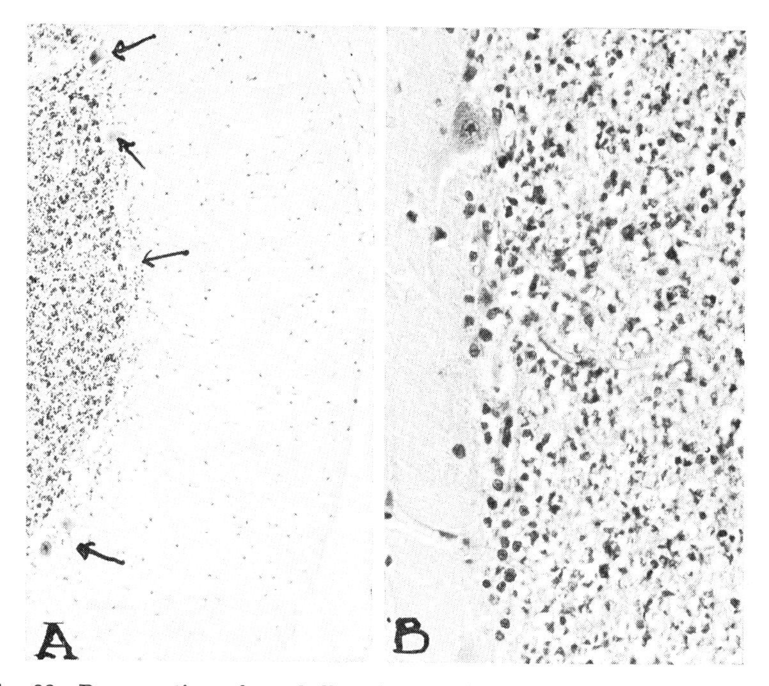

Fig. 88—Degeneration of cerebellar elements in chronic alcoholism. A. Degeneration of Purkinje cells. H & E × 65. B. Degeneration of cells in granular layer. H & E × 250.

with a widespread pyknosis and acute swelling of the various pyramidal cells of the cortical laminae. Korsakoff's psychosis and psychotic manifestations incident to postalcoholic pellagra are accompanied by a precocious and almost universal deposition of lipoid material in the nerve cells of the brain and spinal cord. A frontal lobe syndrome (alcoholic pseudoparesis) results from atrophy of the dorsolateral, frontal, and central cortex. Hemorrhagic encephalopathy of the gray nuclear masses adjacent to the third and fourth ventricles and intervening cerebral aqueduct gives rise to extraocular palsies usually associated with impairment of consciousness and disordered mentation. The peculiar syndrome known as Marchiafava-Bignami disease, with degeneration of the midportion of the commissural pathways (notably the corpus callosum) or symmetrical foci in the frontal cerebral centrum and middle cerebellar peduncles, results from excessive consumption of crude Italian red wine and malnutrition. The sequence of chronic alcoholism and vitamin deficiency is best seen in cases of the more common peripheral neuropathy.

The indirect effects of chronic indulgence in alcohol are typified by degeneration of the posterior and lateral columns of the spinal cord (postero-lateral sclerosis) consequent to atrophic gastritis and anemia.

REFERENCES

1. Umiker, W. O.: The Pathology of Acute Alcoholism. U. S. Nav. M. Bull. 49:744–752 (July-Aug.) 1949.
2. Pick, L., and Bielschowsky, M.: Ueber histologische Befunde im Auge und im centralen Nervensystem mit Methylalkohol. Berl. klin. Wochenschrift. 49:888–893, 1912.
3. Menne, F. R.: Acute Methyl Alcohol Poisoning; Report of 22 Instances with Postmortem Examination. Arch. Path. 26:77-92 (July) 1938.
4. Weil, A.: A Text-book of Neuropathology. Philadelphia, Lea & Febiger, 1933, pp. 190, 191.
5. Patty, F. A., Yant, W. P., and Schrenk, H. H.: Acute Response of Guinea Pigs to Vapors of Some New Commercial Organic Compounds; Secondary Amyl Acetate. U. S. Public Health Rep. 51:811–819 (June 19) 1936.
6. Wright, A. W.: General Pathology and Some Special Complications of Alcoholism. Arch. Path. 32:670–683 (Oct.) 1941.
7. Edmondson, H. A., Hall, E. M., and Myers, R. O.: Pathology of Alcoholism, in Alcoholism, edited by Thompson, G. N., Charles C Thomas, 1956.
8. Petri, E.: Pathologische Anatomie und Histologie der Vergiftungen. Berlin, Julius Springer, 1930, pp. 276–285.
9. Alexander, L.: Wernicke's Disease; Identity of Lesions Produced Experimentally by B_1 Avitaminosis in Pigeons with Hemorrhagic Encephalitis Occurring in Chronic Alcoholism in Man. Am. J. Path. 16:61–70 (Jan.) 1940.
10. Courville, Cyril B.: Asphyxia as a Consequence of Nitrous Oxide Anesthesia. Medicine 15:129–245 (May) 1936.
11. ———: Untoward Effects of Nitrous Oxide Anesthesia. Mountain View, Calif., Pacific Press Publ. Assn., 1950.
12. Jetter, W. W., and McLean, R.: Poisoning by the Synergistic Effect of Phenobarbital and Ethyl Alcohol. An Experimental Study. Arch. Path. 36:112–122 (July) 1943.
13. Shattuck, G. C.: Relation of Beri-beri to Polyneuritis from Other Causes. Am. J. Trop. Med. 8:539–543 (Nov.) 1928.
14. Courville, Cyril B.: Pathology of the Central Nervous System. Ed. 3, Mountain View, Calif., Pacific Press Publ. Assn., 1950.

15. Carmichael, E. A., and Stern, R. O.: Korsakoff's Syndrome: Its Histopathology. Brain 54:189–213 (June) 1931.
16. Gamper, E.: Zur Frage der Polioencephalitis haemorrhagica der chronischen Alkoholiker. Anatomische Befunde beim alkoholischen Korsakow und ihre Beziehungen zum klinischen Bild. Deutsche Ztschr. Nervenh. 102:122–129, 1928.
17. Leudet, E.: Recherches pour servir à l'histoire de la pellagre sporadique et de la pseudopellagre dês alcoholises. Gaz. med. de Paris, 3 s. 22: 319, 339, 399, 1867; also in Compt. rend. Soc. de biol. 4 s., 4:3–29, 1869.
18. Kraepelin, E.: Psychiatrie. Ed. 2, Leipzig, A. Abel, 1887.
19. Tuczek, I.: Ueber die Veränderungen im Centralnervensystem, speziell in den Hintersträgen des Rückenmarks, bei Ergotismus. Arch. f. Psychiat. 13:99–154, 1882.
20. Babes, V., and Sion, V.: Die Pellagra in Nothnagel's Specielle Pathologie und Therapie. Vol. 24, Vienna, Holder, 1901.
21. Singer, H. D., and Pollock, L. J.: The Histopathology of the Nervous System in Pellagra. Arch. Int. Med. 11:565–589 (June) 1913.
22. Ostertag, B.: Zur Pathologie der akuten Pellagrapsychosen (mit Demonstration). Zentralbl. f. d. ges. Neurol. u. Psychiat. 40:127–128, 1925.
23. Winkelman, N. W.: Beiträge zur Neurohistopathologie der Pellagra. Ztschr. f. d. ges. Neurol. u. Psychiat. 102:38–55, 1926.
24. Pentschew, A.: Über die Histopathologie des Zentralnervensystems bei der Psychosis pellagrosa. Ztschr. f. d. ges. Neurol. u. Psychiat. 118:17–48, 1928.
25. Zimmerman, H. M., Cohen, L. H., and Gildea, E. F.: Pellagra in Association with Chronic Alcoholism. Arch. Neurol. & Psychiat. 31:290–309 (Feb.) 1934.
26. Wernicke, C.: Lehrbuch der Gehirnkrankheiten für Aerzte und Studierende. Vol. 2, Theodor Fischer, Kassel u. Berlin, 1882, pp. 229–242.
27. Jacobäus, H. Über einen Fall von Polioencephalitis haemorrhagica superior (Wernicke). Deutsche Ztschr. Nervenh. 5:334–350, 1894.
28. Bonhoeffer, K.: Pathologisch anatomische Untersuchungen an Alkoholdeliranten. Monatschr. f. Psychiat. u. Neurol. 5:265–284, 379, 387, 1899.
29. Hunt, J. R.: A Contribution to Our Knowledge of Polioencephalitis Superior (Wernicke Type). New York, M. J. 83:289–291 (Feb. 10) 1906.
30. Creutzfeldt, R.: Hirnveränderungen bei Gewohnheitstrinkern. Zentralbl. f. d. ges. Neurol. u. Psychiat. 50:321, 1928.
31. Neubürger, K.: Über Hirnveränderungen nach Alkoholmissbrauch (unter Berücksichtigung einiger Fälle von Wernickescher Krankheit mit anderer Atiologie). Ztschr. f. d. ges. Neurol. u. Psychiat. 135:159–209, 1931.
32. Bender, L., and Schilder, P.: Encephalopathia Alcoholica; Polioencephalitis Haemorrhagica de Wernicke. Arch. Neurol. & Psychiat. 29:990–1053 (May) 1933.

33. ———: Myelopathia Alcoholica Associated with Encephalopathia Alcoholica. Arch. Neurol. & Psychiat. 31:310–337 (Feb.) 1934.
34. Campbell, A. C. P., and Biggart, J. H.: Wernicke's Encephalopathy (Polioencephalitis Hemorrhagica Superior): Its Alcoholic and Nonalcoholic Incidence. J. Path. & Bact. 48:245–262 (Mar.) 1939.
35. Bailey, F. W.: Histopathology of Polioencephalitis Hemorrhagica Superior (Wernicke's Disease). Arch. Neurol. & Psychiat. 56:609–630 (Dec.) 1946.
36. Neubürger, K.: Über die nichtalkoholische Wernickesche Krankheit, insbesondere über ihr Vorkommen beim Krebsleiden. Virchows Arch. f. path. Anat. 298:68–86, 1936.
37. ———: Wernickesche Krankheit bei chronischer Gastritis. Ein Beitrag zu den Beziehungen zwischen Magen und Gehirn. Ztschr. f. d. ges. Neurol. u. Psychiat. 160:208–225, 1937.
38. Tanaka, T.: So-called Breast Milk Intoxication. Am. J. Dis. Child. 47:1286–1298 (June) 1934.
39. Környey, S.: Aufsteigende Lähmung und Korsakowsche Psychose bei Lymphogranulomatose. Deutsch. Ztschr. z. Nervenh. 125:129-141, 1932.
40. Davison, C., and Stone, L.: Lesions of the Nervous System of Rat in Vitamin B Deficiency. Arch. Path. 23:207–223 (Feb.) 1937.
41. Jolliffe, N., Wortis, H., and Stein, M. H.: Vitamin Deficiencies and Liver Cirrhosis in Alcoholism. IV. The Wernicke Syndrome. V. Nicotinic Acid Deficiency Encephalopathy. VI. Encephalopathies with Possible Nutritional Involvement. Quart. J. Stud. on Alcohol. 2:73–97 (June) 1941.
42. Marchiafava, E., and Bignami, A.: Sopra un alteraizone del corpo calloso osserota in soggetti alcoolish. Riv. Patol. nerv. ment. 8:544–549, 1903.
43. Bohrod, M. G.: Primary Degeneration of the Corpus Callosum (Marchiafava's Disease); Report of Second American Case. Arch. Neurol. & Psychiat. 47:465–473 (Mar.) 1942.
44. Nielsen, J. M., and Courville, C. B.: Central Necrosis of the Corpus Callosum (Marchiafava-Bignami's Disease). Report of Case in an American Man with Comments on the Pathogenesis of the Disease. Bull. Los Angeles Neurol. Soc. 8:81–88 (June) 1943.
45. Testa, U.: Lesioni del corpo calloso nell'alcoolismo subacuto sperimentale. Riv. sper. di freniat. 52.559–574 (Apr. 30) 1929.
46. King, L. S., and Meehan, M. C.: Primary Degeneration of the Corpus Callosum (Marchiafava's Disease). Arch. Neurol. & Psychiat. 36:547–568 (Sept.) 1936.
47. Lolli, G.: Marchiafava's Disease. Quart. J. Stud. on Alcohol. 2:486–495 (Dec.) 1941.
48. Merritt, H. H., and Weisman, A. D.: Primary Degeneration of the Corpus Callosum (Marchiafava-Bignami's Disease). J. Neuropath. & Exper. Neurol. 4:155–163 (Apr.) 1945.
49. Thomas, A.: Atrophie lamellaire des cellulas de Purkinje. Rev. Neurol. 13:917–924, 1905.

50. Stender, A., and Lüthy, F.: Über Spätatrophie der Kleinhirnrinde bei chronischem Alkoholismus. Deutsche Ztschr. Nervenh. 119:604–622, 1931.
51. Lhermitte, J., De Ajuriaguerra, J., and Garnier: Les lésions du système nerveux dans l'intoxication alcoolique expérimentale. Compt. rend. Soc. de biol. 128:386–388, 1938.
52. ———: Cortical Cerebellar Degeneration. Proc. Roy. Soc. Med. 28:379–390 (Feb.) 1935.
53. Romano, J., Michael, M., Jr., and Merritt, H. H.: Alcoholic Cerebellar Degeneration. Arch. Neurol. & Psychiat. 44:1230–1236 (Dec.) 1940.
54. Courville, Cyril B.: Degeneration of the Granule Cells of the Cerebellar Cortex in Chronic Alcoholism. Its Pathogenetic Significance. To be published, 1964.

1200 North State Street
Los Angeles 33, California

Index

REFERENCES ARE TO PAGES

A

B

C

D

P

Q

R

S

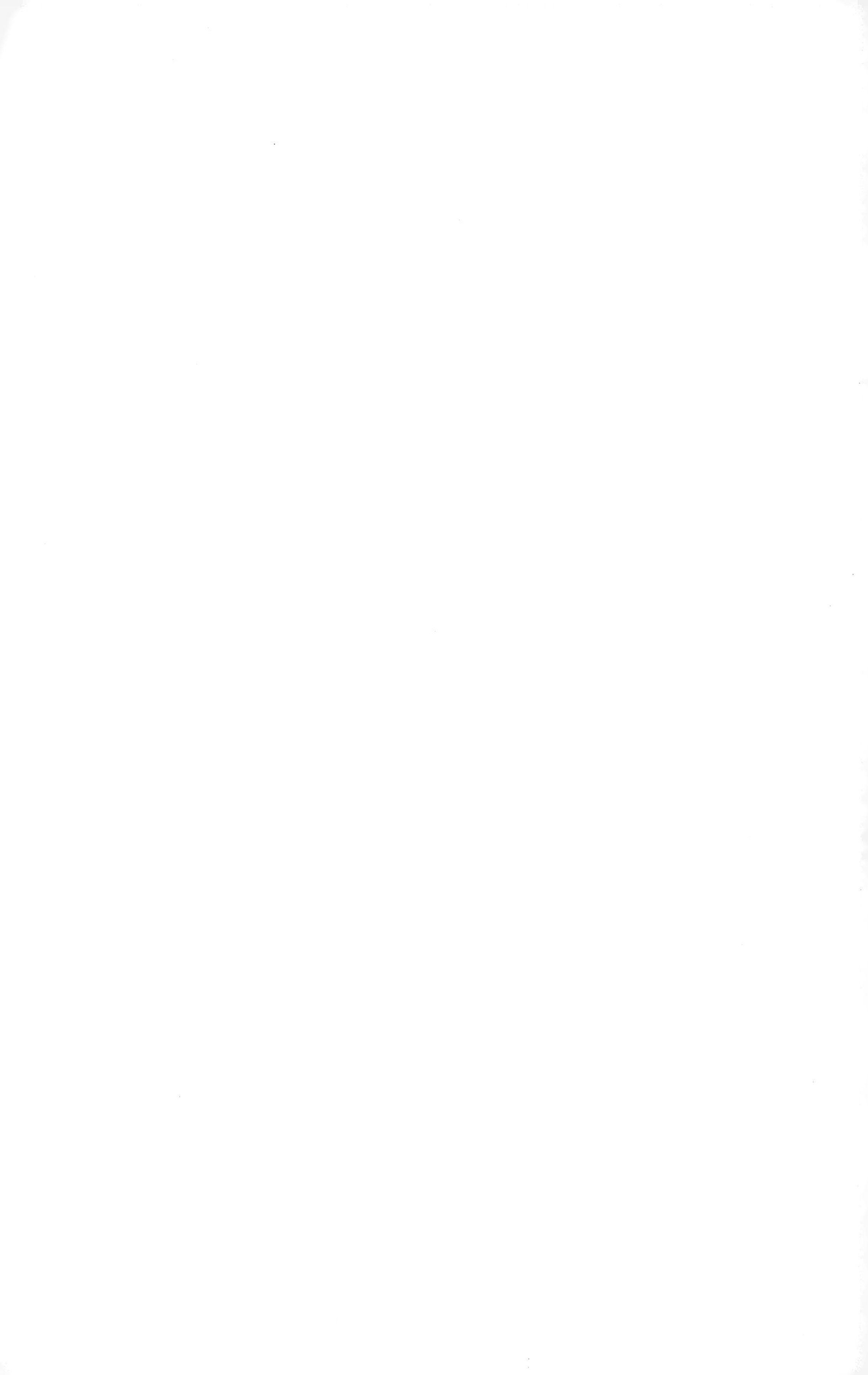